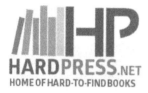

HARDPRESS.NET
HOME OF HARD-TO-FIND BOOKS

Mesmerism and Its Opponents
by George Sandby

Address:
HardPress
8345 NW 66TH ST #2561
MIAMI FL 33166-2626
USA
Email: info@hardpress.net

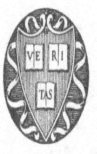

MESMERISM,

AND

ITS OPPONENTS.

BY

GEORGE SANDBY, M.A.

VICAR OF FLIXTON, SUFFOLK.

" All things are marked and stamped with this triple character ; — of
the *power of God*, — the *difference of nature*, — and the *use of man*."
BACON, *Advancement of Learning*, book II.

" Gratia docet de omni re, et in omni scientiâ *utilitatis fructum*, atque
Dei laudem et honorem quaerere."
THOMAS à KEMPIS, *De Imitatione Christi*, lib. III. 54.

Second Edition,

CONSIDERABLY ENLARGED, WITH AN INTRODUCTORY CHAPTER.

LONDON:

LONGMAN, BROWN, GREEN, AND LONGMANS,

PATERNOSTER-ROW.

1848.

LONDON:
SPOTTISWOODE and SHAW,
New-street-Square.

TO

CAPTAIN JOHN JAMES,

ETC. ETC. ETC.

I CANNOT dedicate this little Work more appropriately than to you, through whom I became first acquainted with the great truths of which it treats, and to whose kindness and cordial sympathy I am so deeply indebted.

Believe me to remain,

My dear Friend,

Yours most sincerely,

GEORGE SANDBY, Jun.

A 2

PREFACE

TO THE SECOND EDITION.

In presenting a fresh edition of my little work to the Public, perhaps I shall be pardoned if I submit a few preliminary observations as to its nature and origin; for the earnest part that I take in the promotion of the somewhat unpopular subject of which it treats has probably excited surprise. With many, I appear to be stepping aside from my own vocation, in a cause where far abler men have failed before me, with little other prospect than that of losing the good opinion of the judicious, and of incurring an unnecessary amount of ill-will and misrepresentation. With others, the move is regarded as one, that professionally pursues a wrong, or at least, an unusual direction; and the conventionalist and the fastidious give me, therefore, their cold contempt. For all this, and more I am prepared. *My object is to do good*, great and essential good to the many and to the miserable; and a little odium and ridicule can be easily overborne. And yet (as is the case most commonly in the world) my motives have been rather of a mixed nature; and neither is the matter of the volume so very unprofessional. To treat of the real bearing of Mesmerism on religion and on religious minds; to disabuse the pious but prejudiced Christian of his scruples as to its use*; and to justify my friends and

* A letter from Mr. Symes, surgeon, of Grosvenor Street, published in the 18th No. of the Zoist, shows a melancholy instance of conscientious delusion, arising from ignorance.—p. 171.

A 3

myself for our own practice — this was my original design: other branches of the subject presented themselves incidentally by the way; experience and opportunity enabled me to give information where much was wanted; one thing led to another, till, at last, a little tract, that was commenced with the sole purpose of dealing with a misapplied doctrine of Scripture, swelled into the present heterogeneous table of contents; and the whole aspect of the question passed under review.

Providential circumstances had led me to an acquaintance with Mesmerism, for which I have still the greatest reason to bless God. Superstition, however, has its slaves in every spot; and I was soon pelted with pamphlets through the post, and made the mark for grave and evilnatured censure. Satan and his emissaries were said to have "crept into my house unawares;" and the anathemas of Mr. M'Neile were called arguments in proof. Some slight notice seemed desirable; and I therefore purposed to examine the melancholy bigotry that prompted these reproaches, and show how the very same ignorance had equally assailed, even in recent times, remedies and discoveries, the innocency of which could now be no longer called in question. It was explained to the well-meaning opponent, that phenomena, which shocked his faith and distracted his devotions, were the harmless result of a simple process in nature, and were merely remarkable because they were new.

I was immediately met by the very opposite argument. "If," it was replied, "Mesmerism be neither preternatural nor Satanic, your faith as a Christian is not the less placed in jeopardy; for wonders and cures similar in degree to those which your own science boasts of, are recorded in the Old and New Testaments, and form, in fact, the basis on which all belief in them is grounded: *if the one be only of nature, so also must be the other.*" These

views are more prevalent than it may be at first suspected, and their birthplace will be found in Germany. Richter[*], rector of the principal ducal school at Dessau, when publishing some years back "Considerations on Animal Magnetism," stated that magnetism "solves those enigmas which appertain especially to Christianity;" and added, that all the miracles of the New Testament were performed by this extraordinary agency. The rector declared further, that St. Paul, Luther, and the Saviour were all magnetists. Eichorn and Professor Paulus, with their rationalistic interpretations, may be considered as the originators of a doctrine, which the deistical mesmerists of Germany caught hold of and improved. "It is characteristic of this theory," says a writer of a congenial though different school (that of Strauss) and whose Lectures in London obtained recently some notoriety,—"to regard Christ as a wise man, healing disease by felicitous accident, by medical skill, or by the natural action of his faith;— and in every narrative of miracle to cast about for some supposable germ of fact, out of which the mistake or exaggeration might have innocently grown."[†] Speaking of Eichorn, the same lecturer observes, "While men were *ignorant of nature and her laws,* they made every thing *supernatural and divine.* Useful inventions were deemed special workings of the mind of God. Eichorn considers that there was no fraud in the matter of miracles, only the colouring which fact receives from the opinions of the narrator," and that "the *miracles were natural occurrences,* misunderstood and misreported."[‡] Mr. Justice Coleridge, in his Recollections of his great kinsman, says, "Returning to the Germans, he (Coleridge) said the state of their

[*] Not the famous Jean Paul, nor any relation. He was a man of profound erudition, and a great mathematician and critic, and was well known in Germany. He died about three years back.

[†] Harwood's Anti-supernaturalism, p. 3.   [‡] Ibid. p. 7, 8.

A 4

religion, when he was in Germany, was really shocking. He found professors in the universities lecturing against material points in the Gospel. He instanced Paulus, whose lectures he attended: the object was to resolve the *miracles into natural operations.*[*] German rationalism, as may be seen, therefore, was the school which first applied the wonders of Mesmerism in support of a deistical theory. It was easy for the rationalist to say, that the miracles of our Divine Master were "natural occurrences," but it was not so easy to find a key by which their hypothesis could be explained; and magnetism seemed to offer a ready solution for the difficulty. The suggestion was adopted in all haste by the warm German mind, which so loves the marvellous; the idea spread quickly into France, and took deep root in its infidel soil, as is seen by many of their publications on the subject[†]; and soon crossed over into this country with other continental importations. As a knowledge of Mesmerism gained ground in England, so did this persuasion advance also, and, forming in the Mesmeric world a distinct school, gave serious uneasiness to many pious friends of the cause. Of this it is as idle to pretend an ignorance, as it would be to be blind to the approach of an enemy, and then hope that that enemy had no existence. Neither would it be reasonable to blame Mesmerism for the tenet, and exclaim against its practice as the source of such unhallowed opinions. Which of God's gifts have not been turned against the Giver?[‡] It

---

[*] Coleridge's Table Talk, vol. ii. p. 346.

[†] See particularly the writings of MM. Mialle, and Foissac and Théodore Bouys.

[‡] Mr. Cumming, the eloquent minister of the Scottish Church in London, says beautifully in a charming little tract, called "Infant Salvation,"—"A repugnance to a truth may invent innumerable objections. . . . Evil men can turn any mercy into means of evil. . . . To object to a doctrine because it may be abused, or to reject it because it may be perverted, is just to imitate the man who would cut down a beautiful fruit-tree, because caterpillars find food from its leaves, and spiders weave their webs amid its branches."—p. 34.

was far better to meet the evil at once,—to point out the broad line of separation that runs between the two principles,—and to show with what unexamining haste the theory had been adopted. And this I determined, with God's help, to attempt, and to clear away the cloud of mysticism that hung over the subject. Thus there were two most adverse antagonists to deal with,—those who elevated a newly-found physical influence into the magic of Satan; and those who strove to "retranslate the supernatural back into the natural."[*] I combated both in succession; and have some reason to hope that my labours have not been altogether fruitless.[†]

Again was I met from a fresh quarter with a not unfrequent objection,—an objection, also, more plausible than real. "Mesmerism was immoral; why, then, incur an odium from the advocacy of a system that was liable to grave abuses, and whence painful results had actually arisen?" Here, also, it was requisite to show that the alleged evils were not essential to the practice; that if they existed, they did not counterbalance the far greater advantages; that they *need not exist* at all, if the *conditions and rules* which the leading Mesmerists had established *were carefully observed;* and if not observed, that the opportunities for wrong-doing were scarcely greater than those which accompanied several parts of medical treatment. The use of opiates had its evils; to this might now be added the intoxicating effects from the inhalation

---

[*] Expression in Harwood's Anti-supernaturalism. See also on this subject a recent and popular French work, Salverte's "Philosophy of Apparent Miracles," or *Les Sciences Occultes.*

[†] The late "Charlotte Elizabeth," the editress of the "Christian Lady's Magazine," in her Letter to Miss Martineau on Mesmerism, also places some magnetic wonders on a level with the miracles, though on different principles to those mentioned above. She considers them as diabolical "imitations," "devised by Satan to throw soul-destroying doubts on the miracles" of the Saviour.—p. 18. Hence the increased necessity for distinguishing between them.

of ether, on which, morally, I have never yet heard even the hint of an objection, though every one may see to what vile purposes it might be rendered subservient. But so it is in this world;—give an adversary an evil name, and there is no crime of which he will not be deemed capable. Opium and ether may, according to the proverb, walk within the stable-door, and place their hands on the neck of the animal, and no harm is feared or suspected; while poor Mesmerism cannot even cast a glance within the precincts, but an outcry is straightway raised by these drug-admiring purists, as to all our morals being imperilled by a strange and anomalous remedy!

Thus far, then, the argument of my little work might be regarded as strictly defensive. I had to show, in self-justification alone, that a discovery, from which I had largely profited, was neither satanic, nor immoral, nor subversive of Gospel evidence, nor one which a Christian need fear to encourage; and here the demonstration might have stopped; but, having once adventured into the field, I felt that it was idle to withdraw till the best results of my own practice and observation were offered to the service of the sick room. This, of course, was to pass the professional barrier, and to expose myself to the usual charge of ignorance and interference. But it was a good cause and a righteous. I was able show to the medical sceptic, from my own experience only, that most of the reasons on which he grounded his disbelief were based on mistaken and hastily adopted views, in direct contradiction to the actual workings of nature. I was anxious, also, to encourage the relatives of many a sufferer in their employment of a healing and merciful art, by the relation of what I had myself seen, and done, and studied. For oftentimes, indeed, has some sad invalid been presented to my notice,—the racking agony of his pains,—the wasted helplessness of his form,—the despairing misery of his

eye,—or the fever of his brain have, as the case may have been, given fearful indications of the past and of the future;—hope and relief had in vain been sought through the ordinary appliances:—

> " Soft, gentlest, friendly sleep!
> Sweet holiday! Of all earth's good the help,
> Or origin!"*

had for hours and nights been absent from the chamber! But at length the soothing hand of the Mesmerist is summoned; his gentle, patient, persevering treatment is adopted and pursued; and then, after a time, what a change! what a healthful happy transformation comes over the whole system of one so lately and so fearfully afflicted!

> " A new life
> Flows through his renovated frame;
> His limbs, that late were sore and stiff,
> Feel all the freshness of repose;
> His dizzy brain is calm'd;
> The heavy aching of his lids is gone;
> For Laila, from the bowers of paradise,
> Has borne the healing fruit!"†

That, too, which was the most wanted,—the most courted, the most ardently prayed for, and the most difficult to obtain, is now the first to reappear, and the easiest to be secured. " Great nature's second course, balm of hurt minds, chief nourisher in life's feast," follows readily and peacefully from the composing hand. The magnetist returns, and in a little moment—

> " Day is over, night is here;
> Closed are the eye and ear
> In sleep, in sleep!
> Pain is silent; toil reposes:
>
> • • • •
>
> Neither moan nor weep;
> Dreams and all the race of Fear
> Fade away and disappear
> In the deepest deep!"‡

---

* Barry Cornwall, Fragments, 232.   † Thalaba, book ii. p. 9.
‡ Barry Cornwall, Fragments, 236.

This have I seen over and over again, and with all the attendant blessings of convalescence; and therefore is it, that I am so earnestly, and, perchance, so unwisely enthusiastic in pressing the merits of this marvellous power upon the notice of a numerous and benevolent profession.

The present edition (which I have endeavoured to make a little Handbook of Mesmerism, from its replies to our very opposite "opponents," and from its information under various heads for different inquirers,) contains a large amount of new matter.

An introductory chapter on the opposition of scientific and medical men to the claims of Mesmerism is first given, with tables of surgical operations that have been performed during mesmeric insensibility. Their number will be found to be greater than is generally supposed.

Several recent pamphlets, that have reasserted the charge of irreligion and satanic agency, are examined; and some curious quotations from sermons and tracts, in which the very same accusations against inoculation were published about a century back, are laid before the reader for his instruction and amusement.

The conduct of the Church of Rome in regard to Mesmerism is given in the first chapter. The statement is both interesting and important.

In the seventh chapter, a large variety of fresh instances of natural ecstatics and sleepwalkers will be found. The close relation, or rather identity, of the singular phenomena that they have manifested with phenomena that have since been developed in mesmeric patients, prove the truthfulness and genuine character of the latter. It will be seen, moreover, that the former are not "isolated" cases (as it is asserted in the British and Foreign Medical Review for April, 1845), but extremely numerous; for many more than I have given could be added. The argument, then,

that they furnish is a useful one, and is pressed on the reader's attention. Facts of this description, *which arise in the order of nature*, and agree in the main, and vary only with the accidents of climate, creed, and constitution, show the " conformity of Mesmerism with general experience." They strengthen the reasoning that Mr. Townshend brings forward in his third book, to prove that the magnetic condition is not " an insulated phenomenon, nor an interruption to the universal order, but a link in the eternal chain of things." (p. 184.) And the more that the student of nature shall examine the history of the cataleptic and ecstatic state, as recorded by different religious writers, towards the confirmation of their respective faiths, the more will he perceive a good ground for understanding that Mesmerism is nothing else than a simple reproduction by artificial means of real phenomena and facts that are as old as the creation.

An additional chapter will be also given, embracing practical information for the use of the learner. Instructions in the art of mesmerising did not fall within the original purposes with which this work was commenced, and the subject was omitted in the first edition. But I have been so frequently appealed to by letter for guidance in the management of a patient; and parties, living at a distance, and deprived of the opportunity of personal observation, (the best school after all,) have so often expressed the opinion that information on that head was a *desideratum* in the book, that I have endeavoured to supply the omission. My own experience, which is now neither slight nor superficial, will form the basis of the instruction. But copious information from Deleuze, Elliotson, Gauthier, Townshend, Teste, and other writers and authorities on the subject will be introduced.

If the student wishes to pursue the subject more in detail, the *Instruction Pratique* of the excellent and sober-

minded Deleuze is the first book that I should recommend. There is an English translation, of the merits of which I know nothing.

Gauthier's *Traité Pratique* abounds with information and knowledge of the subject, but it has the besetting sin of many French treatises, being too voluminous and prolix.

Mr. Baillière of Regent Street has published a translation of Teste's " Practical Manual ;" in fact, every book on Mesmerism will be found in his excellent shop.

Last of all, Dr. Elliotson's Letters in the Zoist, containing the narrative of his principal cases, should form an indispensable portion of the medical inquirer's reading. In those valuable papers, nothing is taken for granted, and neither theories nor fancies appear, but facts, carefully observed and well-recorded facts alone, proceed from the pen of one who is the *most cautious* of men in first entertaining an opinion, but the most *conscientious* and *courageous* in maintaining it, when once he is certified of its reality. For,

> " The Truth is jealous: never to the Trite,
> Nor Knowledge to the Wise : but to the fool,
> And to the false, error and truth alike."*

So says Mr. Bailey, in his strange but strikingly powerful poem of Festus ; with whose appropriate words I now commend the following pages to the consideration of the reader.

* Festus, p. 41.

PREFACE

TO THE FIRST EDITION.

The following pages have grown out of a little pamphlet, that was published last summer, called " Mesmerism, the Gift of God."

The favourable reception of that letter by the public, and the demand for a second impression, have induced the Author, at the suggestion of several friends, to enter more fully into the subject, and to meet the various and contradictory objections that are popularly advanced.

This work, therefore, professes, not only to treat of the religious scruples that have been raised in the minds of some Christians, but to discuss with the philosopher the previous question as to the truth of Mesmerism, for a due inquiry into which, circumstances have greatly favoured the writer.

The First Chapter is little more than a reprint of the original pamphlet, in answer to the charge of Satanic agency.

The Second Chapter enters more at large into the same topic ; and showing the tendency of the human mind to see the mysterious in the inexplicable, proves, by example, the periodical re-appearance of this absurd accusation. The Author also examines the unfortunate mistake, which too many of his own profession are disposed to commit, be their religious creed what it may, of thinking that they do God service by depreciating his gifts ; because the parties that employ them hold opposite tenets to their own. —

This feeling is shown to arise, sometimes from a zeal without knowledge, and often from that love of spiritual power, which has disfigured the brightest pages in the history of the Church.

The Third and Fourth Chapters contain an analysis of the common objections against the truth of Mesmerism. Some remarkable cases are adduced from the writer's own experience. An accumulation of other facts is given from the testimony of parties whose standing in society is a pledge for the correctness of what they state. The curative power of Mesmerism in disease is proved by induction and observation. And the medical profession is invited to a reconsideration of their unfavourable verdict.

The Fifth Chapter discusses a common opinion as to the dangers of Mesmerism; — and its fallacy is in great measure exposed.

At the request of a friend, the Sixth Chapter has examined, at some length, the bearing of the wonders of Mesmerism on the miracles of the New Testament. It is notorious, that a feeling is gaining ground that these several facts exhibit an equality of power; and that the divine nature of the one is impaired by the extraordinary character of the other. The consideration of this part of the subject necessarily led to a detailed analysis of the Scriptural events: of course the unbeliever in the phenomena will deem such an inquiry preposterous and laughable; the Christian, however, who knows that Mesmerism is an existing fact in nature, will not regard the examination as superfluous; and even to the philosopher such an investigation *ought* to be interesting.

The concluding Chapter compares the phenomena of natural somnambulism and of Mesmerism with certain modern miracles among the Wesleyans and the Roman Catholics. The latter facts are stripped of the marvellous by a narrative of what occurred in the house of a friend.

Particular allusion is made to those wonders in the Tyrol, with the account of which the Earl of Shrewsbury, in a recent letter addressed to Mr. Ambrose Phillips, perplexed or pleased the Protestant or Romish Churches.

In the Appendix are given a few facts, taken from the history of several natural sleepwalkers, by which it will be seen that the "miracles of Mesmerism" are nothing else than certain phenomena, which have been *often* developed by nature in the spontaneous action of disease.

The author cannot conclude without acknowledging the vast obligations that he owes to the "Isis Revelata" of Mr. Colquhoun, and to "Facts in Mesmerism" by the Rev. Chauncy H. Townshend. Those who are disposed to follow up the subject, cannot but turn with profit to the varied information that those able works afford.

1844.

CONTENTS.

MESMERISM

AND

ITS OPPONENTS.

INTRODUCTORY CHAPTER.

It was one of Fontenelle's sayings, that "*if he held every truth in his hand, he would take good care and not open it;*" a prudential maxim, indicative of that "calculating reserve" with which cotemporaries taxed him; and though its adoption in practice may, doubtless, have contributed to his own ease and interests, such a feeling, if generally acted on, would be fatal to the well-being of human kind.[*]

With so cautious a spirit was the academician afflicted, such a coward was he in his own esteem, that it was observed respecting him, that he always found a pretext for "strangling discussion;" a strange character this for a philosopher! yet Fontenelle was wise in his generation. This indifference for onward investigations, this contentment with admitted truisms, were favourable to his health and popularity. Voltaire called him a universal genius; and his life was prolonged to the exact term of a century.[†]

---

[*] "Le caractère de Fontenelle est * * * une reserve calculée. * * * Il disait souvent que s'il tenait toutes les vérités dans sa main, il se garderait bien de l'ouvrir." — *Biographie Universelle*, art. FONTENELLE.

[†] "La Motte, dans une lettre à la Duchesse du Maine, l'accusait, en plaisantant, d'user de prétextes pour *étrangler les discussions.*" Fontenelle was born in 1657, and died 1757. — *Ibid.*

B

But timidity like this is a sorry counsellor; and a favourite as our author still is for the charm and variety of his writings, this dread of encountering opposition, this slavish suppression of inquiry, lessens, in large measure, our respect for his memory; and it suffers, in the estimation of all generous minds, what Southey calls " an abatement in heraldry."*

Now in this reluctance for the liberation of truth, which Fontenelle expressed in the above often quoted sentiment, there is a something which may remind the reader of the medical profession in regard to their present attitude on the study of Mesmerism. They too seem followers in the same cautious, unrisking, uninvestigating school; they too seem wanting in their usual independence and frank-hearted sincerity; they too seem unwilling, like the philosophic centenarian, to unclasp their hands, and give truth its freest circulation: and yet, while they resemble him in these several points, there is a distinction between them, which is somewhat in favour of the academical secretary.

When Fontenelle said, that though his hand were full of truths, he would not open it for any consideration, his motives were rather selfish than unphilosophical. He had, in fact, no turn for being a martyr in a good cause; he had no wish to be the victim of any fashionable outcry, or held forth as the referee for every doctrine under discussion. If a truth could only be maintained under his championship, the truth must go to the wall. If the public could only be benefited at his inconvenience, the public must forego the advantage. Not that he objected to the knowledge of truth for himself and his own private investigations; it was its escape into the world that he dreaded; he might study it, and examine it in his closet

* See Southey's Letter to William Smith, where he speaks of the present Lord Jeffrey and the Edinburgh Review.

at home; only let him be spared the dangers of a discoverer, and the responsibility of letting too much light upon mankind.

Now in all this reserve and holding back from free investigation, there is much, as we before said, that resembles our medical friends on the Mesmeric question; they are, indeed, all this, and "something more." Fontenelle would not " open his hands" to *communicate* knowledge; but they will not open theirs to *receive* it; Fontenelle would not risk his ease for the instruction of society, but they will not pass from professional routine even for their own. Fontenelle was selfish, timid, and shrinking from consequences; but they are rather illiberal, unphilosophic, and retrogressive. Truth, even for its own sake, or for its benefit on others, seems to have neither charm nor recommendation with them. They close their eyes, they stop their ears, they harden their hearts, they desire not to be informed or set right on this subject, be the advantages or the gratification what they may !*

It may not be without its use to ask, what can be the unexpressed motives on the part of medical men for this strange disinclination for the study of Mesmerism? for that some secret reasons are at the bottom of their conduct, is a point that no longer admits of a doubt. Whilst almost every other educated person is beginning to allow, that there is much more of probability and reality in the representations of the mesmerists, than originally

* Every experienced mesmerist could bring forward some story or other, similar to the following statement mentioned by Mr. Spencer Hall. " It is worth recording, as a feature of the age, that a physician of fashionable practice in the town (Halifax), on being invited to assist in an investigation, protested against it altogether in the most contemptuous terms, on the ground that the fallacy of mesmerism was too apparent to permit him to entertain the thought that it needed inquiry at all; in short, that any such inquiry would be disgraceful to the profession." See Mr. S. Hall's very interesting Mesmeric Experiences, p. 65.

men were prepared to expect, the "profession" still withholds its adhesion. They may, perhaps, not be so loud and offensive in their vituperations and ridicule as they were a few years back; they may have altered their tack, and become more silent and self-distrusting; still, as a body, they openly proclaim an unyielding scepticism; they dislike, if they do not actually reject, inquiry; and seldom voluntarily or with a good grace, either start or pursue the subject in conversation.* In stating this, it is of course remembered with pleasure, that very many have co-operated in our investigations with a most candid and honourable spirit; that the number of those that have openly joined our ranks is increasing every day, and already forms a highly respectable minority; and that the younger men, and more especially the students in the hospitals, are not undesirous of acknowledging the claims of the science to its place among their physiological researches; still it must with regret be confessed that the large majority of experienced practitioners, i. e. those who have secured an advanced standing in their profession, do hold aloof from all serious investigations upon the question, and if they do not give utterance to their feelings by an open expression of contempt, are at least mysteriously dumb or politely evasive on the topic; and it is, therefore, my wish, in a temperate and friendly spirit, to consider closely, what can be the unexpressed reasons for so singular a violation of their general usages.

Of course, they would themselves say, that the reason was a simple one, — that the facts alleged were so monstrous in themselves, and so opposed to the laws of nature, that no inquiry was needed; for that their mere statement carried with them to the medical mind

* In saying this, I am not so much giving utterance to my own experience, as recording the observations of almost all mesmerisers with whom I have spoken on the point in question.

their own refutation.* But this, any one may see, is an assumption of the whole question. It has been over and over again shown, that what are called the "laws of nature" are, strictly speaking, but the results of our present amount of scientific information, which do not preclude, with the progress of knowledge, a further development of hitherto latent principles.† No parties are more aware of this truth than medical men themselves. And for them, therefore, to offer such a plea, is not merely a begging the very point at issue, but a proceeding directly at variance with their own philosophic pretensions; and again, therefore, I respectfully demand, what is the probable motive for this anomaly in their conduct? ‡

The vulgar explanation usually advanced, strange as it may sound to the medical ear, is altogether of a pecuniary nature, and affecting their very character for disinterestedness and integrity. This is mentioned, not for the purpose of expressing my own utter disbelief in its probability, but of pointing out to the public the unreasonableness of such an opinion, and of directing the attention of the profession itself to their position, on this point, in popular estimation.

Though here and there, the jest may goodnaturedly be uttered by one of themselves, that if the claims of Mesmerism were established, their vocation would be perilled and their " occupation o'er," they little suspect how much

* " There is no use in discussing the matter," said an able surgeon to a friend of mine; " the thing is impossible; we know at once that it is impossible." And so it has ever been! It was impossible to prevent the small-pox by vaccination! It was impossible to light the streets with gas! It was impossible to cross the Atlantic by steam! Verily " a little science" is as dangerous as a little anything else.

† Mr. Townshend well remarks, that " such an objection would make our own imperfect observation the measure of Nature's regularity. Are we entitled to conclude, in any case, that, because we have not hitherto been able to assign a law to certain operations, they are, therefore, without law? Is it not wiser to believe that our own knowledge is in fault, whenever Nature appears inconsistent with herself? — Townshend's Facts, p. 14.

‡ Why, for instance, has no detailed notice been yet given, in any single Medical Journal, of the cases recorded in the Zoist?

of serious earnestness is supposed to be lurking at the bottom. They little dream, that their cautious retreat from a participation in the practice is rather attributed to a *clairvoyant* apprehension of a future loss of income, than to a philosophic conviction of scientific superiority. True it is, that the " love of money is the root of all evil:" and that medical men, like other mortals, are not to be regarded as independent of its influence; but the tenor of their general conduct makes a charge of this nature ridiculous and unmerited. My own experience (and I have had but too many painful opportunities of forming an opinion), would lead to the conclusion, that no one profession is so little under the bias of mercenary motives. No men give so much of a gratuitous unbought assistance, or sacrifice so much time and labour without a prospect of remuneration, as do they. And to suppose that a liberal and educated profession like this would oppose themselves to the progress of a great scientific discovery from an ungenerous apprehension of its proving detrimental to their interest, is monstrous in the extreme.[*] They themselves must feel, that a mere defence from such an imputation is almost as insulting as it is unnecessary. But it is necessary,— more necessary than they imagine. If I have heard the opinion once, I have heard it hundreds of times, and not uttered casually or in *badinage*, but gravely maintained and insisted upon, as a matter of certainty. It is, in fact, the all but universal inference; and it would really seem desirable, that the parties thus misunderstood should be made aware of the construction to which their reserved dealing

[*] Dr. Elliotson has well observed, " Some have been hostile from fancy that their pockets would suffer :—but many with abundant means, and more practice than they could get through,—nay, some retired from practice, have manifested the same spirit."—*Zoist*, No. IV. p. 377. Dr. E. agrees, therefore, with me in tracing the hostility to a different cause than the question of income.

has thus rendered them liable. But, in truth, the opinion is itself also founded on a mistake.

Mesmerism must partake much more of the miraculous character[*], before the sanguine anticipations of some ardent partisans can thus be realised. Its effects are indeed great and various, and often most unexpected, triumphing over many of the evils of life in a way delightful for the Christian to witness, — but yet must they be regarded rather as auxiliary to the practitioner, than superseding his attendance, rather as adding a fresh item to the former resources of his art, than dispensing with his kind and necessary care. That Mesmerism is now exercised by non-professional parties, is indeed a fact, but one rather resulting from its present unfixed position, than desirable in itself, or likely to continue. It is because they who ought to be its champions and directors stand coldly aloof, and reject all aid through its influence. But let its claims, as those of an important branch of therapeutic practice, be once fully recognised (and that such a day is steadily approaching, very many indications give certain proof), and a different state of things would then ensue. No longer would a few " incurable " cases, where the despairing physician had taken his leave, be transferred, sometimes at almost the agonies of death, to a mesmerising acquaintance to try if he could procure relief; but the disease would be grappled with at the earlier stages of its development with a more certain assurance of success. No longer would the hesitating patient, through the fear of offending the medical friend, surreptitiously admit into the sick room some amateur magnetist, with a distressing responsibility for all parties; but the treatment would be adopted, openly and more agreeably, by the express direction of professional advice. As it is, Mesmerism is generally employed as the

[*] See the chapter on a Comparison between Mesmeric Cures and the Miracles of the New Testament.

last resource, when every other remedy has been tried and failed; it is employed too, with an unpleasant feeling of risk and uncertainty, if without the sanction of a regular practitioner. And this is a position most painful to the sick person, and one from which he would gladly escape. They know but little of the real invalid, who imagine that he ever desires to rid himself of the visits, or shake off the authority, of the medical man. The sons of Æsculapius are, in essentials, as supreme in the sick chamber, as the Belgian priest in his confessional, or the Wesleyan minister in a Welsh conventicle. It is only when repeated failures have followed the prescription, that their power ceases, or the charm is broken. It is only when the more orthodox systems have lost their effect, that the aid of the heterodox mesmerist is called in. But let the faculty themselves once include magnetic treatment within the legitimate means of relief, and in no very serious case would it be resorted to without their approval. Of course medical men, with large or increasing practice, would not themselves enjoy sufficient leisure to mesmerise extensively; they could but give directions for its use, and supervise its application; still, the treatment itself would in the main be subject to their pleasure, whilst, most probably, here and there, some of the younger members, with peculiar physical and moral qualifications, would devote themselves almost exclusively to the practice: but to suppose that, when once established, Mesmerism would be widely employed without the sanction of the practitioner, or that it would banish the physician from the sick house, is an erroneous view arising from an ignorance of human nature. It is repeated, that the patients themselves would neither wish nor agree to it; nor in very serious diseases would the magnetiser himself be covetous of such anxious responsibility. The druggist, indeed, might suffer from the change; and a large amount of his poisonous doses might

remain unshaken on his shelves; but the power, the influence, and, to come to the point, the income, of the real physiologist and physician would be extended and improved; Mesmerism would take its natural place amidst the other "appliances" of the healing art; and the lecturer and irresponsible manipulator would in great measure disappear.[*]

But, whilst it were almost an impertinence to vindicate the character of professional men from the above illiberal imputation, it cannot be said that a dread of the subject has not in some measure guided their conduct. They have had their fears of Mesmerism, though in a different sense to that intended by the public. For the science is unpopular. Perhaps it would be more accurate to say that it *was* unpopular, since a more favourable estimation of its value has for some little time been gaining ground. Still, it were idle to deny that Mesmerism has laboured under many an unfortunate and odious appellation. The notion of its unreality and falsehood,—the accusation of imposture,—the potent cry of "Satanic agency," so captivating with weak and excitable women, ignorant as they are that the very same clamour has been raised on points wherein such an opinion would be now scouted,—an erroneous idea of the impropriety of the practice,—and, more than all, the novelty of the thing, and the unpleasantness attendant on unestablished theories: all these causes contributed to render the science unpopular, and to attach an

[*] Most mesmerisers with whom I am acquainted rather seek the countenance of medical men, than set themselves up as their rivals. One of the most laborious and benevolent mesmerists has often said, that he only practises the art because the regular practitioner refuses to employ it. The language of Gauthier is the most usual:—" Je pense toujours comme un fait acquis qu'il ne doit point y avoir de traitement, s'il n'est ordonné ou conseillé par un médecin, dont le magnétiseur est le préposé."—*Traité Pratique*, p. 99. See also the language of Mesmer, quoted by Gauthier, p. 697, stating that the physician is alone capable of putting his system into practice. See also Gauthier's own language to the medical world, p. 694. See also some excellent remarks of Dr. Elliotson, in *Zoist*, vol. iv. p. 377.

undesirable reputation to its premature advocacy. The day is not so distant, when it would have been as much a mark of ill-breeding to name the name of Mesmerism to "ears polite" and scientific, as to start the topic of parliamentary reform at the table of a boroughmonger, or to insist on the justice of an increased grant to Maynooth to an Irish Orangeman. Animal magnetism was, in short, tabooed in fashionable circles. And this is what medical men both felt and knew. They felt that, true or false, it was an unwelcome topic; and that to inquire into it would be as unwise, as to practise it would be unsafe. Added to which, there was the dread of ridicule from professional brethren,—the apprehension of being singled out, sneered down, and pointed at, if they meddled, however discreetly, with the "unclean thing." Thus, many causes concurred to render Mesmerism distasteful to the practitioner: a beacon to avoid,—not a light to lead men on; and not many, therefore, ventured on the study. That fine and manly philosophy which shrinks not from following out a fact, let it carry you where it may; that love of truth at all price; that high conscientiousness of principle, which would be ashamed to disown the convictions of the understanding, be the consequences however inconvenient; all these qualifications belong, apparently, but to few.

> " To show the world what long experience gains,
> Requires not courage, tho' it calls for pains ;
> But at life's outset to inform mankind,
> Is a bold effort of a valiant mind."*

These, then, are the reasons, which sufficiently explain the shyness of medical men for embarking in the practice ; the shyness, we mean, of those who had not yet established a firm footing in their vocation, and whose risks would be so far greater than any advantage acquired; and he must

* Crabbe's Borough, Letter VII.

first be well assured of his own moral courage and independence, who would pronounce a sweeping condemnation on such prudential regard to worldly prospects. All this applies, however, exclusively to the rising and younger members of the profession. The question yet remains, what is it that has hindered the leaders of the body, those whose names are too firmly fixed to be damaged by an unpopular novelty,—what is it that has hindered *them* from giving an honest, earnest, impartial investigation to a subject, with such large claims to inquiry, as the science of mesmerism ?

My own impression is, that their resistance has arisen, partly from their being committed to a positive and adverse opinion, and partly from that pride of intellect which belongs so remarkably to scientific men, indisposing them as it does to receive any statements as true which are in contradiction of their own pre-arranged and pre-conceived notions.

That they have committed themselves is certain. In an evil and hasty hour they decided with senatorial authority, that the mesmerical representations were an absurdity, and in the nature of things could not be true. To pass over the declarations of Continental physicians, and the old story of the French academies, it is sufficient to say that the leaders in English practice at once pronounced, *ex cathedrâ*, against the science. Without study, without inquiry, without making a natural comparison between the magnetic appearances and certain analogous facts which had presented themselves spontaneously in several sickly persons, and, being recorded by men of their own profession, might have thrown some light on the question ; with only here and there an occasional and supercilious attendance at an experiment, the most eminent physicians that the metropolis could produce, with one splendid exception, committed themselves at once to an adverse

opinion; and all their provincial brethren followed in their train. This was unfortunate for Mesmerism; but in the end has been still more unfortunate and awkward for themselves. To retrace their ground after so false a step, to own themselves in the wrong, to admit that if greater care had been bestowed, a modified, if not indeed an opposite, opinion might perchance have followed, would of course be painful to men of professional eminence. It would be tantamount to saying that they, the anatomists, the physiologists *par excellence*, had been mistaken in their own vocation, and that ignorant and unprofessional parties had conducted them to the truth. The natural heart kicks against such condescension. Pride, mortified vanity, a dread of reproach, a dread of ridicule, would all be creating an 'uproar in the mind, and forbidding the retractation, however desirable. A younger man might attempt it, but not the advanced and dignified leader. To "stand by his order," however overbearing; to stick by his opinions, however perverse; to look any way but the way that would place him in the right; to appear deaf, blind, absent, or overthoughtful; to be too busy and too absorbed in immediate occupations to find leisure for the study: anything, in short, would better suit his views than a reconsideration of the subject, or a deviation from his positive and primary assertions. A philosopher (says the witty Frenchman) must part with everything sooner than his opinions.* His mind may misgive him as to their truth; he may feel the ground crumbling beneath his feet, and observe signs of an approaching change gathering fast around; no matter for the result; like an angry politician, he must only cry out "no surrender" all the louder for

---

* " Pangloss avouait qu'il avait toujours horriblement souffert; mais ayant soutenu une fois que tout allait à merveille, il le soutenait toujours, et n'en croyait rien."— *Candide*, cap. 30. The same great authority says elsewhere, " Je suis toujours de mon premier sentiment; car je suis philosophe; Il ne me convient pas de me dédire."—Cap. 22.

---

the sight, and with a dogged determination that embraces only one side of the question, postpone the inevitable hour of concession to the latest possible moment, with the worst possible grace.

In that illustrious chronicle which records the doings of the famous doctor of Valladolid, we are told, that the hero of Santillana, troubled in his mind at the frightful havoc which was following their labours, just hinted to his master, in the most delicate way imaginable, the bare possibility as to his being mistaken in his theory. " Let us change," said he, " our practice. Let us, from the idlest curiosity, just give our patients some different preparations, and see their effect. The worst that could happen would be that they could only suffer, as they do at present, and die in the end." Sangrado was staggered for a moment; for something of the same feeling had been passing in his own mind. " My dear friend," he, however, replied, " I would make the trial willingly; but unfortunately it would be attended by an untoward consequence; my opinions are published, and surely you would not have me stultify my own statements?" "Oh, *vous avez raison*," replied Gil Blas, " by no means give a triumph to your enemies; they would say you had found out your error: and sooner than your reputation should suffer by such a step, let patients, people, clergy, and nobility perish in our hands!" *

And even so is it with our medical friends. Their dogmata were given forth hastily to the world; they asserted peremptorily, that mesmerism was an " unreal mockery," and its followers but simple dupes; and although we often most humbly suggest, that peradventure, they *might* be mistaken; that, perhaps, they who *have studied* the question may be *right*, and that they

---

* Gil Blas, livre 2. cap. 5.

who have *not studied* it may be *wrong*; and, like San-grado's pupil, we delicately propose to them, from sheer curiosity, to re-examine the subject — the appeal is idle, — they shake their heads with an imposing gravity for-bidding all reply, for, like their prototype in Spain, their patients may suffer, but they cannot abandon — an opinion!

It may, however, be asked, how is it that we speak so positively as to the feelings of certain members of the profession, and to their being influenced by an opinion, to which they stand thus committed? The answer is one which carries its own proof as soon as it is heard.

Mesmerism *professes* to be a powerful auxiliary to the healing art. It *professes*, right or wrong, to lessen the amount of bodily pain, to induce sleep where sleep is otherwise unattainable, to cure disease where disease is often irremediable. Supposing, for the sake of argument, that the pretensions of the *clairvoyant* were altogether erroneous, and that considerable abatement must be made for the exaggerated expectations of over sanguine mes-merists — still, with these deductions, the claims of this discovery to the possession of a large amount of beneficial properties would yet remain considerable. What then, it might be asked, would be the line of conduct, which, *à priori*, we might anticipate from the friends of human kind on a question of this nature? What would be the language which a philanthropic profession might be ex-pected to employ, to judge them by the test of their usual demeanour? We should say, that, sceptical as they might be as to the establishment of the fact, their uppermost feelings would be those of a *hope that it were true*. On presenting to their notice so unexpected a discovery, of course hesitation and incredulity would be not only natural but proper; still, if they were men — if no sinister influences were biasing their views or warping their

hearts, — their desire would be, that what promised to convey so vast a boon to suffering humanity might not prove a mistake.* Their fears of its failure might be greater than their hopes of its success: they might appre-hend that the anxious wishes of the discoverer had been the "father to his thoughts," and bade him arrive too rapidly at a conclusion; still they would listen with inte-rest, they would examine with care, they would them-selves experimentalise, and do all they could to sift the question, and establish how much of benefit there might be obtained from the treatment; and if the presumed dis-covery resolved itself unhappily into an error, they would sympathise in the disappointment of the suffering patients, and feel a sincere regret for the sad frustration of their hopes. These, do I boldly assert, would be the feelings of benevolent men, if uninfluenced by any counter or in-terested motives. There would be one remedy less for the ills of human life than men's fond expectations had been led to anticipate! Mesmerism would, indeed, be overthrown, but the contemplated relief of thousands would be overthrown also!

Has this, then, or any thing like this, been the conduct of our opponents, medical or scientific? alas for human nature, the very reverse! Their aim has ever been, not to discover the uses, but to detect any fallacies, of the art; not to avail themselves of its resources towards the miti-gation of disease, but to exercise their inventive faculties in starting far-fetched solutions for each result; to fasten on each imagined failure with the most unmitigated glee, to magnify the slightest miscarriage into a defeat of the system itself, to neglect the most important conditions re-quired, and then assume that these conditions were of no moment in the trial: to tax their ingenuity in suggesting

* See, par example, their conduct about ether, and their instant experiment of its value.

explanations that a child could refute; to assert, and re-assert, and assert over again, after their assertions had been contradicted by experiments without number;—this has been, more or less, their line of bearing from the very beginning; and to this, though in a more guarded way, do they still adhere. The maintenance of an opinion would seem to be of greater value than the lessening of human ills; and to show that their first conjecture was correct, a nobler triumph in the fields of science than the chance of relieving one aching throb! If really anxious for truth, and not committed to one party-sided notion, why is it that they do not occasionally venture on a trial? On the contrary, is it not notorious that numbers who have never witnessed a single experiment, who have never at-tempted even half a manipulation, who know nothing on the subject more than what they have read or heard from their fellow-opponents, pertinaciously cling to their original asseverations, without even the apparent wish of being dis-abused of their error? While the sounds of victory, with which they hail an accidental disappointment on the part of the mesmerists, are little consistent with the character of benevolent men, who, if not blinded by their own de-termined views, would readily perceive that the cause of humanity had encountered a temporary discomfiture, and that what was a source of exultation to themselves might prove the death-blow to the hopes of myriads of sufferers!

The above observations apply to one class of opponents; with a second, and, it is believed, a far larger portion, this indisposition for the inquiry may be rather traced to that overweening confidence in their own attainments, which bids men often reject what they cannot explain, and as often qualifies them, in their own judgment, for arriving at a conclusion without incurring the labour of a preliminary investigation.

It might be presumed, in the first instance, that the very

last persons to be influenced by this species of intellectual conceit would be scientific men. We might infer that they whose knowledge is built upon induction and ex-periment, whose every discovery but only carried with it a proof of man's circumscribed acquirements, and that if much had been learnt, far, far more remained behind; that these would be the humblest and most modest of mortals, and the least disposed to fulminate their dogmata, as though they were the omniscient high priests of nature and her secrets. We can well understand, on the contrary, the self-sufficient arrogance of some one-idea'd student of theology. This branch of learning, with all its extensive departments, has its limits; one mind may travel over its main points in a lifetime; and the polemic, who is half blind with poring over tomes of patristic divinity, and has mastered every controversy from the dawning of Luther to the defection of Newman, might well be pardoned for in-dulging in a sneer at the presumed discovery of some un-suspected doctrine in Scripture. But with nature's mys-teries the thing is widely different; here a vast illimitable expanse lies before, here the profoundest knowledge is yet but a "little learning;" and with all that has been dis-closed to the deepest researches, we are, as has been beau-tifully observed, but picking up a few shells beside the ocean of truth. No men are more alive to this fact than the scientific; none would more readily acknowledge it; yet, in practice, few have more frequently forgotten it. Experience has shown, in numerous instances, that they have carried their opposition to novelties in science, not only to an intolerance of the fact discovered[*], but to a

* The Abbé J. B. L., in his curious work called, "Magnétisme devant la Cour de Rome," says truly, "Toujours la science ancienne a persécuté la science nouvelle; et jamais ceux qu'on appelle savans dans le monde, et qui se plaisent à répéter les mots d'intolérance et de fanatisme lorsqu'il s'agit de religion, n'ont été tolérants que pour des opinions qui ne heurtaient pas celles qu'ils avaient adoptées." p. 17.

bitter persecution of the discoverer. Pride, a wounded and angry pride, is, in great measure, the source of this; but there are other causes also at work. Our accurate acquaintance with the details of one department, does not necessarily qualify for a broader insight into general nature. The mind may be full and well stored with matter, and yet rendered only narrower in the process. As Alfred Tennyson remarks, in the finest of his poems,

> " Knowledge comes, but wisdom lingers." *

Knowledge may be poured in upon the mind in an uninterrupted flow; facts from every province in philosophy may be accumulated without end, one on the other; but that large wisdom which generalises from the mighty whole, which can detect a principle where a fact is but partially developed, and travel beyond habitual studies into the analogous and the cognate; this higher wisdom does not necessarily belong to the accredited leaders of the most erudite academy. On the contrary, they are often liberal but in one line, — and philosophers but in one direction. Out of their particular pale, or set, or pursuit, or theory, they can be as bigoted, or as ignorant as the merest tyro in their schools. As our incomparable Arnold most charitably expresses it, speaking of Johnson's fondness for biography, at the expence of a different department in literature : " We cannot comprehend *what we have never studied*; and history (read, mesmerism) must be content to share in the common portion of every thing great and good; it must be *undervalued by a hasty observer*." † In

---

* Lockeley Hall. There are parts of this noble poem, that one reads, as Johnson said of Dryden's Ode, " with turbulent delight."

† Arnold's Inaugural Lecture. See also a very beautiful sermon by the Bishop of Oxford, " Pride a Hindrance to true Knowledge." Among other admirable remarks the Bishop observes, " And so he (the self-satisfied philosophist) will not learn from others, no not even by Nature herself will he be taught. He thinks he knows so much, that his estimate of what is to be known is lowered; *** He has a theory to maintain,—a solution which

---

short, this is a contradiction in the scientific character : masters in one branch of learning, they estimate at an inferior value a knowledge in that of which they are ignorant — they pass it over as of minor moment in attaching an exaggerated importance to their own especial acquirements ; and thus it is, that mesmerism has been refused its " place within the circle of medical sciences," from the usual alliance between ignorance and pride, an ignorance that disbelieves what it has never examined, and a pride that will not stoop to make the needful inquiry.*

As the accomplished author of the " Vestiges of the Natural History of Creation " remarks, " There is a measure of incredulity from our ignorance as well as from our knowledge ; and if the most distinguished philosopher three hundred years ago had ventured to develop any striking new fact which only could harmonise with the as yet unknown Copernican solar system, we cannot doubt that it would have been universally *scoffed at in the scientific world*, such as it then was, or at the best *interpreted* in a thousand wrong ways, in conformity with ideas already familiar." †

Medical men have another cause in their own minds for this dislike of mesmerism, viz. the consciousness that it would upset a large amount of their present presumed acquirements. Foissac tells us in his report, that when it was proposed in the academy to publish the result of the Committee's labours, M. Castel opposed it with energy, exclaiming that if the facts narrated were true, they would

---

must not be disproved,—a generalisation which shall not be disturbed ;—and once possessed of this false cipher, he reads amiss all the golden letters around him." p. 13.

* " Pride is but a fool," said a man of wit : " but," says Tests, " all proud persons are not incorrigible. *** Formerly, I had the *pride of incredulity*, now I have the *pride of faith*. Let our adversaries recollect that *incredulity* is often more *ignorance*." — Tests, Cap. 10. p. 196.

† Vestiges of Creation, p. 187.

destroy *one half of their physiological knowledge.* And M. Castel's alarms are not confined to himself, neither is the feeling peculiar to his own profession. At the Reformation, a distaste for the "new learning," as it was called in contradistinction to the antiquated theology of the schoolmen, whose supremacy it threatened to displace, was a powerful reason with the priesthood for their opposition to Luther's revived doctrines from Scripture. At a certain time of life, men have small relish for returning to school, and passing through a fresh *curriculum* of elementary instruction. And so is it at the present day in Westminster Hall. The leaders at the bar are the natural enemies of any extensive change in matters of jurisprudence. With a new code, old books must be burnt, and practice and precedents sponged from the memory. And mesmerism also would produce so much of a revolution in certain departments of physiology, and so many received theories might have to be overthrown, that the man who has gained a position with his present stock of knowledge hardly cares to begin over again. And so, to release himself from the annoyance, he pronounces authoritatively, that mesmerism *cannot* be true, and that practitioners and their patients are to remain " as they were."

In alliance with much that has been stated above, is the displeasure that medical men entertain at *non-professional* interference. On this point they are always sensitive. Gauthier tells us, that it was a common remark in Paris at one time, " What can we learn from the writings of men that are not physicians?"[†] In a notice of the first edition of this little work in the Medico-Chirurgical Review, it is suggested to the author to "mind his own business," and the

inevitable quotation of *ne sutor ultra crepidam* is instructively introduced. When the benevolent Mr. Hollings took an active part in the first painless amputation at Leicester, by acting as mesmeriser to the patient, there forthwith appeared in a provincial journal a letter from a surgeon conveying " an indirect but not ungentle censure for interference with a subject in which he was in *no ways professionally concerned.*"[*] Nay, Mr. Newman, in his " Human Magnetism," suffers the same prepossession to escape from his pen also. Speaking of Mr. Colquhoun's admirable book, which he very properly terms " the best work " on the subject, he says, it is, however, " written by a barrister, and that before this question can carry weight, it must originate from a *medical person.*"[†] Mr. Townshend's philosophical book, he says, is " liable to the same objection," the facts " being collected by a clergyman who might easily be deceived by the designing." My own far inferior attempt he more naturally considers as open to the same remark. How far Mr. Newman's own publication, assisted by all the adjuncts of professional experience, will supersede the older works of Colquhoun and Townshend, physiologists must determine. But this is from the purpose. The point under consideration is that, of which we have just been giving a few indications, viz. the disposition of the faculty, if not always to denounce, in an open way, what they consider an officious intermeddling with a province exclusively medical, at least to hint, and that not obscurely, at the *incompetency of non-professional* parties,

---

[*] "Mais, dit M. Castel, si la plupart des faits mentionnés dans le Rapport étaient réels, ils détruiraient *la moitié de nos connaissances physiologiques.*"—*Foissac's Rapport de l'Académie.*

[†] " Que peut-on apprendre dans les écrits d'hommes *qui ne sont pas médecins?*—*Gauthier, Traité Pratique,* p. 356.

---

[*] See the masterly Letter of Mr. Hollings in the 2d volume of Zoist, p. 423.

[†] " Human Magnetism," by W. Newman, M. R. S. L., p. 6. The reader, however, should go on to page 11., and see the very curious character given of medical men, whom he at one time considers as the only fitting persons to write on the subject. The contrast is singular. Mr. N. ought to know them. I dare not quote his language, lest I should be supposed to adopt his views.

both for forming an opinion, and for instructing the public. Now, of course, it cannot be denied, that on the great body of facts in any profession, those who have mainly devoted themselves to the study, would be far the best qualified to pronounce a judgment. Common sense teaches it. It is for this that we so highly value the division of labour. And for almost all that is technical, or in detail, it is to the student of his particular department, be he an artist, a lawyer, a theologian, a surgeon, a soldier, or sailor, that we should principally look for information and guidance. But, in admitting this most fully, it may still be a question, how far an indifferent spectator, or one untrammelled by a peculiar routine, may be as well, or even better suited, for taking the more correct observation of a perfectly new object. For he might regard it from a fresh and different point. He might be free from conventional usages. He might not have the prejudices of a particular school. He might be less likely to commence with a "foregone conclusion." He might have a calmer and more philosophic spirit. He might look at it more in connexion with general nature. At any rate we have high authority for disregarding this contemptuous sneer at our incompetency. The lamented Arnold, whose opinions can never be too often quoted, says in his Lectures, "Consider, that no one man in the common course of things has more than one profession; is he then to be silent, or to feel himself incapable of passing a judgment upon the subjects of all professions except that one? And consider farther, that professional men may labour under some disadvantages of their own, looking at their calling from *within* always, and never from *without*. * * * Clearly, then, there is a distinction to be drawn somewhere, — there must be a point up to which an unprofessional judgment of a professional subject may be not only competent, but of high authority; although beyond that point it cannot venture without pre-

sumption and folly."* Burke, too, says almost the same thing in his own forcible way: "While I revere men in the functions that belong to them, I cannot, to flatter them, *give the lie to nature*. Their very excellence in their peculiar functions may be far from a qualification for others. It cannot escape observation, that when men are *too much confined to professional and faculty habits*, they are rather disabled, than qualified, for whatever depends on the knowledge of mankind, on experience in mixed affairs, on a *comprehensive view*," &c.† Here, then, is our answer to the medical sceptic, who tauntingly rejects our testimony as non-professional. We cannot, to please him, give the lie to nature. We cannot, to serve his views, suppress our own facts and convictions. Nay, with all deference be it added, it seems a question, according to Burke and Arnold, whether we, perchance, may not be as well qualified as himself for coming to an opinion. At any rate, as we have studied the subject, and he has not, some little respect might surely be felt for our experience, backed as it is by the strong corroborative proof afforded by some of the ablest in his own vocation.

Apropos of non-professional experience! The medical sceptic, perchance, may have his excuse for thus cheaply estimating our poor untaught judgment; but why does he equally slight the testimony of his well-trained and talented brethren? Turn to the pages of the "Zoist." See who are its main and best contributors? Hospital physicians, one especially whose writings are standard works of reference, and surgeons of large and general practice, giving their cases in detail, with professional, physiological, and scientific commentaries. Now, why is it that none of these cases have been brought forward and examined in any lecture from a professor's chair? Why is it that in

* Arnold's Lectures, p. 194.
† Burke's Reflections on French Revolution.

no journal or review, medical or chirurgical, any notice has yet been taken of any one cure of a marked and striking character? We mean not generally, and with some sweeping dashing sentence of contemptuous discredit, but in detail, and with each fact and passage analysed and discussed in a critical and candid spirit? Why are not the statements denied, if they can, the symptoms explained away, and the cures contradicted? Are the patients unreal imaginary beings? Are the diseases and pains apocryphal inventions? Are the narrators weak uneducated sciolists? Why is it that this silence, so speaking and significant, reigns throughout the pages and the lectures of the opponent? The answer is self-evident.*

Many of us, who are non-professional, might indeed offer a different apology for our obnoxious appearance in the arena. Like Malvolio, " our greatness has been thrust" upon us. We have taken up the inquiry because no one else would. We have been called intruders, but our intrusion has been into an unoccupied room. We are carped at for meddling, but our interference arose from regret at observing a secret of nature continue unexplored. Our scientific opponents bear a certain resemblance to the ungracious animal in the fable. They neither investigate themselves, nor suffer any one else. But, again we say, the prominency has been none of our own seeking. Most of us would be willing to retire from the responsibilities of the superintendence, and leave the trained physiologist to enjoy his due precedence and prerogatives. To be administrators, not advisers, is what we rather aim at. Only let the faculty not neglect the study themselves, and the non-professional advocate would cease to be consulted, and fall back into his natural and more consistent position.

* I am told that not a single notice or examination has yet appeared in any medical gazette or journal of the striking cures recorded by Dr. Elliotson in the Zoist.

One of the strangest reasons in the world for professional disbelief of our Mesmeric cures, was once given me in an off-hand way by a London physician. As he is a man of a certain mark, and seemed to be expressing the conventional views of his brethren, perhaps his speech may be worth a notice. "You," said he, "are not aware of the *vis medicatrix naturæ.* We, however, who are *behind the curtain,* and know how very generally cures, for which we receive the credit, are altogether owing to the power of Nature, have our reasons for being sceptical as to the presumed efficacy of Mesmerism." The reader will, I hope, give me credit for being too well-bred to receive the gentleman's observation with any thing else but a polite smile. But I thought his speech funny at the time, and I think so still. Without commenting, however, upon what first presents itself to the mind after such a remark, let us observe to what an *argumentum ad absurdum* his reasoning arrives. Supposing that unassisted nature had been the sole agent in several of his own cures, would he assert that nature, and nature alone, had been the agent *in all?* If so, to what good purpose was his attendance? *Cui Bono?* Supposing, for instance, that three or four aguish patients out of ten had thrown off their disease without the aid of quinine, would he deny that quinine had been the main remedy with the remainder? And so is it in fevers, and so in other diseases; nature and a vigorous constitution, of course, have often done the work, while the doctor had been receiving the fame and the fee; still, neither the doctor nor his doses are exploded or expelled. For though our friends are "behind the curtain" as to the true cause of many of their most successful results, they are still actively alive to the great importance of judicious treatment, and of well-applied remedies in the sick room.

And the very same reasoning, in like manner, applies to Mesmerism. If, indeed, our cause only rested upon a handful of cases, the subtle sceptic might talk of the coincident operation of nature, and pause before he gave in his adhesion to our science. But again we say, what has been said over and over again, that our argument is not built upon one, or two, or twenty successful cures, but upon an accumulation of them,—upon cases without number occurring in England, in France, in Germany, in the United States, and elsewhere; and therefore it is that we reply to the incredulous practitioner, who would refer our success in Mesmerism to the *vis medicatrix* of Nature's simultaneous action, that as neither he would allow, in his own treatment, that *all his* cures were to be placed to a lucky coincidence, the same argument holds good in Magnetism, and that our cures are too numerous to be disposed of by such an off-hand assertion.*

Doubtless our medical friends have very reasonable grounds for suspense and caution, before they lend an over-credulous ear to the first marvels that are told them of Mesmerism. For, in their own practice, they meet with so much that is counterfeit,—so much that can be traced to imagination, or is exaggerated, or laid to a wrong cause, that, not unnaturally, they expect to find in every startling novelty but an old acquaintance under a new face. It is but Proteus, they think, appearing again with a fresh trick and a varying form. And distrust of this kind is not so irrational. Human nature is always the same; and he who would delude in one case, is not likely to be a pattern of simple dealing in another, and Mesmerism is, of course, not exempt from its own temptations

* See Mr. Kiste's Letter " Facts against Fallacies " (Baillière), giving an account of the interesting case of the late Hon. Mrs. Hare, where, at p. 45, another favourite explanation, the *post hoc non propter hoc*, as it regards Mesmerism, is fully met.—As Mr. Kiste says, " It is not an isolated case that proves the power; it is not the publication of one or two narratives that settles the question; it is the number that gives authority."—P. 44.

and its own deceits. All this is but self-evident; and we can afford to allow that all our patients may not be free from the suspicion of over-acting, and that many cases, true in their commencement, have had somewhat of the unreal and of the doubtful superadded in their progress; and therefore can we grant to the slowly-judging practitioner a large indulgence for circumspection and delay. But circumspection is one thing, and uninquiring scepticism another; and to confound the natural with the artificial,—the simple untaught villager * with some well-exercised *somnambule*, whose object is gain and not instruction, is equally unphilosophical and uncharitable. Enough can be spared, from our long list of cases, for the pleasant charge of imposture, enough for imagination, and enough for nature and its simultaneous action, and a large residuum of curious phenomena will yet remain for the consideration of the student; or, to employ the often-quoted language of Coleridge, after ample deductions for " Collusion, Illusion, and Delusion," animal magnetism must yet continue a puzzle for the wisest.

These are the reasons that we venture to suggest, as explanatory in some degree of that strange reluctance for the recognition of Mesmerism, which the leaders of the medical profession exhibit.† And to examine their motives

* " Persons, who have been frequently mesmerised, may be charged with having been well practised in their parts: but they who exhibit for the first time the mesmeric characteristics, without even having heard them previously described, stand aloof from all suspicions of the kind. There is neither habit, nor imitation, nor duplicity to be charged upon them, and, therefore, the phenomena they display may be regarded as eminently genuine. But, on the other hand, it should be considered that such phenomena, if more to be relied on, are also humbler in degree than those belonging to a more advanced stage of sleep-waking, &c."—*Townshend*, p. 92.

† I have purposely omitted another reason, which is sometimes advanced in explanation,—viz. *a fear of the trouble that Mesmerism would occasion*,—because I do not believe that such a motive would actuate men. The same reason is also given for the diminished application of ether in the hospitals. The notion is idle. Mesmerism would scarcely give more trouble than many of the present medical arrangements; but even if it did, the labour would fall on the nurse or assistant,—not on the medical man, whose duty would be simply to advise and superintend the treatment

in the manner that has been attempted, has, for the cause of truth, become expedient. For so small a fraction of the public ever actually judge for themselves, and it is, moreover, so much men's habit to receive their opinions on medical subjects from the favourite family physician, whom they elevate into a species of Esculapian Pope, that it is needful to show when he is pronouncing with contemptuous sneer against the virtues of Mesmerism, that his own claims to infallibility are not so conclusive. The oracle, after all, may not be oracular, the judge may incur the suspicion of partiality. This, I say, it had at length become desirable to point out, and having thus explained the feelings which we suppose to have hitherto biassed the heads of the profession, we will now proceed to a more pleasing task, and observe what is the present attitude of the body at large, more especially that of the younger and rising members.

To use a modern and fashionable phrase, I should say that they are in a state of *transition*. Their tone is no longer what it was a short time back. With the exception of one or two noisy writers, who placed themselves prominently forward at first, and now, for the sake of consistency, feel compelled to keep up a clamour, the language of scientific and professional opponents has, in general, assumed an altered character. While very many (far more, indeed, than the public generally suspect,) are directing an active attention to the science, the larger number are silently marking its progress, offering but a passive spiritless resistance, or, at the utmost, venting their feelings of annoyance with a subdued smile of cautious consideration. The loud laugh, the open, assured, triumphant sneer, the scornful charge of ignorance and credulity, the attempt to put the thing down at once by an overbearing system of insolence and ridicule, all this has, in great measure, passed away; and now we are condescendingly

informed, if any thing at all be said on the subject, that "*perhaps* there is a something in Mesmerism, that *perhaps* this asserted power is not altogether a pretence, and that though, unhappily, they themselves have not the leisure to prosecute the study fully, they begin to suspect that we have a portion of truth for our foundation," or, in other words, are not the dupes and knaves that they so recently represented us. This, or something like this, is now the usual admission, if circumstances extract an opinion, and so far there is a material change; but, left to themselves, left to their own willing and more agreeable choice, the course that opponents now take is that of *silence* on the subject, a guarded, calculating, timid, embarrassed silence.[*]

The above, then, it may be stated, is the present and all but universal course of the opponent. It seems tacitly understood to be the order of the day, and thus marks what may be called a state of "transition." Silence furnishes a convenient escape from untoward admissions, prevents an awkward commitment to a premature opinion, and enables the cautious follower of undisputed truisms to bide his time, and wait the upshot of events. But silence, however desirable, is not always practicable, and circumstances will occasionally occur, compelling the adversary to speak; and then what inevitable concessions ooze out! what faint denials! what shiftings of argument! what a change of language to that which would have been held but six years back? The deep sleep, the cataleptic

[*] Many persons have noticed to me this significant silence which sundry stories could be brought to prove. A friend was lately narrating some striking mesmeric cases he had performed, in some that had hitherto been treated as hopeless. "And what do the medical men say to all this?" was the reply. "Stop,—why say nothing at all!" Another acquaintance from a different part of the kingdom was giving much the same statements: "and what do the doctors say?" was the question. "Oh, they say it is most extraordinary; but the moment that they quit the room, they drive the matter from their head, and take no further notice than if the most ordinary occurrence had just transpired." The experience of all mesmerisers confirms this observation.

condition, the alteration in the sensibility, and various other phenomena, which lately would have been rejected with scornful hardihood, are now feebly contradicted, and oftentimes half confessed to be real; while the whole force of the antagonist is directed against clairvoyance, and clairvoyance alone, as if that were now the sole remaining point for discussion! Sometimes, too, a restless feeling, created by the "pressure from without," (as was lately hinted by Dr. Engledue to a learned professor,) will not allow the uneasy semi-believer to sit still, but sends him, like an unhappy moth, to flutter wantonly against the light, to retreat with singed wings and a damaged reputation. See, *per exemple*, the flounderings about the truth which Mr. Kiste, in his pamphlet, lately brought before the public notice.[*] A medical gentleman at Lymington, in an unquiet state of mind at an interesting case of relief which occurred in his neighbourhood, writes, in a hasty moment, a letter to the Hampshire Advertiser, with the earnest desire of turning the science into ridicule. He there pronounces Mesmerism to be an "absurd innovation;" he is "gratified to find distinguished members of the profession entertaining the same ideas as his own on the subject." He offers to wager 500*l*. at Tattersal's, that clairvoyance and community of sensation are not proved. Still, with all his jestings and carpings, our anti-mesmerist knows not how to avoid making very important admissions:—

He allows that "it is true" that some persons "are capable of being put into a kind of sleep or stupor through the medium of the nervous system."

He allows that in this state persons can hold a conversation.

And he allows, that "in this state, which can be occasionally in certain individuals produced, persons appear to

[*] "Facts against Fallacies," by Adolphe Kiste,—(Bailliere).

be much *less susceptible* of *acute* pains, and perhaps in some instances *might undergo a surgical operation without being conscious of it.*"

Here are brave admissions from a professed opponent! here are curious proofs of the "absurdity" of the "innovation!" "A man might undergo an operation without being conscious of it," and this, too, before the late splendid discovery of the uses of ether! Think of such a confession emanating from a provincial surgeon, in the year that Dupotet concluded his lectures in the metropolis! Why, our practitioner, after such a letter, would have been placed under the ban of the College. His patients would have fled, like the thanes from Macbeth! he would have been an excommunicated man! one of the martyrs of science! the jest and bye-word of every Hampshire apothecary!

Mr. Kiste's opponent would have acted more wisely had he practised the conventional reserve. But his admissions prove the progress of the cause, and are only re-stated for the purpose of instructing the reader as to the marked advancement that has been made.

Look again to the undisguised acknowledgments, which the leading quarterly journal of medicine and surgery has lately felt itself compelled to utter. The British and Foreign Medical Review comes forth under the auspices of Dr. Forbes.[*] Our learned editor is well known, among other things, for certain enterprising attempts to "put down" clairvoyance—quite an Alderman Cute in his way,—one who is hasting about the town to any spot where a fresh somnambulist offers himself, and ever and anon publishing the results of his visit in a small pamphlet for the edification of the curious. This uneasy activity, however, is useful in its way, and looks plausibly to the spectator, but is often attended by embarrassing incidents.

[*] It is said, whether truly or not, that Dr. Forbes is about to retire from the management of the Review.

Truth, in the place of falsehood, will provokingly present itself; in the midst of the assumed imposture, strange puzzling phenomena appear and disturb the convictions; an uncomfortable consciousness creeps in, that all is not delusion and trick. The bold knight that had armed himself for certain victory over a wicked sorceress, finds a virtue and strength in his enemy that he little expected, and his weapons of attack recoil upon himself. And to do the Doctor justice on an occasion of this kind, he is honest enough "as this world goes." "An honest soul, i'faith, sir, by my troth he is, as ever broke bread; as honest as any man living, that is no honester." That is, in the pursuits of science, he loves truth after a way of his own, and will not suppress it when he encounters it, but he does not, like a genuine philosopher, love it with all his heart and all his soul. He loves truth, much as a man might love some poor relation, who is apt to involve him in responsibility and expence, not as an idolised mistress, whom he could follow with devotion over half the globe. He will not disown her when he meets with her, and can even give her a respectful shake of the hand, and an encouraging pat on the shoulder; but he will not of his own accord go to the house where she is known to dwell, nor to the company where he is most likely to find her. His mission seems to be to hunt down the first mesmeric adventurer, French or German, that may land upon our shores — to resolve himself, for the protection of the public, into a general supervisor of each advertising *somnambule*, — and then magnifying clairvoyance into the "be-all, and end-all" of the whole inquiry, to lead the unreflecting into a mistaken estimate of the value of the science, in proportion to any blunders he detects, or any failures of the fatigued and over-worked performer. But does he make experiment of the art in his own practice? Does he try its uses in private families? does he watch its effects among simple, ignorant

patients? Does he study the cases of scientific and professional magnetists, and mark the progress of a cure, and the phenomena that develop themselves? This, it would appear, he does not do, and therefore he is but a one-sided and most inefficient investigator. Clairvoyance is not Mesmerism, but *only a part of it.* Still what he does, he does in good faith. I have myself met him at a mesmeric examination, and can vouch for his candid straightforward dealing, and therefore it is that his admissions are of some value. He is a prosecutor, as it were, that pleads the cause of the defendant, a witness who gives evidence against himself; and more than all, his statements prove the growing influence of our facts upon the rising medical generation, and the successive phases, if we may so speak, in which the science has appeared, and still advances in its orbit. It is to this point that the attention of the reader is now requested.

In 1839, the British and Foreign Medical Review, of which Dr. Forbes was the editor, contained the following statements and expressions in an article intended to put down Mesmerism at once and for ever:—

"The empire of medicine has just passed through one of those unaccountable paroxysms of credulity, to which, from time to time, it seems ever to have been subject." * * * "Considering the high sanction, which even a temporary belief in the powers of animal magnetism has obtained in this country, we look upon its recent rise and progress, and its abrupt and shameful fall, as calculated to degrade the profession." We then read of "the great delusion,"—"the last complete and melancholy explosion,"— "*dreaming physicians,*" and "diverting and degrading scenes." And to crown all, comes this decisive sentence, "to elevate an article to the consideration of animal magnetism, now that the English practitioners are one and all *ashamed of*

its very name, would be a work of *supererogation*, if the delusion," &c. &c.

These and similar phrases are to be found in the Review, and so triumphant was deemed the article for the confutation of the science, that it was afterwards published in a cheap and separate form, and extensively circulated among the medical fraternity.

Time now brings us on to the second period of our history; and we are to suppose that, in the interim, " all went merry as a marriage bell" with the anti-mesmerists and laughers, and that their ignorant ridicule carried all before it.

In 1845, however, exactly six years after the British and Foreign Medical Review had placed this final extinguisher on the subject, the defunct science is seen walking and stalking abroad, and to all appearance in a healthier and stouter condition than ever; and now what is the language of the lately crowing periodical?

In the April number of that year, these are some of the paragraphs:—

" Animal Magnetism, however encompassed with error, is the abuse of a truth rather than an absolute fiction."* " Mesmerism has hardly received fair play at the hands of many of our professional brethren. * * * Its pretensions are too well supported to justify an opposition made up almost exclusively of ridicule and contempt." " We think it is proved, or to say the least, we think it to be made in the highest degree probable, that *there is a reality in the simple phenomena* of Mesmerism, meaning hereby, the sleep, the coma, altered sensibility, &c., as provoked in certain constitutions by the manipulations, &c."† And after a long and detailed examination of several points, the article closes with again asserting, " that there is a

* P. 430. † P. 440. The italics are as in the Review.

reality in some of the facts," * * and that the writer " has not dreaded the ridicule of his brethren, in declaring his *full belief in the reality of some* of the facts, which have been often set down as sheer delusion or imposture."*

Behold a mighty revolution in the editor's apprehension! What a wondrous " change has come o'er the spirit of his dream!" Six years, six little years! and the " great delusion" contains a "reality in some of its facts," and " has not received fair play at the hands of our brethren!"

> " Quantum mutatus ab illo
> Hectore!"

The Hector that in 1839 was ready to break a lance with " dreaming physicians," and who triumphed so joyously over the " abrupt and shameful fall" of the " exploded" science!

Again " the magic car moves on;" again, with its revolving wheels, time brings forward fresh admissions and fresh views. In October, 1846, after an interval of only eighteen months, the steady progress of our science once more demands the notice of the Journal. In a review of Dr. Esdaile's interesting work, " Mesmerism in India," and in an article written in a fair and impartial spirit, are the following passages amongst others of a similar character.

" In the volume before us, we have a well-informed surgeon telling us that, within a period of eight months, no less than 73 surgical operations were performed by himself, without there being any indications of suffering on the part of the patients; * * and for our own part *we feel confident*, that, in the instances adduced, there exists, at the very lowest estimate, a *basis of fact*."†

" On every sound canon of evidence, we must admit

* P. 445.
† British and Foreign Medical Review, October, 1846, p. 478.

the existence of *some* reality in Dr. Esdaile's facts. Let us remember that the statements involve nothing that we should deem *to be impossible,* even as *natural occurrences.*[*]

This is the language that Mesmeric writers have always used. But formerly we were laughed at, now our very expressions are adopted.

And then comes this crowning and atoning passage:—

"We conceive, that the evidence attesting the fact of certain abnormal states being induced by Mesmerism, is now of such a character that it can no longer be philosophically disregarded by the members of our profession, but that they are bound to meet it. * * * Indeed, we hesitate not to assert that the testimony is now of so varied and extensive a kind, so strong, and in a certain proportion of cases so seemingly unexceptionable, as to authorise us, nay, in honesty, to *compel* us to recommend that an immediate and complete trial of the practice be made in surgical cases."[†]

Such are the strong and weighty admissions which the onward movement of Mesmerism has extracted from our editor in his *third* notice of the subject, and in the teeth of his first unqualified denouncement. And these contradictory passages are adduced, not with the paltry purpose of earning a cheap triumph over the writer, but to furnish the non-medical world, who seldom procure professional journals, with an insight as to the present posture of our science, and the threatened divisions in the surgical camp. As for Dr. Forbes himself, so far from being taunted with this modification of opinions, his change of language entitles him to the highest credit. Away with the old cuckoo cry about consistency and ties of party. Honour, all honour be to any and every man,

* P. 480. † P. 485.

---

who, questioning the soundness of first impressions, gives a subject fresh consideration in his mind, and manfully expresses his altered views before a legion of scoffers. Be it on politics or trade, medicine or Mesmerism, he who freely thinks for himself, and acts on his convictions, is worth fifty poor pretenders to wisdom, who cling to their party for no other reason but because it is their party, and whose narrow foreheads are incapable of estimating at its real value a generous assertion of truth and of new intentions.

> " The slowly judging eye,—the doubting ear,—
> The holy love of truth,—the reverent fear,
> The philosophic brain, that loves to scan,
> May make a Sage,—but *spoil a Partisan.*"

But the above is not the only recantation that marks our progress. The Medico-Chirurgical Quarterly Review,—that Journal which has been so systematically coarse and offensive in its language and matter, shows signs of a preparation for striking its colours, and of admitting the folly of the contest. These are its own words. " Without agreeing with our author (Esdaile) in the general favourable estimate he gives of Mesmerism, we may state that we believe the cases we have alluded to are *entitled to our belief,* and that the subject is one of such vast importance as to call for a searching investigation!" The perusal of this startling paragraph nearly took away my breath. Those only that are acquainted with the unworthy expressions that have sullied the pages of this Review on the subject of Mesmerism, can fully estimate the force of that evidence, which could wring such admissions from the writer.[†]

Mr. Allison, late a surgeon in the East India Com-

* " Rhymed Plea for Tolerance," by John Kenyon (Moxon) p. 114, a work which breathes the best spirit of real religious liberty in a fine poetic flow of masculine sense.

† Medico-Chirurgical Review, October, 1846, p. 533.

pany's service, has also written certain strictures against the science, in a small pamphlet, called " Mesmerism and its Pretensions physiologically considered." With the exception of one or two unimportant passages, his remarks are expressed in a liberal spirit, and therefore mark that change in the language of the opponent, that the reader should notice as one of the signs of our progress. He *admits*, for instance, the deep sleep or coma, and only differs with the magnetist as to the cause which induces it. He *admits* the cataleptic condition, of which, however, he would have spoken with greater accuracy had he termed it " rigidity " instead, between which and catalepsy there is an essential distinction. And then he comes to the " curative effects of the system," of which he appears to doubt, " because Mesmerism," he says " is inadequate to restore an altered composition and a structural derangement, and the consequent loss of power, of which they are the antecedents." * The fallacy of this reasoning it is scarcely necessary to point out. It will be noticed in its proper place. Mr. Allison may, however, be mentioned as an honourable opponent, whom a little more inquiry and practical experience would, in all probability, soon range on our side.

With the above exceptions, then, and that of Mr. Estlin, a surgeon at Bristol, who delivered to the Medical Association " an address on Mesmerism;" and that of some occasional letters in provincial newspapers, principally anonymous, and often vulgar and coarse in the extreme; and with that of the usual tirades of the Lancet and of certain medical and chirurgical journals, whose character for consistency is at stake, it may be repeated that the present tactics of the profession have led them to a wary and general silence. It is not the silence of indifference, nor the silence of contempt, as they might

* P. 60.

pretend in reply, (for their anxious, angry manner, when the subject is forced upon their attention, proves that our facts have established a hold upon their memory,) but the silence of a discreet and worldly wisdom. They are, in short, biding their time, and watching at a distance, what course their leaders may take, or what conduct public opinion may compel. This, we need scarcely remark, is not very magnanimous; and the philanthropist might arraign this want of sympathy for a study that promises so much relief to their suffering patients, while any lawyer would demonstrate that sufficient evidence had been adduced to constitute much more than a *primâ facie* case: still we must concede a large indulgence to their position. *It is poor human nature, and nothing else.* Those who are most hasty in condemning their caution, should pause, and ask themselves, what might be their own bearing, if placed in the position of many a hardworking practitioner, with prospects in life altogether dependent on the measured opinion of a neighbourhood? It is not every one that feels himself born with an impulse for advocating great and unpopular truths, or for risking the sacrifice of himself and family at the shrine of what he deems an unwelcome novelty. Some clever lines in Douglas Jerrold's admirable magazine but too faithfully paint the common feelings of the far greater majority of our species.

" Opinions current in the world
Adopt with deep respect :
New-fangled thoughts and things at once,
My prudent son, reject." *

Or to apply the language of Brougham, when speaking of a favourite literary hero, " *his brave contempt of received*

* " The Last Words of a Respectable Man,' vol. ii. p. 385. The whole of the little poem is worth reading, as a pleasant exposé of that very but contemptible wisdom, which regards success in life as the first object of exertion.

opinions, and his deep-rooted habit of judging every proposition by its own merits" is the fortunate characteristic of a select few. And so much for the present disposition of the great bulk of the profession.

But a more gratifying statement remains to be told. Human nature has its bright and noble aspects on every question. Though the magnates of the College thus cling to their original and perverse assertions,—though the major part of their brethren hold back in reserve or affected indifference, an increasing number is passing over from their ranks every day. Each year, each month, has been adding fresh converts to our views, and augmented strength to our division. The minority keeps swelling, and advancing and spreading around; and let it only proceed for a short period longer in an equal ratio, and it will soon threaten to disturb the present disparity of forces. That love of truth, and that fearless disinterested contempt of consequences which so proudly distinguished Elliotson and the other first champions of the cause, have not been without their effect, or without their reward. Society is not so hopelessly corrupt, or so slavishly submissive to established views, that high-minded examples are utterly thrown away. The same independence of action, the same conscientious expression of opinion, the same adherence to nature, her laws and her developments,

> " Nature—deep and mystic word !
> Mighty mother—still unknown,"†

are re-appearing at different localities and on divers occasions, and commanding observation and respect from those around. My mesmeric friends report the names of several recent and firm adherents. Mesmeric publications give evidence to the same fact. Miss Martineau, in the Preface

* Brougham's " Men of Science," &c., p. 63.
† Barry Cornwall, p. 194.

to her Letters, says that she "was not prepared for what she now knows of the spread of Mesmerism." Letters from medical men, "from various parts of the country, each believing himself almost the only one who has ventured upon the practice," had poured in upon her, and given what she calls "hard work" in the answering. And she adds that she is "persuaded that if these, and the many more who must exist, *could find some means of greeting each other, in order to put their facts together,* they are strong enough to take possession of high and safe ground, and bring the profession,—at least the rising medical generation,—up to their own standing."*

I am myself, also, constantly receiving letters from strangers, and from the most opposite quarters, narrating some interesting case, and its satisfactory effect on a medical friend. The pages of the Zoist confirm the same fact; and it, at length, may be confidently said, that an impression has been made,—that the leaven is fermenting and working into the mass; or, to use Cobbett's homely but expressive illustration on political subjects, "the straw is moving," and gives evident indication of a "coming event."

Among other favourable signs may be mentioned the recent progress of Mesmeric literature.

For instance, the increased sale of the Zoist, a Quarterly Journal of Mesmerism, gives indisputable evidence. Some of the later numbers have been crowded with interesting matter.

Dr. Esdaile's "Mesmerism in India," has come down upon the sceptic with an embarrassing impetus. "The experience, which he has given to the world in this book," says the critical Forbes, "is assuredly not a little startling."†

* Preface, p. viii.
† I observe that it is stated in some of the Indian Papers, that the government in India is so impressed with the value of the new agent, as to have

Dr. Storer's "Mesmerism in Disease," with "its few plain facts," is found on the table of many a sick-room.

The immense demand for Miss Martineau's delightful "Letters," is in the memory of every one. Her appearance in the field marked an era in our history.

Mr. Newman's "Human Magnetism," is another important contribution. As a professional man, with extensive provincial practice, he demands a hearing from the most incredulous.

"Vital Magnetism, a Remedy," by the Rev. T. Pyne, is a little work that may be read with profit by the Christian and the philosopher.

Mr. Spencer Hall's "Mesmeric Experiences" is full of information. As a lecturer and philanthropist, this gentleman has attained a deserved celebrity. He has, perhaps, succeeded in producing converts to the science almost as much as any man in existence.

"Animal Magnetism," by Mr. Edwin Lee, another medical advocate, furnished additional evidence of progress among the profession.

Mr. Kiste's "Letter," containing the striking case of the Hon. Mrs. Hare, narrated by herself, should not be omitted in our list.

Mr. Colquhoun's "Isis Revelata, or History of Animal Magnetism," and Mr. Townshend's "Facts in Mesmerism," still retain their deserved pre-eminence. The former gentleman has lately added to his many claims on our respect by a translation of Wienholt's "Lectures on Somnambulism," a book full of curious matter.

Mr. Lang's "Mesmerism in Scotland," &c. is well known, and has been before noticed.

Issued an order, that "all passed students of the Medical College should study practical mesmerism for two months under Dr. Esdaile before receiving any appointment in the public service." What a lesson for those at home! and what an awkward contrast with the interdict, enforced at the London University!

Some smaller Tracts could be mentioned, such as "Animal Magnetism," by a surgeon;—"The Curative Power of Vital Magnetism," by Mrs. Jones, of Salisbury; and several lectures and pamphlets, all indicating the direction in which the wind begins to blow.

Several little pamphlets on the Satanic and Anti-Satanic question have also appeared. These prove the progress of the science. People do not cry out about the diabolic and supernatural, unless they are previously persuaded of the reality of the system.

The German and French press teems with volumes on the subject. They would alone constitute a considerable library.

The publication of Reichenbach's "Researches on Magnetism and certain allied Subjects," by Professor Gregory of Edinburgh, is so pregnant with weighty consequences, that it is impossible to foretel the results of his experiments.

The delivery of the Harveian Oration, by Dr. Elliotson, before the College of Physicians, in June, 1846, notes another epoch. While his nomination to the office reflects credit on Dr. Paris, the distinguished and talented President,—the full attendance of Fellows, and the enthusiastic reception of the orator at the close of the speech, and as I hear also, at the dinner, all foreshadow most significantly the coming change. It was my good fortune to be present; and I shall not soon forget the manly and dignified way in which this successor of Harvey, speaking of certain mesmeric phenomena, asserted their reality before his distinguished brethren. "Vera esse affirmo," was the proud language of the orator. To hear this uttered on such an occasion, and before such an audience, was no small or immaterial advance.

These, then, it may be said with confidence, are symptoms of progression. They prove that our facts

have made no small lodgment in public opinion; they prove that a large array of intelligence and education is enlisted on our side. And what, therefore, can be thought of those, who, without a moment's examination, reject a subject thus advocated, and turn aside from so copious a body of evidence with but a smile or a sneer? How different, indeed, has been the conduct of two most remarkable men of our day, in whose footsteps every one might, in turn, be proud to tread! Coleridge, for instance, said in 1830, that his "mind was in a state of philosophical doubt as to animal magnetism." * He had declared elsewhere that " *nine years* the subject of Zoo-magnetism had been before him;" that he had " traced it historically," —had " collected a mass of documents " on the subject,— had " never neglected an opportunity of questioning eye-witnesses,"—and "without having moved an inch backward or forward," his conclusion was, that the evidence was " *too strong and consentaneous for a candid mind* to be satisfied of its falsehood or its solvibility on the supposition of imposture or casual coincidence." † These, then, were Coleridge's opinions on this disputed question; and are we all alive to the high value that attaches itself to the views and statements of that deep-thinking man? Southey says in a letter to William Taylor, "I am grieved that you never met Coleridge: all other men, whom I have ever known, are mere children to him." Again, " It grieves me to the heart, that when he (Coleridge) is gone, nobody will believe what a mind goes with him." ‡ And yet this giant in intellect was occupied during *nine years* in exploring a subject, which does not take our sciolists and sceptics as many *seconds* to dispose of! Oh, how perpetually are we reminded of the presumptuous ignorance

* Table Talk, vol. i. p. 108.
† Note in Table Talk, vol. i. p. 104.
‡ Life of W. Taylor, vol. i. pp. 454. 462.

of small and second-rate men! Sixteen years ago, the mind of Coleridge was in a " state of philosophical doubt;" —he then thought that the "evidence was too strong for a candid mind" to reject upon the usual solutions of imposture and delusion; what would he have said now, had he lived to be an eye-witness of phenomena that have since developed themselves, and observed the mighty advancement of the science, in its mitigation of disease, and the extinction of pain in surgical operations?

The incomparable Arnold was, also, warmly interested in the question. In the most charming of modern books, he says in a letter to Dr. Greenhill, "I shall like to hear any thing fresh about animal magnetism, which has always excited my curiosity." * And in another letter he adds, " What our fathers have done, still leaves an enormous deal for us to do. The philosophy of medicine, I imagine, is almost at zero: our practice is empirical, and seems hardly more than a course of guessing, more or less happy. The theory of life itself lies, probably, beyond our knowledge. * * * We talk of nerves, and we perceive their connexion with operations of the mind;—but we cannot understand a thinking, or a seeing, or a hearing nerve. * * * Here, and in a thousand other points, there is room for infinite discoveries; to say nothing of the wonderful phenomena of animal magnetism, *which only Englishmen with their accustomed ignorance venture to laugh at*, but which no one yet has either thoroughly ascertained or explained." †

In addition to inquirers like Arnold and Coleridge, several living names could be mentioned, men high in intellect as in station, whose adherence would shed a lustre on any cause. It would be invidious and unwarrantable to drag their testimony before the public; but those that

* Arnold's Life, vol. ii. p. 90.   † Ibid. p. 97.

are enjoying a silent sneer at our credulity, might blush, were they but conscious whom they included in their ridicule.

What chapters, indeed, could history unfold on the blunders of scepticism. Barron mentions, in his life of Dr. Jenner, that "on Monday, the 28th of March, 1808, the following question was discussed at the British Forum," (a literary and scientific debating society,) 'which has proved a more striking instance of the *public credulity*, the gas-lights of Mr. Winsor, or the cow-pox inoculation?' The result of the discussions was as usual announced, and *both vaccination and gas-lights* were handed over to *scorn and ignominy.*" * What a pleasant resemblance have we here to the discussion by the Royal Medical and Chirurgical Society, on the 22d of November, 1842!

Let the subject, then, be viewed how it may, Mesmerism presents certain difficulties to the philosopher.

If it be false, its reception among so many able, cool-judging, close-reasoning inquirers, is a moral phenomenon, almost as marvellous as the statements that are narrated.

If it be true, its rejection by so large a proportion of the learned and the scientific, appears, at first sight, a phenomenon also.

There is, however, one solution to the latter puzzle. The vast majority of disbelievers have never personally, or with *adequate perseverance*, pursued the inquiry.

As men, therefore, will so rarely investigate for themselves, it is to the evidence of others that we must continue to appeal. We repeat, then, that testimony in favour of the uses of Mesmerism towards the alleviation of disease is increasing in importance every year. Facts upon facts, cures upon cures, from all quarters and all classes, are being received and recorded without cessation.† I pass

* Jenner's Life, vol. ii. p. 111.
† See the Zoist, passim.

by, for the present, the consideration of clairvoyance and of the higher phenomena, as points that have less immediate bearing on the exigencies of a sick-room. For the same reason, the strange connexion between mesmeric action and the organisation of the brain, may be referred to the studies of the cerebral physiologist. The part of the inquiry that interests myself as a minister of the gospel, whose calling so often brings him into acquaintance with the numerous ills that flesh is heir to, is the unquestionably vast remedial power of the art. And viewing it in this light only, I cannot but regard mesmeric influence as a rich provision of nature, or, to speak more meetly, as a bounteous gift of the all-merciful Creator, for the relief and preservation of suffering man.

Tiraboschi, in speaking of Andrea Vesalio, that "great light of modern anatomy," who flourished at Padua in the middle of the sixteenth century, describes him as one who, like another Columbus, discovered a "new and till then unknown world in the human body." * Surely, in calling to mind the mighty influences on our nervous system that the magnetic discovery has produced, and may be made still more capable of producing, we should rather say, that the appellation "Columbus of the human frame," would, with far greater propriety, be applied to Anthony Mesmer!

In truth, what regions of fresh health and unsuspected blessings may not this bounteous gift of Providence be destined to disclose for the succour of the miserable! By what boundary shall we narrow our hopes about its uses or their consequences? For the extinction, indeed, of sensibility in surgical operations, in the case of a healthy subject, Mesmerism may probably be superseded by the more active

* E quasi un altro Colombo scoperse un nuovo ed finallora incognito mondo nel corpo umano." Tiraboschi, tom. 7. p. 915. Vesalio was a native of Brussels, though he resided at Padua.

properties of ether. I say, in the case of a healthy subject, because with patients liable to affections of the heart, of the brain, or of the lungs, or with a constitution impaired by long-continued illness, the deleterious and depressing effects of ether render its inhalation extremely hazardous. Doubtless, it acts far more rapidly and readily than Mesmerism; still the latter, I suspect, will be found, with a large number, the safer remedy *in the end.* And even were it not so, the inestimable powers of that science for the cure and alleviation of disease, yet remain unapproached; while I still believe, that in the production of insensibility for lengthened operations, especially where there is a sickly and enfeebled frame, the mesmeric treatment will retain its old pre-eminence.*

Apropos of the inhalation of this potent drug! there is one use to which that splendid discovery may also be converted, even if it be not so extensive a boon as we all sanguinely anticipated.† *It supplies a singular and unexpected argument towards the confirmation of Mesmerism.* Perhaps few readers, except those that closely study the subject, are aware of the extent to which painless operations under the

---

* It is now observed, that ether is not so much used in some hospitals as it was. Mr. South, the well-known and able operator, in his " System of Surgery," says, that he has " great doubt of the propriety " of employing it, and " has not made up his mind to try it at all." Dr. Pickford has published a solemn warning against its use, stating that it tends to produce tubercular consumption, and recording some of its fatal effects in the Dublin hospitals. In spite of all this, I cannot but believe, that for lithotomy, amputations, and severe cases of midwifery, where the patient is in other respects sound and healthy, etherisation must prove an inestimable boon. To my thinking, mesmerism and ether will not clash, but rather be applied respectively to a different class both of operations and patients.

† In the Lancet for October 16th, it is now said, in a review of Dr. Snow's work on the inhalation of ether, when speaking of its "ultimate success" where the operation itself has prospered, " we think it is still questionable whether etherisation tends to induce favourable terminations!" Cautious language this; especially when the editor in the same article speaks of the " high hopes, enkindled by the novelty and brilliancy of the discovery, having subsided."—P. 410. Mesmerism, therefore, is not so much " superseded," so proved by etherisation.

---

influence of Mesmerism have been carried. Mesmerists and mesmeric publications, record about *three hundred* well-authenticated instances. Some of these operations have been of a most formidable kind, amputations, removal of enormous tumours, cancerous excisions, &c., and all claiming equal unconsciousness of suffering, and equal success with those performed under the newer system of inhalation. The characteristics of both conditions are the same, and the proofs common to each. Both under mesmerism and under ether, the patients " during the operation show no sign of resolution, neither grasp any thing, clench their hands, close their mouths, bite their lips, nor hold their breath; neither talk, laugh, nor sing, make no muscular effort or any other kind of effort to prevent themselves from attending to their pain, nor display the physiognomy of determination, but lie placidly sleeping and breathing, perfectly *relaxed* and motionless from head to foot."* In a mesmeric operation that I have related, the operator said that " there was no more movement in the patient than there would *have been in a corpse.*" In a *procès-verbal,* which records an operation at Cherbourg for the removal of a tumour, it is said, speaking of the mesmerised patient, " she showed no emotion, no muscular contraction, and even when the knife penetrated deeply into the flesh, she was *like a statue.*" The circumstances, then, in both systems, are identical, with this important distinction: whilst the inhalation of ether, it is said, alters the vital constituents of the blood, or acts injuriously upon the brain and lungs, and impairs the power of rallying with the debilitated when the operation is over—serious results, which are but poorly compensated by a temporary cessation from pain; the mesmeric coma actually produces a healthy influence, greatly supports the nervous energy of the

---

* Zoist, No. 17, p. 44.

patient both before and after the operation, is capable of repetition again and again when the wound requires dressing, or when ease and sleep are desirable, and has never yet been charged with causing death, or raising a fear through any dangerous symptom!

This, then, was the state of the question before the new mode of preventing pain by the inhalation of gases had been introduced into the hospitals.* *Three hundred* surgical operations, performed when the patient was equally insensible under the influence of Mesmerism, had actually taken place! *Three hundred* well-authenticated facts, with competent and trustworthy testimony! And what, it may be asked in reply, was the notice taken of these startling occurrences by the surgical world? Either, according to usage, there was no notice taken at all, or, if men condescended to make a remark, it was said that the patients were *three hundred impostors*, who, to please their Mesmeric patrons, pretended to feel no suffering, when oftentimes their sufferings must have been acute; or that they were *three hundred cases of peculiarity of constitution*, under which, through the vagaries of nature, but a small amount of pain or sensation were known; or that our representation of a painless condition was childish nonsense, opposing common sense and the laws of physiology; or, lastly, that it was a melancholy delusion, for that the *three hundred* tricksters did not stand alone, but had given birth to many more than *three hundred* dupes!

Sometimes, moreover, the actual existence of the patients was denied. A list, therefore, of such operations as have fallen under my own inquiries, and have taken place since the year 1841 is herewith appended.†

* Etherisation is extensively used at the George's and St. Bartholomew's: but I understand not at the London or University college, unless demanded by the patient. Neither is it much used in the two Borough Hospitals; at least it was quite discarded there a short time back.

† I have not gone back to the well-known operation on Madame Plantin,

The *first* operation, however, that took place in England, was the introduction of a seton into the back of Elizabeth Okey, under the direction of Dr. Elliotson, in the spring of 1838.

The *second* operation of the same kind in England, was the division of the tendons at the back of the knee-joint in a young lady of the age of 17, by Dr. Engledue, of Southsea, August, 1842.

Then followed the famous Nottinghamshire amputation, under the management of Mr. Topham, of the Temple, that case which will be the grand *opprobrium* of the Royal Medical and Chirurgical Society for some years to come.

Eight Amputations in the Mesmeric State.

The leg of James Wombell, by Mr. Ward, at Wellow, Nottinghamshire, October, 1842.

The finger of John Marrien, by Mr. Dunn, of Wolverhampton, 1844.

Leg of Mary Ann Lakin, by Mr. Tosswill, at Leicester, August, 1844.

Leg of Elizabeth ———, by Mr. Paget, at Leicester, November, 1844.

Arm of Mrs. Northway, at Torquay, by Mr. Jolly, May 16. 1845.

Leg of Thomas Dysart, by Dr. Fenton, at Alyth, Perthshire, June, 1845.

Leg of Mademoiselle D'Albanet, at Cherbourg, France, October, 1845, by Dr. Loysel.

Leg of John Pepperal, at Bridgewater, by Mr. King, August, 1846.

Miscellaneous Operations.

Removal of large excrescence from eyebrow, by Dr. Arnold, of Jamaica, August, 1842.

for cancer in the breast, at Paris, in 1829, as it is reported in so many mesmeric publications; nor to an operation in the upper part of the thigh, near the crural artery, of a farmer, which is mentioned in Chardel's *Psychologie Physiologique*.

2 2

Severe operation on the jaw of E. Gregory, at Chatham, by Dr. Charlton, June, 1842.

Opening of large abscess, by Mr. Carstairs, Sheffield, November, 1842.

Venesection, by Dr. Elliotson, 1844.

Venesection, by Mr. Symes, Grosvenor Street, 1844.

Introduction of a seton by Mr. Symes, 1844.

Establishment of issue by Mr. Tubbs, of Upwell, 1844.

Excision of wen, at Upper Alton, U. S., 1843.

Removal of tumour, at Lowell, U. S., 1843.

Seton introduced, by Mr. Culledge, of Chatteris, 1844.

Incision under a nail, by Mr. Smith, of Portsea, 1844.

Incision into an abscess, by Dr. Mason, of Dumfries.

Operation for squinting, by Mr. Tosswill, Leicester.

Removal of tumour, at New York, by Dr. Bodinier, January, 1845.

Removal of tumour, by Professor Ackley, May, 1844, at the Cleveland Medical College, America.

Removal of breast from Mrs. Clarke, by Dr. Ducas, Professor, &c., Georgia, U. S., January, 1845.

Removal of polypus from nose, at Boston, U. S., by Dr. Wheelock, July, 1843.

Removal of cancer from breast, 1845, by Dr. Ducas, Professor, &c., Georgia, U. S.

Incision into tendon Achillis of Mademoiselle A. S., at Cherbourg, France, December, 1845, in presence of M. Delente, Director of M. Hospital, &c.

Application of caustic to eye, by Mr. Parker, Exeter, March, 1846.

Removal of large tumour, Dr. Loysel, at Cherbourg, May, 1846.

Removal of large tumour, at New York, by Dr. Bostwick, May, 1846.

Removal of tumour, at Bermuda, by Dr. Cotes, March, 1846.

Removal of tumour from neck of Mademoiselle Le Marchand, at Cherbourg, by Dr. Loysel, 19th September, 1846.

Removal of a tonsil by Mr. Aston Key, October, 1846.

Three operations by Dr. Loysel, June, 1847, at Cherbourg[*], with one man and two women, being incisions into the neck, and extirpations of a bulky mass of glands, &c.

Extractions of Teeth.

5 by Mr. Nicholls, of Bruton Street.

1 1841, in Paris, by M. Talbot.

2 1841, by Mr. Martin, dentist, of Portsmouth.

25 by Mr. Prideaux, of Southampton, in 1842.

1 by Mr. Dias, dentist, of Jamaica, 1842.

2 by Mr. Carstairs, Sheffield, 1842.

3 by Mr. Webb, Bungay, 1844.

2 by Mr. Tubbs, of Upwell, Cambridgeshire, 1844.

1 in Hinckley, Leicestershire, June, 1843, from James Paul.

1 by Dr. Tuthill, Jamaica, February, 1843.

1 by Mr. Nasmyth, Edinburgh, May, 1843.

2 by Mr. Grattan, dentist, Newry, January, 1843.

10 at Middlesex Hospital, by Mr. Tomes, dentist, March, 1844.

1 by Mr. Case, Fareham, 1844.

1 by Mr. Shew, Cheltenham, 1844.

2 by Mr. Heath, of 123. Edgeware Road, 1844.

4 at Barnstaple, by Mr. Weekes, ditto, 1844.

1 by Mr. Lintot, of Welbeck Street, 1844.

1 by Mr. O'Connor, March, 1844.

1 by Dr. Arnott, of Edinburgh, June, 1844.

1 by Mr. Curtis, Surgeon, of Alton, July, 1845.

2 by Mr. H. S. Thompson, of Fairfield House, York, 1845.

1 at Plymouth, by Mr. Brendon, S. D., March, 1846.

8 by Professor Bell, of King's College, London, June, 1846.

1 by Mr. Fox, of Plymouth, April, 1846.

2 by Mr. Edwards, Bath, June, 1846.

1 at the London Hospital, by a senior student, August, 1846.

---

[*] These operations complete the twelfth performed at Cherbourg, by means of Mesmerism, since October, 1845.

1 by Mr. Bell, December, 1846; and, lastly,
94 by Mr. Purland, surgeon-dentist, of Mortimer Street, Cavendish Square, whose zeal and experience in the good cause of humanity are so great and unremitting.*
Total of extractions of teeth in the Mesmeric state, 178.

To this catalogue must be added 95 operations performed by Dr. Esdaile in India, of which cases Dr. Forbes (as before quoted) has said, that "the evidence is of such a character, that the question can no longer be disregarded by the profession."†

Many more extractions of teeth, and minor operations could, doubtless, have been given, had I applied to different Mesmerisers for their returns; but, with the above facts, thus stands the question:—

Operation by Dr. Elliotson - -	1
Operation by Dr. Engledue - -	1
Amputations - - - -	8
Miscellaneous operations - -	29
Extractions of teeth - - -	178
Operations in India by Dr. Esdaile, principally of a most formidable character -	95
Total of surgical operations without pain under Mesmeric influence - -	312‡

* Mr. Purland, who has been so successful in mesmeric operations, is no bigot to one method, but has also employed Etherisation in upwards of 150 cases of teeth-extraction, without accident. From his experience we should infer that ether, by its greater readiness of application, would supersede Mesmerism for minor operations, were there no *secondary effects* to dread.

† Seventy-three of these operations are recorded by Dr. Esdaile in his work: the rest are to be found in subsequent reports sent by him to England.

‡ Yet it is of a science that has produced all this benefit to man, that a London physician lately uttered the following *[illegible]*.—In the Minutes of Evidence taking before a select committee of the House of Commons on Medical Registration, Dr. Seymour pronounced, that in patronising the Mesmeric Hospital (where operations of the kind reported above are to take place), "a person of great rank in the state showed a great disregard to the acquirements of the College of Physicians, to common sense, and to every thing else."—P. 118. Quære, what is here meant by *every thing else?* It may mean a disregard to electric telegraphs, to Jenny Lind, or to the Bank Restriction Act, but surely not a disregard to humanity? It is to be hoped, for the sake of his patients, that our Doctor knows more of medicine than of logic.

Here, then, is at least a respectable collection of facts,—respectable from their number, from their bearing on physiology, and from the testimony of the reporters;—and yet Sir Benjamin Brodie, the great authority in surgery, in a recent lecture which is given in the Medical Gazette, spoke with a sneer about this "*new principle in pathology*," for the adoption of which he added that the mesmerists had not yet furnished the "*requisite data*;" and then this experienced surgeon presumed to tell his auditors, "that it seems to be in *the power of almost any one under the influence of excitement or a strong moral determination to sustain bodily suffering without any outward expression of what he suffers.*"*

If this monstrous dogma of Sir Benjamin Brodie were true, our *three hundred* painless operations might have reached to *three thousand*, and still the "*requisite data*" to satisfy an anti-mesmeric mind would have been wanting, for every one of the three thousand sufferers might only have been "under the influence of excitement or a strong moral determination to sustain" pain, for the sake of giving pleasure to the magnetist. The Zoist might thus have gone on piling operation upon operation, like Pelion upon Ossa, and yet the proof of our "new principle in pathology" would have been as far off as ever! But suddenly and happily, the merciful discovery respecting ether startles the world with a joyful intelligence, and our loudly-contradicted assertions stand forth verified to the letter.

* *N.B.* Sir B. Brodie had unfortunately committed himself to an opinion, in an article against "Animal Magnetism" in the 61st vol. of the Quarterly Review, p. 273., which appeared in the year 1838. *Sed revocare gradum!*

From the Land's End to John O'Groat's House, one loud shout of congratulation is heard, proclaiming the truth, that insensibility in operations is procurable for the sufferer. Almost every hospital in the land gives some proof of the fact. The surgical world, and certain surgical periodicals are in a delirium of delight.* Every leading operator in town and country fastens on the report with avidity, sends for the apparatus forthwith, at railway speed, and realizes the truthfulness of the representations within but a few days after his first notice of the plan. Whether this consentaneous rapidity of action arose (as some maliciously assert) from the hope of passing Mesmerism by with a side-wind†; or whether (as others more slyly suspect) from an eager anxiety of demonstrating to the world that the faculty can yield a fair trial to a *new* system, especially when that new system happens to be so accessible of proof to the meanest capacity;—or whether (as it would be far

---

* A writer in the Lancet (March, 1847, p. 265,) who had passed over in silent neglect the three hundred mesmeric operations, suggests that "public acts of thanksgiving" should be offered up to the Almighty for the discovery of etherisation. I agree with the writer that this great boon should, indeed, call forth our deepest gratitude to the Giver of all good: but why this one-sided piety? Was there no other gift which might equally have excited our thankfulness? Mr. Liston, too, the *facile princeps* of modern surgeons, writes a letter (which appears in the Lancet, January, 1847, p. 8.) "*thanking for the early information,*" and adding "it is a very great matter to be able thus to destroy sensibility;" yet Mr. Liston had been present when some earlier information had been given, but there was no thankfulness then! In No. 15. of the North British Review for May, 1847, there appears a letter from Mr. Liston to Professor Miller of the University of Edinburgh, beginning as follows:—

"Hurrah!

"Rejoice! Mesmerism and its professors have met with a heavy blow and great discouragement!" Rejoice, not because humanity has received a signal service,—but because Mesmerism has suffered a heavy downfall! And he concludes with a second "Rejoice! and thine always, R. L." Can this letter be really genuine?

† The editor of the Lancet says, in January, 1847, p. 16., "We suppose we shall now hear no more of Mesmerism and its absurdities as preparatives for surgical operations. The destruction of one limb of the mesmeric quackery will be one not inconsiderable merit of this most valuable discovery." Unluckily, however, for the Lancet, Etherisation has rather confirmed the truthfulness of the mesmerism.

more agreeable to believe) from a noble professional desire of diminishing the amount of human misery; what was the cause of this electric and *quasi* masonic movement in favour of ether is foreign to our argument: the point to be noticed is this,—that in spite of the philosophising explanations of Sir Benjamin Brodie,—in spite of the scientific argumentations of Dr. Marshall Hall*,—in spite of the learned reasonings of one part of the College, and the sneers and silence of the other, INSENSIBILITY TO PAIN in surgical operations, as *originally maintained by the mesmeric minority*, is now a confessed fact in nature, and admitted and *proved* by the chirurgical sceptics themselves.

This, then, is the argument to which the attention of the medical world is now requested with every deference and respect. They are entreated to place their adverse feelings for one little moment in abeyance. They are reminded that this asserted condition of insensibility to pain was but lately flouted by themselves with scorn,—that it was denied to be possible,—or that it was explained away by reference to strong mental volition or peculiarities of *physique*. Whether mesmerism were or were not the medium, was not the question with them;—the insensibility itself was the fact called in doubt, the point previously to be proved. Now, however, this disputed condition of nature is found to be easily procured through a different agent, the vapour of sulphuric ether, and that controversy is at once closed; may we not, therefore, ask with some little confidence, whether an unexpected argument has not presented itself in corroboration of Mesmerism, and whether the assumptions of the magnetists may not be felt to be true?

Be it remembered, then, that these now successful and observing students of nature, who thus maintained before

---

* See Elliotson's Pamphlet on "Surgical Operations without Pain" and Dr. M. Hall's "Physiological Proofs against their Truth," p. 15.

a scoffing majority this fact of insensibility to pain — are the same men, who equally maintain the curative powers of mesmeric treatment, and its marvellous efficacy in disease.

These same men equally maintain, from observation and experiment, the truth of clairvoyance, of intro-vision, of community of taste and sensation, and of sundry other phenomena.

These same men equally maintain the frequent connexion between Mesmerism and Phrenology, and the strange action of the former on the cerebral organisation.

It is contended that their assertions now merit the amplest credit and consideration. The data on which they build their conclusions are the same, or similar, in quality and character to those on which they founded their belief in that "new principle of pathology," which, discredited as it was by the first operators of the day, is now as notorious and common as any fact in physics.

For the sake of humanity, for the sake of a large proportion of their own suffering patients, the evils of whose condition might possibly be lessened by the auxiliary hand of Mesmerism, the medical profession is once more urged to cast behind them their unworthy slanders and suspicions, and to give nature and nature's votaries the benefit of a fresh trial. One of our most startling phenomena, insensibility to pain, has been verified by themselves; why must the remainder be still regarded as impossible?* If

* Dr. Radclyffe Hall, in 1845, wrote a series of elaborate but temperate papers in the Lancet against Mesmerism, in which he seemed to ground his disbelief of the science on the contradictions between mesmeric writers, — not understanding that these apparent contradictions related to different stages of the mesmeric condition, — or arose from the different effects on opposite constitutions. However, in 1845, he was an unbeliever. In March, 1847, he writes a paper in the Lancet, narrating some curious effects on a patient from the inhalation of ether, effects corresponding in character with what I have seen repeatedly in Mesmerism, such as freedom of manner, smartness of repartee, increased intellectuality, &c., which in mesmeric patients have been considered false or "assumed from some craving for effect," but of

one fact be established, surely a fair inference is formed in favour of others. The remembrance of this should, in good truth, render the sceptic more humble in himself, and less disposed to question the experience of his brethren. "The secrets of Nature," says the profound Pascal, "are hidden: although she be always at work, we do not always perceive the results: time reveals them from age to age, and though *always equal in herself, she is not always equally known.*"* Emerson, the accomplished American essayist, has a passage, which the most advanced student might read and remember with profit: "Our life is an apprenticeship to the truth, that around every circle another can be drawn; that there is no end in nature, but every end is a beginning; that there is always another dawn risen on midnoon, and under every deep a lower deep opens. * * * *New* arts destroy the *old*. See the investment of capital in aqueducts made useless by hydraulics; fortifications by gunpowder; roads and canals by railways; sails by steam; steam by electricity. * * * There is not a piece of science, but its *flank may be turned to-morrow.*"†

which, in his ether-patient, Dr. Hall is "*perfectly satisfied that nothing is feigned.*" This is one move in advance. The Doctor then adds, "I was formerly led to conclude, after examining the statements of the mesmerists, that insensibility to pain, as the result of influence on the nervous system, was possible, *but not very probable*. The discovery of the effects of ether has furnished additional data; and we are now warranted in acknowledging that sensibility may be entirely suspended for a time by artificial means." Here is then, a second move towards Mesmerism. Why, then, does this candid opponent conclude his letter with talking of his "incredulity in the sublime absurdities of clairvoyance?" Perhaps, ere long, we shall read of an ether-bed clairvoyant.

* " Quelque toujours égale en elle-même, elle n'est pas toujours également connue."—Pensées de Pascal, P. Partie, art. 1.

† Emerson's Essays, Circles, 55, 56.

CHAPTER I.

PROGRESS OF MESMERISM.—OPPOSITION TO MESMERISM.—CHARGE OF
SATANIC AGENCY.—SERMON PREACHED AT LIVERPOOL.—REV. HUGH
M'NEILL.—MESMERISM AND ELECTRICITY.—MESMERISM NOT SUPER-
NATURAL.—WHY GENERAL LAWS OF MESMERISM NOT STATED.—WHY
MESMERIC PHENOMENA NOT UNIFORM IN ALL PATIENTS.—SERMON
UNWORTHY OF MR. M'NEIL'S REPUTATION.—MESMERISM AND THE
COURT OF ROME.—MESMERISM AND CHARLOTTE ELIZABETH.—" MES-
MERISM TESTED BY THE WORD OF GOD."—" DIALOGUE BETWEEN A
MESMERIST AND A CHRISTIAN."—MR. BICKERSTETH AND MR. CLOSE
ON MESMERISM.

THE decided advance that Mesmerism has made[*] in this country
within the last two years,—the number of cautious and practical
men that maintain its reality and utility,—the variety of diseases to which it has been successfully applied,—all lead the
friends of truth to hope, that the public mind has taken a turn
on the subject. In spite of the discredit under which it is often
compelled to labour, through the vanity or ignorance of
itinerant lecturers[†], the good cause is making a steady and
certain progress. For it is not by public exhibitions at a
theatre, that delicate experiments on the human frame can be
conducted in due compliance with the conditions, which are

[*] Miss Martineau, in the preface to her Letters, says, " Of the knowledge
gained since these Letters were written, no part is more striking to me
than that of the *great extent of the belief and practice of Mesmerism.*"

[†] Of course, such experienced and excellent lecturers as Mr. Spencer Hall
form exceptions to this observation. Still, my opinion is, that even with so
able a man as he is, a public exhibition is the last place for studying Mesmerism. And the same reason applies to a lecture in an hospital. " Lorsqu'on réfléchit aux conditions nécessaires aux succès de ces expériences, on
ne peut assez s'étonner qu'il se soit rencontré quelqu'un pour les tenter dans
cette occasion. En effet, tous les promoteurs de la doctrine recommandent
la tranquillité, l'ordre, la patience, la confiance &c. et les salles de l'hôpital
ne présentaient ici qu'une foule inquiète, turbulente, déhante entre mesures,"
&c.—*Rapport Confidentiel,* p. 44. See also L'Abbé J. B. L., in his " Magnétisme devant la Cour de Rome," p. 204, in his remarks on the attacks
against Mesmerism.

---

essential to their success. Those conditions can only be fully
appreciated by men, that are accustomed to the niceties, which
the demonstration of the simplest phenomena in chemistry and
electricity requires. The failures, therefore, that arise from
the disturbing influence of a crowded audience on the nervous
system of the patient,—the disgust occasioned by the disputes
between the lecturer and the spectators,—the suspicion, and
perhaps occasionally the detection, of imposture, are constantly
checking, in different quarters, that tide of public opinion that
is gradually rising in favour of this science.[*]

Still, in defiance of these drawbacks, it keeps advancing. Men
almost universally begin to think that *"there is something in it,"*
and on further investigation they find that that small "something" is a very powerful reality. No one, not even those who
make inquiries on the subject, are aware of the great extent to
which the practice of Mesmerism is carried on, quietly and
unobtrusively, in private families. Having corresponded much
on the subject, I have been astonished at finding the numbers
who apply to it for relief. Men's minds are evidently ripening
for its reception. They have clearly reached that state, in
which an impression can be made. Till that state has, to a
certain degree, arrived, it matters not what may be the subject-
matter, no new truth can be successfully established. Be it in
religion, or politics, or natural philosophy, or medicine, all the
books and arguments in its favour fall unheeded on the public,
till the facts and statements have been for some time well
shaken together in men's minds, and other and external circumstances predisposed them towards its acceptance. No undue
exertions can force this period forward, nor bring it prematurely into being. Prejudice, ignorance, bad education, and
self-interest will have their triumph and their day. But when

[*] " Fabsence de faire des expériences publiques a été un des grands prin-
cipes de M. Deleuze, parce qu'elles compromettent souvent la santé de malades ;
mais cette raison n'a pas été la seule, et il n'est pas douteux que M. Deleuze
connaissait parfaitement les causes du trouble dans lequel se trouve habi-
tuellement un somnambule en présence de multitudes opposées au magnétisme."—
Gauthier, Traité Pratique, p. 542. The whole of Gauthier's 7th book, from
p. 542 to 561, deserves to be read, for its full exposition of the effects of
the presence of anti-mesmerists.

once the signs of vitality have shown themselves, we may accelerate the growth. We may then hasten the progress very materially. It is my conviction that Mesmerism has at length reached this critical point;—that it has obtained a considerable lodgment among reasoning people;—and that from opportunities with which I have been eminently favoured, it is in my power to promote its establishment very essentially. It is then the purpose of this work to combat those arguments which are most generally advanced against Mesmerism, to strip the subject of those marvels with which popular ignorance has surrounded it, and to show that animal magnetism is nothing else than the employment of a common and simple agent, which the Supreme Intelligence has provided in mercy for his creatures, and of which nothing but prejudice or superstition can decline to make use.

I shall begin with that view of the question to which accidental circumstances more strongly, in the first instance, directed my attention,—I mean the opinion that Mesmerism is a mysterious and unholy power, from the exercise of which good men and Christians ought to keep aloof. It is needful to make our commencement hence: for the class of readers to whom I more particularly address myself, must be first assured that the practice is neither presumptuous nor sinful, before we can expect them to study its phenomena, or be witnesses of its effect as a sanative process.

The opinion, then, of the irreligious character of this science has been mainly promoted by a Sermon, that appeared in one of the numbers of the *Penny Pulpit*, and has been actively circulated through the country, entitled "Satanic Agency and Mesmerism," and which is alleged to have been preached in Liverpool by the Rev. Hugh M'Neile.

This sermon, however, was not published with the sanction of the preacher, and so far he is not responsible: but inasmuch as its sale is a matter of notoriety in the town wherein he resides;—and as no steps have been taken by him for a disavowal of its contents, though an opening for that very purpose was good-naturedly afforded him;—and as the short-hand writer, from whose notes the sermon was printed, is ready, we

are informed, to make affidavit of the accuracy of his report, —it may fairly be inferred, how incredible soever it may sound, that *that sermon*, with perhaps some little variation of language, was *actually preached* by Mr. M'Neile.

Now a sermon put forth, even in this unauthorised manner, with the *prestige* of so popular a name, certainly deserves every respectful consideration. The number, moreover, of Mr. M'Neile's admirers, and the zeal [*] with which they distribute this publication among the thoughtful and the religious, give additional importance to its pages;—and it having come to my own knowledge, that several parties had been prevented from adopting or witnessing the curative effects of Mesmerism, through scruples of conscience raised by this very discourse, I was prepared to bestow upon it a much more careful perusal than intrinsically it requires.

Believing, then, as I do most firmly, that Mesmerism is a mighty remedial agent, mercifully vouchsafed by the beneficent Creator for the mitigation of human misery—a remedy to be employed, like every other remedy, prayerfully, thankfully, and with a humble dependence on the will of Him who sent the chastisement, and can alone remove it,—having daily reason, too, to bless God for the introduction of this very remedy within the circle of my own family, it is difficult for me to express the amazement, the regret, the feelings akin to something like shame, with which I first read this most deplorable publication. And knowing the delusion under which so many labour on this question—a delusion which the unfortunate language of this sermon has tended so greatly to strengthen amongst the ignorant and the superstitious, I feel it to be nothing short of a sacred Christian duty laid upon me to use

[*] My readers may judge of the activity with which anti-mesmerists and their emissaries circulate this sermon, when they learn that some thousand copies have been sold, and a reprint called for. It was sent, for instance, to my own house by some anonymous neighbours, with the intention, it is presumed, of deterring us in our course at the very moment we were receiving the most providential benefit; and it was in answer to this well-meant impertinence, and to the weak or wicked nonsense that was elsewhere muttered about a minister of the gospel permitting diabolical practices under his roof, that I was originally induced, somewhat in self-defence, to take up the subject.

my endeavours to lessen the error. And if these pages should be the means of removing the prejudices of but one family, or of alleviating the pains of but one afflicted sufferer, through his adoption of Mesmeric aid, the knowledge of it would give me a gratification which I would not exchange for many of the most coveted distinctions of eloquence and power.

To much, however, of the earlier passages of this sermon no Scriptural reader can offer any objection. Where it presents from the Bible a digest of the evidence for Satanic agency, and of the condition of the fallen angels, and of their power over the race of man; where their fearful spiritual influence on our depraved nature and deceitful hearts is laid bare in all its deformity; to all this the well-instructed Christian tremblingly subscribes. When, therefore, Mr. M'Neile is alleged to state "not only that there did exist such a thing as Satanic agency, but that it continued to exist after the incarnation of Christ; that it continued to exist amongst men after the resurrection of Christ; that it is predicted to exist until the second coming of Christ;" to all these and similar positions I am not prepared to express any dissent. *But* when, from these premises he goes on to assert that certain peculiar facts, recorded in *Chambers' Edinburgh Journal*, and of the reality of which he does not appear to doubt, are*, "beyond all question, beyond the course of nature," or, in other words, supernatural and the result of some miraculous or diabolical agency, what thinking mind does not see that such a conclusion is most illogical and absurd? Is there no other alternative? Is nothing else possible? Is nothing else probable? Before so strong and momentous a decision were thus peremptorily pronounced, should not a fair and candid man at least stoop to inquire, to

---

* Merie Casaubon, son of the learned critic Isaac, says well in a work called "*A Treatise concerning Enthusiasm, as it is an Effect of Nature, but is mistaken by many for either Divine Inspiration or Diabolical Possession.*" " When in matter of diseases, we oppose natural causes to supernatural, whether divine or diabolical, as we do not exclude the general will of God, without which nothing can be, so neither the general ministerie and intervention of the Devil who, for ought I know, may have a hand in all or most diseases."—Cap. 3, p. 61. This whole treatise should be read by the religious opponents of Mesmerism. Merie Casaubon died 1670.

investigate, to consider calmly, whether some better explanation were not admissible? Should a lover of truth—should a friend to whatever might alleviate suffering humanity, thus hastily, and, *ex cathedrâ*, deliver an adverse opinion upon a science which, to say the least, is at present only in its infancy? If we cannot admire the reasoning faculty that this sermon evinces, can we on the other hand, praise its charity? "In forming a judgment of this," says Mr. M'Neile, "I go, of course, on what I have read. *I have seen nothing of it*, nor do I think it right to tempt God by going to see it. I have not faith to go in the name of the Lord Jesus, and to command *the Devil* to depart." Really, any one would suppose that he were reading the ignorant ebullition of some dark monk in the middle ages, rather than the sentiments of an educated Protestant of the nineteenth century. What is this but a revival of the same spirit that called forth a papal anathema against the "starry" Galileo? What, but an imitation of the same objections which pronounced the doctrine of Antipodes as incompatible with the faith, and maintained that the theory of Columbus threw discredit on the Bible? Verily the University of Salamanca, which opposed the dogged resistance of theological objections to the obscure Genoese, and the Inquisition at Rome, that condemned the philosopher of Pisa, might claim a kindred associate in the minister of St. Jude's! For, according to Mr. M'Neile, Mesmerism must be "nothing but human fraud for gain sake," or something "beyond the power of *unassisted* man to accomplish." Is my brother-divine, then, so intimately versed in all the mighty secrets of Nature? Has he so thoroughly fathomed her vast and various recesses,

---

* In the time of Elizabeth, there was a strong feeling and prejudice against the use of forks. One divine preached against the use of them as "an insult on Providence, not to touch one's meat with one's fingers." Probably the eloquent preacher would not enter a room where a fork was held for dinner, in order to boast that "*he had seen nothing of one.*" The "Illustrated London News," for May 24, 1845, from which the anecdote is taken, unfortunately does not give the text, on which this sermon was preached. The text for one of the famous sermons against inoculation was Job, ii. 7. : "So Satan went forth from the presence of the Lord, and smote Job with sore boils." Mr. M'Neile's text against Mesmerism was, 2 Thess. ii. 9, 10. Forty years after the sermon against forks, they were still a novelty.

F

that he ventures to pronounce everything that may be contrary to, or beyond his own knowledge and experience, as the invention of evil spirits, or the contrivance of evil men? Is there nothing new to be discovered? Are the regions of light and life exhausted and laid bare? Have we at last reached the *ultima Thule* of art and science? "*It is not in nature* for any one to bear to be so treated," says Mr. M'Neile authoritatively; introducing at the same time and in the midst of the same sentence this evasive and contradictory exception, "*so far as we have yet learned.*" And having previously assumed the sinfulness of Mesmerism, and rather regretted that he had not "the faith to bid the *Devil* to depart," he again goes on, and says "*there may be some power in nature.... some secret operation.... some latent power in nature, which is now being discovered .... something like the power of compressed steam .... or like .... electricity.*" *Why, this is the very point in question.* This is the very subject of the controversy. This *is* the very fact which the large and increasing body of believers in Mesmerism confidently assert. And "if there *may* be such a power in nature," why does he prematurely denounce it as diabolical, and the act of Satan, before the truth has been fairly and fully established? Why not wait, and examine, and patiently and prayerfully study the statements, the experiments, and the results that present themselves, and with a serious thinking spirit revolve the evidence of the whole matter, and say whether perchance it may not be "the gift of God?" (Eccl. iii. 13.) "Be not rash with thy mouth (says the royal preacher), and let not thine heart be hasty to utter any thing before God; for God is in heaven and thou upon earth; therefore let thy words be few." (Eccl. v. 2.) Surely it were the part of a wise and sober Christian, who remembereth that "nothing is impossible with God," to weigh a great and curious question like this in a humble posture of mind, and not rashly to pronounce of his fellow-men, who, for their faith and their attainments in grace, may, for aught he knows, be as acceptable with the Saviour as himself, that they are agents and instruments of the evil one. Washington Irving[*] tells us, that when Petro Gonzales de

[*] *Life of Columbus,* vol. i. book 2.

Mendoza, Archbishop of Toledo and Grand Cardinal of Spain, became first acquainted with the views of Columbus, he feared that they were tainted with heterodoxy, and incompatible with the form of earth described in sacred Scripture.[*] But we read that "farther explanations had their force," and "he perceived that there could be nothing irreligious in attempting to extend the bounds of human knowledge, and to ascertain the works of creation;" and the great cardinal therefore gave the obscure navigator a "courteous and attentive hearing." Even Mr. M'Neile, with all his Scriptural attainments, might find a wholesome lesson for instruction in the example of this great Roman Catholic prelate, when listening to the novel theories of the unknown Columbus. For, with one breath to say, that there *may* "be such a power in nature," and with another to describe men, who simply make use of that power, as those who deal with "familiar spirits," does appear the most monstrous instance of inconsistent condemnation we ever met with: it is a begging the whole question with a vengeance; it is a summary judgment without appeal; it is a decision affecting papal infallibility. And yet this competent juryman says, "I *have seen nothing of it,* nor do I think it right to tempt God by going to see it."

After certain criticising observations, however, as to the scientific character of some Mesmeric proceedings, on which we will speak presently, he refers to the well-known "magnetic experiment" of the operation for a cancer in France, which a

[*] How sad it is thus to see religious minds shrinking from the exposition of facts, and placing all the stress on a theological interpretation! The same feeling still lives. We must all remember the late explosion on geology by the Dean of York, before the British Association, and the admirable rebuke from Mr. Professor Sedgwick. In the memorial of the Roman Catholic Bishops of Ireland, of May, 1845, presented to the Lord Lieutenant upon the subject of the Government Bill for Colleges and Education, they professed a willingness to co-operate with the Legislature, provided "certain means for protecting the faith of the students were secured;" and they state that "pupils could not attend lectures on *logic, geology,* or *anatomy,* without exposing their faith or morals to imminent danger, unless a Roman Catholic professor be appointed for each of those chairs." Thus it is that men do not so much seek *facts,* as *conclusions* from those facts, — conclusions, as in Mesmerism, to which they had arrived by preconceived notions.

lady underwent without feeling any pain in its progress, and mentions it as "recorded in a report made by the Committee of the Royal Academy at Paris." And so determined is he to discover the evil spirit at work in the business, that he says— "If this be a falsehood, there is something almost *supernatural in the fact,* that we have a whole academy joining to tell the public this lie. If it be a truth, if the fact be so, then here, beyond all question, is something *out of the range of nature — out of the present power of man,* unless this is a new science." In this age of discoveries and marvels, surely a thinking mind need not deem it so very incredible*, that some large addition to scientific knowledge, or even a "new science," as he calls it, should be brought to light. We have of late seen so many of the wonders of God's providence made manifest to our view— wonders, of whose existence our forefathers had not the shadow of a suspicion, that the Christian, while he contemplates them all with thankfulness and awe, might rather be expected to adopt the apostolic language, and say, "*we know but in part,*" and we "*see but through a glass darkly.*" "Lo!" (said the patient Job, while he was acknowledging the power of God to be infinite and unsearchable)—" lo, these are *parts* of his ways; but how *little a portion* is heard of him? but the thunder of his power who can understand?" (xxvi. 14.) But, says Mr. M'Neile, on the contrary, "*we know* what sleep is, and *we know* what pain is!" Does he, indeed, "know" what sleep is? Is he so accurate a physiologist that he is acquainted with all its varieties†, its appearances, its modifications and actions, ac-

* This was written before the recent discovery of the merciful properties of ether. By Mr. M'Neile's logic this must be satanic also,—" something out of the range of nature, or the power of man!" As Miss Martineau observes, " while we have hardly recovered from the surprise of the new lights thrown upon the functions and texture of the human frame by Harvey, Bell, and others, it is too soon to decide that there shall be no more so wonderful, and presumptuous in the extreme to predetermine what they shall or shall not be."—*Letters,* p. 2.

† Does Mr. M'Neile, for instance, who so well "knows what sleep is," know and understand the nature of somnambulism? Can he explain its peculiarities or its causes? Yet this is sleep under one of its variations;— but how strange, and with what singular diversity of effect! Still it is not so uncommon but that most persons, at some period of their lives, have known an example or two of it amongst their neighbours; and we con-

cording to the changes and conditions of the human frame? Does he too "know" what pain is? Is he so deeply read in pathology that he is prepared to state unerringly its effect upon the body of man under every possible contingency? Why, he himself says—"We *do not know* all the properties of matter certainly, and there *may* be some occult property in matter which these men have discovered, and which may have the effect, when applied to the human frame, of rendering it *insensible* to pain." Again, I say, this is the point at issue. Why may there not be such an "occult property in matter," the beneficent "gift of God" for the use of his creature man, without calling up a diabolical machinery to explain the difficulty? In an admonition that *he* gives to the medical profession, he quotes Shakspeare, and begs respectfully to suggest to them, that there are "more things in heaven and earth than are dreamt of in their philosophy." *They* might, with a beautiful propriety, fling back upon him his own quotation, and request him to apply it to this very question. A Christian minister, however, would rather go to

stantly meet with a paragraph in a newspaper, headed "*Somnambulism,*" giving a tale of wonder for the curious. As Mr. Townshend says in his "Facts," "there are many who remember to have heard tell of some sleep-walker, who has been known to rise from his bed, and to display in slumber even more than his ordinary activity, balancing himself where the waking eye would sicken. Who does not believe in the existence of such a state? Doctors have descanted upon it with the precision of medical lore; metaphysicians have examined it as a curious feature of humanity; and the light and gay, regarding it as a mere matter of amusement, have flocked to see its mimicry in dramatic representation, enhanced by all the charms of music, and the fascinations of genius."—(P. 190.) Now, can Mr. M'Neile explain this state of natural somnambulism? Can he doubt its occasional existence? Has he studied its very singular phenomena? And if he have studied them, will he deny that they bear a close, nay, the very closest resemblance to the phenomena of Mesmerism,—so much so, that they appear to arise FROM THE SAME STATE OF THE HUMAN ORGANISM,—with this difference, that the former arises spontaneously, and that the latter is produced artificially by the magnetic process?

The reader is referred to that most philosophical, yet strictly practical work, the "Isis Revelata" of Mr. Colquhoun. The student, who wishes to investigate this very peculiar state, should also consult the "Traité du Somnambulisme et des différentes Modifications qu'il présente," par A. Bertrand, Docteur de la Faculté de Médecine de Paris;—a curious work, full of singular and well-authenticated facts. See also the "Instruction Pratique" of Deleuze, cap. 5.; and see also an account of a very striking case in the "Encyclopædia Britannica," art. *Sleep-Walker.*

the inspired Volume, and say—"Who is this that darkeneth counsel by words *without knowledge?* Gird up now thy loins like a man, for I will demand of thee, and answer thou me. Where wast thou when I laid the foundations of the earth? Declare, if thou hast understanding ..... Have the *gates of death* been opened unto thee? or hast thou seen the doors of the shadow of death? Hast thou perceived the *breadth of the earth?* Declare if thou *knowest it all.* Where is the way where light dwelleth?—and as for darkness, where is the place thereof? That thou shouldest take it to the bound thereof, and that thou shouldest know the paths to the house thereof?" (Job, xxxviii. 8, &c.) The Almighty Father, whose judgments are unsearchable, and whose ways past finding out, hath hidden from the curious eyes of man the reasons and explanations of many of his gifts, and left us to grope ignorantly in the dark upon subjects the most familiar, and which are for ever present around us. But is this outside and superficial acquaintance with the works of nature * to shut out from our remembrance the ever-present agency of the hand of God? To condemn Mesmerism as an abomination of the devil, because little or nothing is yet known respecting it, is a line of argument which, if pressed to its absurd conclusion, would ascribe half the wonders of creation to the care and contrivance of the spirit of evil. What, for instance, is our life— the bodily life of man? In what does it consist? What is its immediate and secondary cause? What produces it—what terminates it—what gives it vitality and continuance? I believe that the best physiologists are not prepared with any positive opinion on the matter. Some consider (and with great show of probability) Electricity to be analogous to the principle

---

* The eloquent author of the "Vestiges of the Natural History of Creation" says truly, "How does this reflection comport with that timid philosophy which would have us to draw back from the investigation of God's works, lest the knowledge of them should make us undervalue his greatness and forget his paternal love? Does it not rather appear that our ideas of the Deity can only be worthy of him in the ratio in which we advance in a knowledge of his works and ways; and that the acquisition of this knowledge is consequently an available means of our growing in a genuine reverence for Him?" p. 233.

of life. Some consider Electricity to be *the* principle of life. We are aware that all nature abounds with electric matter—it is here and everywhere; perchance, under God, in it we "live and move and have our being." We hear of Galvanism and and Magnetic-electricity, or Electro-magnetism, and its efficacy through machines, upon the human body, in relieving paralysis and rheumatism, and different neuralgic disorders. Why might not Mesmerism, or Animal-magnetism, as it would appear to be appropriately called, be Electricity under a different character? * Its results are often the same, or rather very similar. Why might not the electric fluid of the operator unite itself under various modifications with the electric fluid of the patient, and thus act with a curative influence upon the principle of life within us? It is Mr. M'Neile himself, who in this very sermon has referred to Electricity, and to the shock of the Galvanic battery; and I would, therefore, just remind him, that in the study of

---

* In our present imperfect knowledge of Mesmerism, and before its facts are generally admitted, it may be premature to adopt a theory: still I cannot help expressing an opinion that electricity, under some modification or other, is the immediate agent to which the Mesmeric action must be referred. The Germans are so satisfied of this fact, that they have given to Mesmerism the new and appropriate name of "Electro-Physiology." Kant, it is well known, in one of his earlier works, gave it as his opinion, that the causes of common magnetism, of electricity, of galvanism, of heat, &c., were all the product of one common principle, differently modified. To these, of course, might now be added the immediate cause of Mesmerism. And thus we should have one simple and single principle uniting animated and inanimate nature in one common and connected operation, *i commend viewsh.* There are several facts which show this strong analogy between Electricity and Mesmerism. Here is one: the electric fluid escapes most readily from a *point.* Dr. Lardner, in his treatise, introduces several illustrations to prove this fact. He says, "the increase of electrical density, at the angular edge of a conductor produces still more augmented effects at its corners: .... this effect is still further increased if any part of a conductor have the form of a point." (Lardner's "Cabinet Cyc." *Electricity,* p. 272.) Now all mesmerisers have found by experience that the mesmeric medium is most powerfully conducted by the *tips of the fingers,* analogously to Lardner's illustrations. In regard to the resemblance between animal magnetism and mineral magnetism, I have seen, over and over again, the hand and head of the sleeper following the hand of the mesmeriser, in the same way as the needle follows the loadstone. This subject is treated most ably in the Rev. Chauncy Townshend's admirable work, "Facts in Mesmerism," in the chapter on the Mesmeric medium. See also Colquhoun's "Isis Revelata." See also a clever letter in No. ii. p. 169, of "The People's Phrenological Journal," by Mr. F. S. Merryweather.

this very subject there is yet much darkness; that there is yet much to learn; that we do not yet know how far its action is connected with the principle of life—and certainly we would defy him to prove that Mesmerism or Animal-magnetism is not an essential portion of the system.[*]

And this brings us to Mr. M'Neile's main argument, upon which he appears to plume himself most confidently, for he repeats it over and over again under various phases:—"I would wish (says he) that the professors of this science should state the *laws of nature* by the *uniform action* of which this thing is done.....Let them put forward the elements of the science in a scientific manner.....It belongs to philosophers, who are honest men, and who make any discovery of this kind, to state the uniform action.....We hear of these experiments—but hear nothing of a scientific statement of the laws.....Let us have the laws of the science.....I consider that no Christian person ought to go near any of these meetings, or *hear any of these lectures*, until a statement shall be made, grounded on a scientific assertion of the laws by which this thing is said to act." And so on *passim* to the end of the sermon.

Now this argument, perseveringly as it is repeated, may be disposed of very easily.

First, in regard to his demand, that "the laws of this science be stated" clearly and "in a scientific manner." To this there can be no objection. This is a just and legitimate challenge. Nay, we would say in his own words, "Science is open and above-board to all who will examine it—it courts examination; let us not listen to it, so long as they keep it secret, and hide the nature of it." True, most true. But who keeps it a secret? Who hides the nature of it? The believers in Mesmerism are earnestly solicitous that the most open, public, free, and full examination of the subject and its details should be constantly

taking place. They invite its enemies and impugners to be present. They call upon the most prejudiced and the most partial to come with their prejudices and partialities, and witness *facts*. All they require, on the other hand, is an honest and candid conclusion out of an "honest and good heart." But are Mesmerists to be blamed for not stating the laws and principles of this system, when they do not know them themselves? Does Mr. M'Neile remember, that Mesmerism is yet but in its cradle? That, *practically*, it has been but little known except within a few short years? In saying this, we are of course aware, that those who have looked farthest into the question, maintain that for centuries back, the Egyptians[*], and, perhaps, the Chinese, have been acquainted with it; and that, at intervals, it has been always more or less known. To me the great wonder is, that an art within the reach of everybody, should have remained so long a secret: however, the fact is, that publicly and philosophically the system has only been recently studied.[†] At this very moment, numbers of cautious, observant men are noting down facts as they arise, with a view to a safe and surer conclusion. On the great Baconian system of induction, they are recording the experiments, the variations, the modifications, as they present themselves; and when these shall be well established, they will come to the theory. Would Mr. M'Neile have the *theory first* declared, and *the facts* collected *afterwards* to prove it? This might be convenient, but hardly philosophical. Our opponent must be content to wait patiently a few years, before his demand of having the general laws of the science scientifically stated, can be properly complied with. Mesmerism is yet in its infancy. We cannot yet state "*how a pass of the*

---

[*] See in 12th cap. of "Magnétisme devant la Cour de Rome," a good deal of information collected on the analogy between the two systems, from the experiments and "Études Physiques" of M. Charpignon. Baron Von Reichenbach's important treatise on "a supposed New Imponderable," and the most recent researches of Professor Faraday, relating to electricity and magnetism, introduce us to a new class of facts, and show, as Professor Gregory observes, how "much remains to be discovered" on these subjects.

---

[*] In Mr. Warburton's interesting work, "the Crescent and the Cross," it is said, "Magnetism appears to have been well understood by the Egyptian Hierarchy; not only from some of the effects we find recorded, but in one of the chambers, whose hieroglyphics are devoted to medical subjects, we find a priest in the act of mesmerising. * * * The patient is seated in a chair, while the operator describes the mesmeric passes, and an attendant waits behind to support the head, when it has bowed in the mysterious sleep."

[†] Only recently in this country; but in Germany there have been many admirable and philosophical works published some time, for example, Wienholt's, who died in 1804.

thumb*, or a movement of the fingers, acts on human flesh"—
we cannot yet state "*how* it stops the circulation of the blood
so as to resist the strengthfulness of the human frame"—we
cannot yet state "*how* it prevents the delicate touch being felt
in the cutaneous veins." But because we cannot yet give a
scientific statement of the matter, are we to forbear its use as a
remedial agent, or to ascribe these unknown properties to the
"devices of the devil?" In the cognate or analogous science
of mineral magnetism, the peculiar cause of union between
magnetic pyrites and iron had been for years altogether inexplicable—and perhaps, with all our knowledge of electricity, is
not even yet satisfactorily explained. But was the mariner to
deny himself the use of the compass in the stormy and trackless
ocean, or to attribute the influence of the loadstone to the contrivance of Satan, because the "*how*," and the "*why*," and the
"*wherefore*" had not been philosophically accounted for? All
he could say was, that the needle was guided by the finger of
that Divine Being, whose ways were in the great deep, and
whose footsteps are unknown. And all we can say is, that
Mesmerism is the good "gift of God" for the use of his creature
man, though its immediate and secondary causes are at present
inexplicable—the good gift of that merciful and Almighty
Father, who is "always, everywhere, and all in all."

And, secondly, as to his expectation that the laws of this
science should act "*uniformly*."..... "It is a part (says he) of
all nature's laws that they shall act uniformly....If it be in
nature, it will operate uniformly, and not *capriciously*. *If* it
acts *capriciously*, then there is some *mischievous agent* at work."
Of course in this implied charge of capriciousness, or want of
uniformity, he refers to a variation of the symptoms or phenomena exhibited respectively by different patients. And in
consequence of this variation, which must be admitted, his
hearers are taught that the "sin of witchcraft" has ensnared
the operators, and that some mocking, juggling fiend has taken
possession of the patient. Now in regard to nature's laws, we
at once agree that they are fixed, consistent, and unalterable.

* See the Sermon, p. 152.

The physical world abhors "capriciousness." "Comets are
regular," and nature "plain." It is for this reason that
sciences are called "exact." To take an instance or two at
random, we know that in the process of crystallisation, certain
bodies invariably assume certain specific forms; and that in
electro-magnetism, the mutual attraction or repulsion of electrified substances is directly proportional to the quantity of
electricity conjointly in each of them. All these facts fall
under the category of general laws. And does Mr. M'Neile
imagine that the laws which govern Mesmerism are not equally
fixed, consistent, and uniform, though *phenomena vary* when
the *accidents differ?* Does he imagine that a seeming "capriciousness," or eccentricity, is not in reality a sure unalterable
result of some unknown or inexplicable cause? We would lay
it down as an unequivocal position, admitting of no exception,
that where the accidents are the same, where the relative
circumstances of the operator and the patient are precisely
similar, the effects or phenomena would be as certain and
regular as in any of those sciences termed exact. But the
difficulty is to find this precise undeviating resemblance—this
absence of all difference, and hence the *apparent* want of
uniformity. In so sensitive, delicate, varying a frame as the
human body, so subject to "skyey influences"—so affected by
diet, clothing, lodging, and climate—so changed by a thousand
minor incidents, could the same uniformity of action be expected as in inert matter or mechanical substance? Is it probable, that a patient, wasted by years of depletion and violent
medicines, and with whom blisterings, and cuppings, and
leechings had gone their round, would exhibit the same symptoms as some robust and hearty sportsman, whose constitution
had been tried by nothing of the same order? Would not a
diet of port wine or porter produce a very different habit of
body from that created by blue pill and Abernethy's biscuits?
We are taking certain extreme and opposite conditions; but
when we reflect that the circumstances of constitution, of
custom, of food, of disease, admit of as many varieties as the
human face divine; that these varieties form the habits of body;
and that it is upon our bodies so modified, that Mesmerism acts,

common sense must see that perfect uniformity of result is hardly probable.* For instance, with one party, the mesmeric sleep is obtained at the first sitting; with another, not for several days or weeks. One patient recognises the hand of the operator, and cannot endure the touch even of a relative; with another, to be touched by either is a thing indifferent. One only hears the voice of the operator; another, without preference, answers any speaker. Nay, with the same patient the symptoms vary at various sittings.† Still, in spite of all this, we say, that in main essential points, the resemblance or uniformity is very remarkable; that the properties, as thus developed, have an evident affinity; but if Mesmerisers are not able to lay down broad general rules, predictive of positive results, the fault is to be found in our imperfect acquaintance with a new study, in the difficulty of the science and the delicacy of the human frame, which is its subject. But is there any thing strange in this? Surely we might find something very analogous in our favourite illustration from natural philosophy. The nature of electricity, for instance, is not so perfectly known, that a law could be laid down by general reasoning, so as to foretel of a certainty the manner in which electrified bodies would act, in any position, in which they might be respectively placed. Do we, therefore, say that there is no uniformity; or, as Mr. M'Neile might say, that there is no electricity, or rather, that the whole is determined by the accidental caprices of Satan? No: we answer, that the distance

* The pages of the "Zoist" confirm this observation. See some remarks in vol. iii. p. 52. by Dr. Elliotson in a "Cure of Hysterical Epilepsy." The Report of the French Commissioners, signed by Bailly, Lavoisier, and Franklin, says, "Les malades offrent un tableau très-varié par les différents états où ils se trouvent. Quelques-uns sont calmes, tranquilles, et n'éprouvent rien; d'autres toussent, crachent, sentent quelque légère douleur, une chaleur locale, ou une chaleur universelle et ont des sueurs; d'autres sont agités, et tourmentés par des convulsions." (P. 5.)

† The effects of Mesmerism, however, are not more various than are the effects of etherisation. The Lancet says that the latter "varies considerably in different individuals" (January, 1847, p. 75.); and a lengthened description is there given of the very great difference in the results on different parties. The passage in question should be consulted by those medical men who reject Mesmerism on account of "its want of uniformity in its action on the patient."

of the positive and negative bodies being known, and no derangement arising from other or accidental causes, their uniformity of action is certain; [but we add, that as philosophers could not determine a just theory of all this from the physical principles of electricity, it was necessary to proceed by observation and comparison of phenomena before the law of variation could be fully established. And so it is in Animal-magnetism; it will be by observation, by induction of various and numerous particulars, as exhibited in individuals of various constitutions and habits, that any approach to a consistent theory of action can be established. All this will require much time, and many and tedious experiments; and my own opinion certainly is, that in the operation of this system on so sensitive a subject as the human frame, it will be almost impossible to lay down specific and positive rules of its effects, in all cases, and under every modification of temperament.*

And this, forsooth, is the foundation on which the weighty charge of Satanic agency is attempted to be built! These the reasons on which Christian men are warned against going near Mesmeric meetings, or hearing any Mesmeric lectures! I would not speak with harshness of any language or conduct that appeared to take its rise from motives of piety, however misdirected; but where so mischievous a delusion has taken root, both justice and humanity require us to say, that never in the history of the human mind has an idle and miserable bugbear been created from more weak and worthless materials. If there be any thing supernatural in the matter, it is that a man of Mr. M'Neile's acknowledged abilities could have given utterance to such puerilities; and that when they were published, any parties could care to distribute them to their neighbours; and that when read, any single mind could have been influenced by the perusal. I have felt sometimes ashamed at encountering this solemn trifling with earnest argument—but even since this work has been commenced, I have met with

* Mr. Townshend says, admirably, "The reader surmises that the new science is not in unity with itself, confounding diversity with discrepancy. While there is much that is different in our facts, there is nothing whatever that is contradictory."—Introductory Epistle, p. 9.

several additional instances, in which a superstitious awe on the subject of Mesmerism, produced exclusively by this sermon, had seized the minds of the unhappy sufferers, and deterred them from employing a remedy peculiarly adapted to relieve them. It seems incredible—yet such were the facts; truth is stranger than fiction; and so I resumed my pen with an increased desire of doing some little good in abating the folly. I hoped to remind the admirers of Mr. M'Neile, that powerful as he is, his power rather lies in the command of language than in the strength of argument—that he carries more sail than ballast; and, certainly, that when he scattered around him such words as "witchcraft" and "necromancy," and called down, as it were, a fire from heaven on the heads of benevolent lecturers, the minister of St. Jude's had altogether forgotten "what spirit he was of."*

But there are ignorance and bigotry with men of every creed; and a few heated fanatics are able by their noise and gesticulation to raise the semblance of a serious resistance, and thus rouse the scruples of a numerous following. We have seen what occurred at Liverpool, with the leader of a section in the Church of England. The Church of Rome can also present its alarmists; and thus show, for the hundredth time, how extremes and opponents are constantly uniting.

As the Heads of the Romish Church have acted with much prudence and reserve respecting Mesmerism, and as much misapprehension still exists in the minds of many Roman Catholics as to what their duty may forbid or permit, the real history of what has occurred shall be briefly unfolded.

* Mr. Close of Cheltenham, who is a rival authority with Mr. M'Neile in the same theological school, and whose words, therefore, will obtain a hearing from the admirers and auditors of the other, says in his Lecture on Miracles, "he was certain that there was no interference of the evil spirit in Mesmerism. Satan had nothing more to do with Mesmerism than he had to do with us in every thing else. Never would he grant this vantage ground to the prince of darkness, or suppose that he had exercised mesmeric power. True, we could not explain the phenomena; but therefore to conclude that they are diabolical, appeared to him the most inconclusive argument," &c. —Lecture, p. 25.

This language is very straightforward and manly on the part of Mr. Close, and, we hope, will obtain the attention that his character deserves.

Mesmerism, it is well known, has taken extensive hold in different parts of the Continent. At first, it only occasioned disputes between the faculty and the believer, as to the truth of certain phenomena; but when those points were, in great measure, determined, the religious consideration, as usual, stepped in. In different places, one or two over-anxious members of the hierarchy addressed a petition to the Court of Rome to learn what their conduct should be, in the direction of souls, in reference to magnetism. It would appear that one of those applications emanated from Belgium, and another from Piedmont; though this is uncertain: but that which is certain is, that the answers from the General Congregation of the Roman Inquisition were cautious documents, carefully eschewing an opinion as to the nature of a remedy, on which their Eminences, the Referees, knew little or nothing,—dealing principally with hypothetical conditions, and stating expressly in one, that the "*simple act of employing physical means*, provided that there was nothing wrong in the intention or in the manner, and that no evil spirit, &c. were called in with its influence,— *was not morally prohibited.*"

Either these two answers were not generally known,—or, if known, were not deemed satisfactory, for in the course of a few months a third application followed, and as the answer to that application is supposed to settle the question definitively, as far as Roman Catholics are concerned, it is desirable, for their satisfaction, to explain the real meaning of the letter.

It appears, then, that in Switzerland a young ecclesiastic raises the cry of "magic," or "satanic agency," in consequence of certain mesmeric benefits that had occurred in his neighbourhood. He communicates his feelings to his diocesan, the Bishop of Lausanne and Geneva, desiring to learn whether a confessor or curate might safely permit his penitents and parishioners to exercise the art as supplementary to medicine. The Bishop, instructed by the curé as to all the marvellous details, directs his Chancellor, M. Xavier Fontana, to apply to the Sacred Penitentiary at Rome for information. A long missive, therefore, is sent forth from the Episcopal palace at Fribourg, on the 19th of May, 1841, in relation to this "new witchcraft," as the Tablet

terms it. This epistle contains a lengthened enumeration of mesmeric effects. And the Bishop, having given it as his opinion, that he "saw valid reasons for doubting, whether such effects, *the causes of which is shown to be so little proportioned to them*, could be *simply natural*," [*] — prays to know whether, "*assuming the truth of his statement*," he might permit animal magnetism *thus characterised* (illis caracteribus aliisque similibus præditam) to be practised in his diocese?

Among the facts, on which the Bishop grounds his argument that the agency seemed supernatural, was the *insensibility to pain* in the patients, their sleep being so deep that "a violent application of fire or the knife was unable to arouse them." This also is a Liverpool argument: "who has power over the flesh of man's body, to place it in such a condition as that the ordinary applications which cause pain, *produce no pain?*" (Sermon, p. 149.) Mr. M'Neile and his coadjutor, the Catholic Bishop, must now direct their attention to the *diablerie* of Etherization: but this is by the way.

The Sacred Penitentiary, assuming Mesmerism to be what the Bishop describes it ("*thus characterised*"), returns the following cautious and brief reply through his Eminence, the Cardinal Castracane:—

"The Sacred Penitentiary, having maturely weighed the above statement, considers that the answer should be as it now answers:

"The use of Magnetism, *as set forth in the case* (prout in casu exponitur), is not permissible.[†]

"Given at Rome, 1st of July, 1841."

Nothing could be more temperate and guarded than this response. No violence of language, no ignorant vituperation, no pandering to vicious prejudices. The decision amounts simply to this. "We know nothing more of Mesmerism than such as you describe it, and we come to no general conclusion

---

[*] "Validas censeo rationes dubitandi an simpliciter naturales sint tales effectus, quorum occasionalis causa tam parum cum iis proportionata demonstratur."

[†] "Sacra Penitentiaria mature perpensis expositis respondendum censet prout respondet: usum magnetismi, *prout in casu exponitur*, non licere."

---

on its merits. But *if* it be, what your exposition represents it, *i. e.*, if the apparent cause be not proportioned to the effect, and that something *out of nature* be at work in the action,—why, then, *in that case*, the use of the remedy, 'so characterised,' is not permissible." In other words, if Mesmerism be satanic and preternatural, it is a treatment which every Catholic Christian is forbidden to employ:—if it be simply a newly-discovered action in nature, the court offers no opinion whatever as to its use.

The Roman Catholic reader, therefore, who may have been misled by certain statements in the Tablet newspaper[*], and elsewhere[†], in reference to this decision from Rome, may perceive on examination that the general question of Mesmerism is still left open, and that the Holy See has only pronounced hypothetically; and as to a particular case.

But there is much more for the guidance of the obedient Catholic, than the negative evidence which the above correspondence offers. In July, 1842, the Archbishop of Rheims also consulted the Holy See, forwarding several explanatory

---

[*] About the time that Miss Martineau was publishing her "Letters on Mesmerism," the "Tablet" newspaper came out with two articles on the subject, the one contradicting and upsetting the other. On December 14, 1844, the "Tablet" hastily said that "so much of Mesmerism as is not positive deceit or the work of an excited imagination, is really and truly of a *diabolical nature*." "No person, who was not mad, would have any connexion with it." * * * * But this is not all; the Archbishop of Lausanne applied to Rome for information whether Mesmerism was allowable under any circumstances, and received for answer, a most emphatic negative." As this was rather a strong way of interpreting the circumspect reply of the Grand Penitentiary (prout exponitur), on the following week the editor showed himself better informed. "That there is any thing diabolic in Mesmerism, that we know what it is, or what it is not, we are very far from affirming." * * * "We do not positively say that this Mesmerism is an unholy act; we do not say that this response of the Sacred Penitentiary is actually binding in England; we are not competent to speak on these points," &c. In fact, the retractation in the number for December 21, is as complete as could be fairly expected after the startling assertion of the week before; and the "emphatic negative" of Rome dwindles down to a recommendation from the editor to consult a spiritual director before the remedy be adopted.

[†] Miss Martineau has unintentionally added to the misconception, for she says, "the Pope has issued an edict against the study and practice of Mesmerism in his dominions," p. 68. It will be seen that the Pope has done nothing of the kind.

documents, and desiring to know whether, without reference to any *abuses* with which it might be charged, the *use* of the system itself was a thing permissible ?

No official judgment was returned to the Archbishop : but the Cardinal Castracane answered by letter in 1844, saying that "the general question had not been decided yet, *if ever it would be* : that an opinion had only been given as to *particular cases* (à quelques cas particuliers): and that a premature decision on the whole bearing of such a subject could only compromise the honour of the Holy See."

The Archbishop placed this letter in the hands of the Vicar General of the diocese, that those interested in the question might know how to proceed.

Here, then, is a complete refutation of the erroneous opinion entertained by many members of the Church of Rome, that the practice of Mesmerism has been forbidden by the Supreme Pontiff, on account of its satanic character. The Pope has not been guilty of any such absurdity. He has been too wise to fulminate oracular sentences on a physical question of which he knew but little ; and too charitable to censure his fellow-men for the study of an art, which they exercise in the humble hope of being serviceable to their brethren. All that has occurred comes simply to this : certain questions are raised by young and officious zealots ; and an imperfect representation is forwarded to Rome, and the very point at issue assumed in the statement. On that statement and those representations a conditional judgment is given ; but beyond that, the answers neither advance nor decide. Abuses in this, as in every other science, are naturally forbidden,—but the use itself remains free for the conscience of the individual. Satan is to be expelled in any shape that he presents himself ; but that Mesmerism is satanic is a point not yet concluded.

The Catholic, therefore, who feels anxious to introduce the healing powers of Mesmerism within his household, may venture on the practice with an assured conscience. For if such were the wise and benevolent decisions of his Church under the presidency of the late Pope, who can doubt what judgments would be given by his enlightened and admirable successor?

for Italy is, indeed, breathing the air of life and regeneration ; and science, and truth, and freedom are hoping to meet once more, in harmonious strength, on its classic and delightful soil ! "

But the Bishop of Lausanne and the eloquent preacher at Liverpool are not the only parties who have seen something preternatural in this useful science. A lady has mingled in the mêlée, and added to the confusion. The late Mrs. Tonna, better known under the appellation of " Charlotte Elizabeth," the authoress of some religious works, and the editress of the " Christian Lady's Magazine," stepped forth as an opponent in 1845, and addressed a letter to Miss Martineau. Several papers, also, on the topic have appeared from her hand in the Magazine. And her opinions have, unfortunately, carried considerable weight with a numerous section in the religious world, especially with her own timid and excitable sex.

This letter has been so completely answered, in a cheap pamphlet, by a gentleman resident at Brighton, that it is scarcely needful to analyse its contents.† It is assertion and assumption from beginning to end, without a pretence at an argument or a proof. She says, in the first page, that " her business " is not " with the medicinal effects," but " with the supernatural manifestations." And she adds, that she calls them " supernatural," because " the effects produced are beyond the scope of any existing agencies in nature, unless operated upon by some power altogether superhuman." For this assertion she offers not the remotest reason : she gives no evidence why such " agencies " cannot exist in nature — all this is taken for granted ; and having thus settled the very point at issue to her heart's satisfaction, she uses this assumption as a convenient peg, whereon she may hang up the remainder of her observations.

---

* Most of the above facts are derived from a recent work, " Le Magnétisme devant la Cour de Rome," &c., by L'Abbé J. B. L. Copious information on other mesmeric points is also to be found in the book. As the French works on this subject contain too often a substratum of irreligion, it is pleasant to be able to recommend this volume for its piety and right feeling.

† " Mesmerism,—A Reply to a Letter addressed by Charlotte Elizabeth." (Sampson Low.)

There is, however, such a strange and self-refuting inconsistency in the following passage, that it merits consideration : " *I am ready to admit*, that so far as the *simple* phenomenon is concerned, of alleviating bodily pain, and of so lulling into repose the nervous system as to induce a torpid state, there may be nothing supernatural ; influences not yet fully discovered by the investigations of philosophy may exist, and be communicable from one individual to another, operating perhaps by electricity, to an extent hitherto unsuspected. The marvellous conformation, the surprising power, acting by deliberate volition, in the electric eel, confirm this theory ; but I beseech you to mark the limit of my admission, — it is strictly confined within the boundaries of physical and mental operation." (p. 8.) And why this admission? And why stop here, and go thus far, and no farther? *It is a merely arbitrary line, drawn by her own will and fancy, without rule or reason.*

What ground has she for terming one phenomenon "simple" and not another? What does she know more about the one than about the remainder? If the writer " admits that influences not yet fully discovered by philosophy may exist, and be communicable from one individual to another," it is no more than what the staunchest Mesmerist advances. Her admissions, she says, are "confined within the boundaries of physical and mental operation." Good : — but Mrs. Tonna forgets to tell us what those boundaries are ; she forgets that this is the point under discussion ; she forgets that the " *simple* phenomenon of lulling pain " was regarded as supernatural and beyond the boundary but a year or two back ; and she forgets that " the unsuspected influences" of which she here speaks may also be, in the most natural way, the causes of those " superhuman and diabolical " manifestations which frighten her readers now. No boundary line can be drawn by her on the subject. For, to apply her own language, the whole action of Mesmerism is, at present, " utterly inexplicable," one part as much as another.

Phrenology tells us truly, that it would be a waste of time to attempt to reason with a brain that could be influenced by the unproved and unsupported assertions of this letter. The hapless man or woman must be so organized as to suffer from a cerebral

disqualification for apprehending an argument. Facts alone could produce an impression : and with a fact, and that a very curious one, shall the asseverations of Charlotte Elizabeth be now met.

Lord Mahon, in his agreeable History of England, mentions in a note, that " a project to connect Madrid and Lisbon by water-carriage had been formed under Charles the Second ; but the council of Castile, after full deliberation, answered, that if God had chosen to make these rivers navigable, he could have done so, without the aid of man, and that therefore such a project would be a *daring violation of the Divine decrees,* and an impious attempt to improve the works of Providence." In the opinion, therefore, of the Castilian council, to make an unnavigable river navigable was to pass the "boundaries" of a becoming "physical operation." Change the date and the scene, and the people and the subject ; and what is mesmeric treatment to similar minds but an " impious attempt to improve the works of Providence," — not a pious and humble acceptance of a merciful gift ! *

Of a somewhat different character to this last " letter " is a small pamphlet called " Mesmerism, examined and tested by the Word of God." This tract is published at Sidmouth, has circulated † largely in the South-west of England, and is supposed to be written by one of the Plymouth brethren. Its religious effect in some parts of Devonshire is stated to be considerable.

In regard to its tone and spirit, there is not much to condemn ; and it also possesses a better claim to be considered argumentative, than all the other productions which have appeared on that side of the question ; still, on a close inspection, it follows the fate of its predecessors, and its more formidable objections fade away into nothing.

It takes Mesmerism as it is described by some eager, ill-

* Vol. I. p. 466. Lord Mahon refers for this fact to " Letters " by Rev. E. Clarke, 1763, p. 234.

† It has reached to a *fourth* edition. This at least shows that the believers in Mesmerism must be numerous in that district.

judging enthusiasts, raises up an imaginary and unscriptural monster, and then demolishes by a copious collection of texts this creation of its own brain, or of the brain of some wild and unrecognised advocates.

For instance, its main and longest argument is taken to prove that Mesmerism does not bring man to a knowledge of God, nor restore him to that image of his Maker, which he had lost by sin, as it would appear, that some ardent "practitioners" pretend that it does.

In answer to this, I would first say, that "the high standing here assumed, and the exalted place thus given to Mesmerism" (p. 4.) is a position that I have never yet heard advanced, nor remember to have seen put forth in any mesmeric publication whatsoever. The doctrine is a chimera, and one not generally, if at all entertained.

Secondly, the passage which is quoted in proof (p. 4.) does not, to my apprehension, assert the above doctrine very clearly. "God in his goodness has given man Mesmerism, to help him the better to discern himself (God)." At the best, this sentence is very vaguely expressed: and, perhaps, is not intended to mean more than that the Almighty Being has purposed by this gift, in common with his other gifts, to bring man to a fuller knowledge of his goodness and love. But if it do go the length of upholding an anti-scriptural knowledge of the great Creator, who is the writer? Where is the context? Is the writer or lecturer a fair sample of the mesmeric public, that such serious importance should attach itself to his notions, and that a page or two of arguments and quotations from Scripture should be drawn together to refute them?

That some Mesmerists believe in the doctrine of man's advancing perfectibility, and that Mesmerism is considered one of the signs of its approach, is probable; but this it shares in common with the other marvellous discoveries of the day. Steam, railways, etherisation, electric telegraphs, and other modern wonders in nature and art are all named by a particular school as evidences of progression on the part of man towards some utopian existence of complete knowledge and power; but who rejects the assistance and application of those other gifts to the purposes of life, from disbelief in the day-dreams of a

handful of visionaries? And why is Mesmerism to be reprobated any more than those other discoveries on account of the idle fancies of a few imaginative "practitioners?"

If, then, it be said, as this writer assumes, that any number of Mesmerists entertain the opinion that their science is capable of superseding the "*one only way*," whereby a guilty world may be brought to a "knowledge" of the great God and Father of all (p. 5.), it can only be stated in reply, that the thing is not true, that such an opinion is not generally held, and that a long array of texts to controvert it, is a fighting with an unreal ideal enemy, and an uncandid attempt to load Mesmerism with an obloquy that ought not to belong to it.

The more serious charge, therefore, of this pamphlet, that the science is "directly contrary to the Word of God" (p. 1.), falls to the ground: the science has not been elevated on the unchristian pinnacle which this writer imagines.

Of a similar character is the charge, that it must be by "some superior intelligence," *i. e.* supernatural and diabolical, that the "mesmerised person becomes so gifted in his sleep, that with precision and promptness he answers learned and scientific questions:" that "untaught persons in the trance explain the causes of earthquakes and volcanoes — say what electricity is, and its effects on the sun and planets," travel in thought "many billions of miles to the stars Sirius, and Aldebaran," and state "with confidence what God did in this globe many thousands of years ago." (pp. 1, 2. and 11.)

Is this a fair description of Mesmerism? Supposing that a narrative were to be published of the improvement and effects of modern gunnery, could Captain Warner's "Long Range" be correctly set forth as a leading instance of what has been accomplished? Could the historian build up his tale of artillery achievements from the promised result of that invention? And so in Mesmerism; that certain patients led on by a growing love of creating wonder have, in their excited state, *pretended* to "dream mighty dreams, and see marvellous visions," is perfectly true, and much to be lamented: but are their nonsense, or impostures, or hysteric credulity just specimens of the effects of magnetic influence?

Would the writer of this Pamphlet deem the visions of Swedenborg and his "*actual observations* of what was occurring in Heaven and Hell" any argument against that pure creed of the Gospel, which walks "by faith and not by sight?" or that the monstrous worship of the bones of dead men militated against a worship "in spirit and in truth" of the Father of light and love?

The real point is, how does Mesmerism appear, as delineated by the best authorities and its sober-minded advocates,—not what is its character, if estimated from some extreme and isolated cases?

That there is, in certain peculiar constitutions, a very remarkable *transference of thought* from the Mesmeriser to his patient, (out of which the extravagant pretensions, narrated above, have taken their birth,) is true, and is also one of the most striking things in the science. But there is a limit to this action. That which is in the mind of the Mesmeriser, or may be latent in his brain, is communicated by some connecting and sympathetic medium, most probably of an electric character[*], to the mind of the sleeper, and developes itself by outward manifestations, more or less perfect. Sometimes this communicated knowledge mingles with some older information that is lying dormant in the mesmerised brain, and brings out a result that partakes still more of the seemingly miraculous.

[*] In expressing my belief in the electric theory, or in that of some cognate "imponderable," I am aware that I am somewhat contradicting a previous observation as to the imprudence of a premature hypothesis. But Dr. Jenner says truly in one of his letters, " If there were no theorists in the world, how slow would be the advance of science ! * * * Such is the nature of the animal economy, that there are a thousand processes going forward, which can never be stared full in the face ; but there is no harm in a *plausible guess*." Baron's life of Jenner, vol. ii. p. 369. The most learned Bishop of St. David's says kindly, when speaking of the earliest philosophers, in language that may apply to mesmerising theorists : " It is scarcely possible to refrain from smiling at the boldness with which these first adventurers in the field of speculation, unconscious of the countless of their resources, or of the difficulty of the enterprise, rushed at once to the solution of the highest problems of philosophy. But, to temper any disdainful feeling, which their temerity may excite, it should be remembered that *without the spirit* which prompted this hardihood, philosophy would probably never have risen from its cradle."— Thirlwall's History of Greece, vol. i. p. 132.

Still nature is at work, and nothing more. Not rarely too, the wonder-loving somnambule superadds certain marvellous creations of his own to the former reflected images, and thus exhibits in the end a sad mixture of falsehood and reality. But there is a line to be drawn, to which the actual power extends, though that line is established with difficulty :— but it is confined, in my judgment, to the active or latent knowledge, that is possessed by the Mesmeriser, or the patient, or some parties present or in connexion. All this is wonderful enough, and proves the strange influence of the mesmeric fluid " on the chambers of the brain ;" but there is a wide difference between the possession of this rare and circumscribed action and "an intuitive discernment" about volcanoes and earthquakes, and as to what is now taking place " in Jupiter and the sun." [2]

But, argues our opponent next, " Now let us suppose, that by some sudden transition, an ignorant man is thrown into a position, where he instantly becomes learned : he is *ever afterwards learned*. This must be so : it would be absurd to conclude otherwise. We may as well assert that nature has a retrograde tendency, &c. But this is not the case with those who have undergone the mesmeric influence : all their wonderful knowledge departs with all their wonderful sleep ; therefore the learning cannot be the unlettered individual's own acquired learning," but the whisperings of some "superior intelligence" (p. 3.). The argument is, that because the knowledge exhibited by the sleeper in his sleep is *forgotten* by him when he wakes up, the knowledge so conveyed is not "according to nature," and "cannot be supported by sound philosophy," but must be communicated by some *extra-natural* agent,—or, in other words, by an evil spirit. " When the sleep is over, he is precisely the same man as before." What he once knows, " *he never loses.*" Now it so happens that our friend is wrong as to the "soundness of his philosophy," and in his knowledge of nature, *setting Mesmerism and Mesmerisers altogether aside.*

[*] To show that the above is the confined and practical view entertained by Mesmerists in general, respecting this power, it may be as well to add, that it is commonly called " thought-reading," and by the French *pénétration de la pensée.*

Analogy and observation lead to a very opposite opinion. The natural Sleep-walker, who in his trance has been performing some marvellous feats, and frightening or amusing his relatives and friends, *knows nothing* of all that he has said or done on returning to his waking state. He had passed into a new and different world, and is oblivious of all that had occurred whilst he was there. This is invariable: and so also very constantly under etherisation. Medical men report, that their patients, on restoration from the intoxicating or benumbing effect of ether, have often shown themselves utterly unconscious of what had taken place under its influence. Now the mesmeric condition is an abnormal one, the same, or very similar to that, into which the natural somnambulist spontaneously falls. And therefore, oblivion or ignorance of what occurs in the magnetic sleep, is precisely a state of things which we should be led to expect from comparing it with its kindred condition, and so far from being a proof of the extraordinary influence of a diabolic spirit, is rather a satisfactory and conclusive argument as to the *natural* action of the whole proceeding.

The condition, indeed, of *double consciousness*, as it is termed, with instances of which medical and physiological works abound, is a complete refutation of this writer's argument. Dr. Dyce, of Aberdeen, has detailed a remarkable case in the *Edinburgh Philosophical Transactions.* Dr. Abercrombie, in one of his admirable works, mentions a similar instance, where a young girl, in a state of somnambulism, "showed astonishing acuteness;" but was, "when awake, a dull awkward girl, and did not appear to have any recollection of what had passed during her sleep." [*] Mesmerism had nothing to do in producing these cases. And the author of this pamphlet, if he enter more deeply into the inquiry, will find that his views on this point are based on an error, — for that this cessation of "the perceptive or reflective faculties" is strictly "according to nature," and agreeable to "sound philosophy and good common sense." [†]

[*] Abercrombie " On the Intellectual Powers," p. 296.
[†] Dr. Moore, in his " Power of the Soul over the Body," mentions a Dr. Haycock, professor of medicine in Oxford, who would give out a text, and

The only other argument in the Tract requiring notice, is the assumption of the satanic character of Mesmerism from the perversion of its use (p. 9.). When the writer shall have specified which of God's gifts are not perverted to evil purposes by evil agents of some kind, we will enter on the objection. Our health, our strength, the best faculties of our understanding are often so employed, that "the result is only evil" (p. 10.): would the writer have us therefore infer, to use his own language, that "it must be evil to practise" or employ them? (p. 11.) In a certain sense, indeed, Satan may be said to be the "*secondary cause*" of much that exists in the world, by his permitted use of divinely-created materials to his own malicious ends: and Mesmerism, of course, forms no exception; for I agree with a writer in the British Magazine, that "whether this power originally be satanic or not, Satan has often learned to turn it against men." [*]

The writer of " Mesmerism tested by the Word of God," has not written in an unfair or illiberal spirit; and with very many of his observations I cordially concur: but he has not shaken me in my firm faith, that this power, against which he contends, is yet "of God:"—and in spite of the earnest and important nature of his arguments, his Pamphlet will be found, on close examination, to be in the words of the poet, —

> " Like a tale of little meaning
> Though *the words are strong.*" [†]

Another specimen of these "paper bullets of the brain," under the charitable title of " *A Dialogue between a Mesmerist and a Christian* [‡]," has also been forwarded to me by some anonymous opponent.

The writer of this diatribe, "*founded on actual conversation*," has taken care to have the lion's share of the argument, and to put his adversary at all convenient disadvantage.

The tirade is founded on the old unproven affirmation, which

deliver a good sermon on it, in his sleep, but was *incapable of such discourse* when awake."
[*] See a short but sensible Letter on Mesmerism, in " British Magazine " for September 1844, p. 301.
[†] Tennyson, " Lotos Eaters," vol. i. p. 184.
[‡] Published by Nisbet and Co., Berner Street.

is here affirmed over and over again, that " Mesmerism is super-natural *because* it *must* be supernatural;" a short and easy way of disposing of a question.

It is penned in such an illogical style, and proceeds so benevolently on the assumption implied in the title-page, that a Mesmerist cannot be a Christian, that an examination of such melancholy bigotry would be an abuse of reason.

For instance, to apply his own weapons of offence, what would the writer say of a " Dialogue between a Vaccinator and a Christian?"—" A Dialogue between a Student of Scripture and a Student of Astronomy?"—" A Dialogue between a Disciple of the Lord Jesus and a Practiser of the Devilish Art of Inoculation?" as if the two things were incompatible. Yet we know what feelings have once existed against these different subjects.

I have a pamphlet by me, published in 1754, of 195 pages in length,—which speaks of inoculation as a " practice incon-sistent with the duty to the Creator,"—as " an audacious attempt to take ourselves out of the hands of the Almighty," —as " an unnatural practice,"—"insulting our Maker,"—and as " a human invention,"—" throwing" the party inoculated "into a *state full of presumption and rebellion* against God." *

The language of this ignorant pamphlet *against inoculation* so completely the language of this present writer *against Mesmerism* (the date of its publication being taken into con-sideration), that, *mutatis mutandis*, its arguments might be borrowed by our very original opponent for the next edition of his " Dialogue."

Mr. Bickersteth, the truly admirable and pious Rector of Watton, has been represented as one of the opponents. In his " Signs of the Times from the East" he had hastily observed, that he was "compelled to view it as possible that a super-natural, and therefore diabolical, power may be engaged in producing some of the wonders of Mesmerism, and that he would not for any supposed benefit have any thing to do with

<hr>

* " A Vindication of a Sermon, entitled ' Inoculation an Indefensible Practice, &c.'" by the Rector of St. Mildred's, Canterbury.

it." In a most honourable and Christian-like letter, however, to the editor of the Zoist *, he " frankly admits that his language was unguarded and improper ;—that his " words conveyed an idea far from his mind,"—and that he " has seen enough to make him think that though Mesmerism may be fearfully abused, it may yet be *one of those powers which God gives for the benefit of the human race*." Similar, too, is the language of Mr. Close of Cheltenham in his " Lecture on Miracles," before referred to. When, therefore, the scrupulous Christian perceives two such able and evangelical exponents passing over to the other side, his conscience may surely feel more at ease respecting a remedy, from which he once turned away in superstitious dislike under the teaching of those that ought to have known better. A division of opinion, at least, exists in one influential section of the Church. And if the authority of Mr. M'Neile and "Charlotte Elizabeth" are relied upon by one side, the honoured names of Mr. Bickersteth and Mr. Close may be quoted as far more than a counterpoise on the other.

After all, the whole controversy lies in a nutshell. *Omnia immundis immunda;* "unto the pure all things are pure"—as the Apostle teaches ; "but unto them that are defiled and un-believing " is *nothing pure;*"†—and Mesmerism is satanic or otherwise, according as we receive it or use *it*.

<hr>

* * Zoist, No. 17, p. 71.   † Titus, i. 15.

CHAP. II.

MESMERIC AGENT INVISIBLE. — GRAVITATION. — ANECDOTE FROM WEST
INDIES. — NEW SYSTEM OF REMEDIES MARVELLOUS. — POWER OF CLERGY,
AND SPIRITUAL TYRANNY. — WITCHCRAFT. — BARK INTRODUCED BY
JESUITS. — INOCULATION. — VACCINATION. — SIN OF ARRAIGNING GOD'S
BOUNTIES. — WHAT SCRIPTURE DOCTRINE OF EVIL SPIRITS. — CHARGE
BROUGHT AGAINST MESMERISERS. — LINES "ON HEARING MESMERISM
CALLED IMPIOUS."

DEPLORABLE as are the rhapsodies which the last chapter examined, there is nothing new in the state of feeling, of which
they are but the index. There is a tendency in the human
mind to refer every thing that cannot be explained to the influence of Satan; and though this idea of the supernatural has
been refuted over and over again by subsequent discoveries,
men still continue haunted with the same restless fears of the
mysterious, and suppose the man of science to have signed a con-
tract with the spirit of evil. But the one thing in Mesmerism
that so especially disturbs the imagination of the timid, and
produces so much of painful feeling, is the fact, that the immediate agent is *invisible*. It is this that throws so mystical a
character over the subject. Superstition then comes to the aid
of ignorance; for when men cannot perceive all that exists, it
is an easy way of solving the difficulty, by assuming that the
whole transaction is beyond the boundary of nature. "If I
could but *see* what causes all this," said a fair disciple of
M'Neile's one day, "I should be easier." "The devil," observes the sermon, "works here unseen."[*] These reasoners

* Maxwell, a Scotchman, and the famous predecessor of Mesmer, in his
treatise "De Medicina Magnetica," published in 1679 at Frankfort, asks,
"how men can refer the best gifts of God to the worst of creatures, the devil,
because the secret nature of them is not perceived?" "Anne maxima Summi
Boni dona, in pessimum creaturarum diabolum, tanquam auctorem referre
aequum putatis? Verum hoc humani erratis ingenii proprium est, et la-
tentis naturae secreta non perspecta condemnat."—Praefat. This remarkable
treatise will be noticed again: it is in the British Museum.

require a visible patent fluid to pass before their eyes to clear
the practice of its sinfulness. In demanding this, they forget
that there are other agents in nature which are outwardly imperceptible. For in accordance with this argument the evil
spirit must be at work in the air we breathe, and in the wind
by which our navies are wafted, for it is only through *their
effects* that we discern them;—and the Christian passenger
should refuse to embark on any vessel but a steam-ship; and
enter a solemn protest to the captain, if he presume to consult
his compass as a guide to the destined haven.

But the power that thus directs one of the extremities of the
magnetic needle to the north, is not the only invisible influence
in nature. "We may suspect," says an able French writer[*],
"that there are in the world several subtle fluids, and certain
concealed properties, of which we have yet no notion; and this
is the reason why we find many phenomena inexplicable." But
I cannot do better than give the words of a friend on this subject, in one of his powerfully written letters:—"How senseless
(says he) is the objection of those who demand the explanation
of a cause, as though there were one power of any description
that ever was or ever can be explained. We register effects,
and the course of these effects; of the nature of a cause we
know nothing. Gravitation is perhaps of all powers the most
universal and the best understood, but who can explain this?
We see the stone fall to the ground, and smoke rise up aloft,
the storm rushes by, and the mountain torrent dashes over the
precipice into the gulf below—but of the cause of all these
various and apparently opposite effects, we know nothing—but
that the power is simple and uniform; it is attraction, a sympathy between bodies, but which is no explanation. We cannot
see it, for power is an action beyond the sphere of our perceptions; we know it in the effect of matter on matter, and can
trace the course of these effects through all material nature, but
nothing more—we observe the conditions under which each
effect is made manifest, but beyond which all is mystery; of the
cause we know nothing. It is the same with the phenomena of
animal life which we perceive through the action of Mesmerism,

* M. Virey, in "L'Art de perfectionner l'Homme."

the results of which are uniform under similar conditions, but vary with all the changes observable in the living body ; and so far as we are acquainted with these changes, can we calculate upon the result of Mesmeric action ; and it is the same with the effects which follow in the course of every other power by which the living body is influenced ; the laws of action are but the recognised material conditions under which any effects take place, and nothing more. Could we even perceive a medium of communication between acting bodies, as the wire which conveys electricity, or the air which communicates all the exquisite harmonies of sound to the sensitive nerve, or really witness a visible tangible fluid passing out from one body into another, the difficulty and the mystery would be the same ; for a fluid is not a power, nor a medium of communication a cause of the influence which it communicates ; these are but the different chains in the links of material appearances, which for convenience we call causation ; but which in truth explain nothing ; they are but means to an end, the filling up of the links in the chain. Gunpowder explodes by the near approach of flame,— but which the circumstance of the slightest damp will prevent. Now, who can the least explain these phenomena ; or tell us what is light, or heat, or the nature of this repulsive power,— which is the explosion ? In all matters on which we are ignorant, we should suspend our judgment ; for experience alone can lead to knowledge, and the wisest of men have ever been the most humble before truth, and the most careful in giving judgment ; for their experience has shown the folly of human wisdom in giving judgment without knowledge ; that knowledge which *is* power : for the ignorance of the indolent is not bliss : 'for though all knowledge,' says Lord Bacon, 'is valuable and connected, the knowledge of man to man is the most important, and ought to be the foundation of every system of education.' Let us then, with pure humility and an earnest spirit, seek to know ourselves, that we may be wise unto salvation,— praising God for all that he may reveal to us, and not in the pride of intellect, without inquiry, presumptuously reject the light which is from Heaven, and ascribe the ways of God to the agency of Satan.'

After all, this dread of the mysterious depends altogether upon the accident of our experience. Habit reconciles us to every thing.* What is as a miracle in one century, is a matter of course in another. And if our eyes be but accustomed to a particular result, though the cause may transcend our senses, it never enters into the thoughts of the large majority of men to ask whether the actual agent be unseen or visible. There is a curious story mentioned in that amusing little work, "Six Months in the West Indies," which strikingly illustrates this remark. When a steamer was first started at Trinidad, Sir Ralph Woodford took a trip of pleasure in her through some of the Bocas into the main ocean. "When they were in the middle of the passage, a small privateer was seen making all sail for the shore of the island. Her course seemed unaccountable ; but what was their surprise when they observed that, on nearing the coast, she ran herself directly on shore, her crew at the same time leaping out over the sides of the vessel, and scampering up the mountains !" This was so strange a sight, that, to discover the cause, Sir Ralph went on board of the privateer, and found only one man there with a broken limb, in a posture of supplication. "He was pale as ashes, his teeth chattered, and his hair stood on end, and 'Misericordia, Misericordia,' was his only reply." The explanation at last was, that "they saw a vessel steering *without a single sail,* directly in the teeth of the wind, current, and tide ; that they knew no ship could move in such a course by *human means ;* that they concluded it to be a supernatural appearance,"—"and that when he himself heard Sir Ralph's footsteps, he verily and indeed believed that he was fallen into the hands of the evil spirit." Here, now, was a state of terror, as in Mesmerism, the result of novelty alone. This Spaniard had been accustomed

* Meric Casaubon, whose "Treatise concerning Enthusiasm" has been already quoted, says in another work, " *On Credulity and Incredulity,*" " Another great cause of wondering is the power of use and custom, which they, who by the report of others, or by their own experience, have not been acquainted with, must needs ascribe to *magic* and *supernatural* causes many things which are *merely natural.*"—p. 14. This was written about two centuries back ; strange, that with all our discoveries, we should have yet advanced so little !

all his life to steer his little vessel through the aid of an unseen magnetic power, and by the invisible action of the wind; and there was nothing wonderful to him in these ordinary properties of nature;—but when a ship was propelled by the means of human machinery, by paddles, and boilers, and steam that were open to the eye, this unusual spectacle filled the poor sailors with a dread of approaching evil,—they "concluded it to be a supernatural appearance,"—while the real object of mystery remained unheeded in the cabin through the simple effect of daily habit.[*]

The turn, however, which the fears of the superstitious so frequently take, is in an uneasiness on the subject of medical treatment, and at the application of some new and unwonted remedy. This fact can be corroborated by writers without number. It is not the disease that so much alarms, as the cure that subdues it. It is hence that the populace takes affright; on this that preachers preach, and the learned bestow their wisdom. Old Burton, in his well-known work, the "Anatomy of Melancholy," has a whole chapter on the "*rejection of unlawful cures.*" He gives us a catalogue of writers, who affirm that cures are perfected by diabolical agency. "Many doubt, saith Nicholas Taurellus, whether the divell can cure such diseases he hath not made, and some flatly deny it, howsoever common experience confirms to our astonishment, that magicians can worke such feats, and that the divell without impediment can penetrate through all parts of our bodies, and cure such maladies by meanes to us unknown." "Nothing so familiar," adds Burton, "as to hear of such

* Sir Joshua Reynolds, in one of his charming "Discourses," says, "It is very natural for those, who are unacquainted with the cause of any thing extraordinary, to be astonished at the effect, and to consider it as a kind of magic. * * * The travellers in the East tell us, that when the ignorant inhabitants of those countries are asked concerning the ruins of stately edifices yet remaining amongst them, the melancholy monuments of their former grandeur and long-lost science, they always answer, that they were built by magicians. The untaught mind finds a vast gulph between its own powers and those works of complicated art, which it is utterly unable to fathom, and it supposes that such a void can be passed only by supernatural powers."—*Disc. 6.*, p. 147. How completely this applies to Mesmerism, which the untaught mind, in its routine practice, finds itself "unable to fathom," and therefore calls it, in one moment, impossible, and, in the next, preternatural!

cures:"—"we see the effects only, but not the *causes* of them:"—"sorcerers are too common, who in every village will help almost all infirmities of body." "Many famous cures are daily done in this kind," he adds again, "*and the divell is an expert physician.*" And after a little farther discussion of the question, he decides, that it is "*better to die than be so cured.*"[*]

Galen, who has been termed the Prince of physicians, and whose name is as a proverb in the profession, was accused of sorcery by his cotemporaries in reward for his unequalled success. "They turned against him even the credit of his cures, by the charge of having procured them through *magical means*,"[†] Paracelsus, his distinguished successor, was subject to the same imputation. A physician named Sennert, born at Breslaw in 1572, suspected that Paracelsus had tampered in the *black art*, and seriously asserts that extraordinary cures can only be performed by a compact with Satan. For he says, that "the devil has a competent knowledge of physic, but as all his favours and promises are deceitful and destructive to soul and body, no benefit, but much evil was to be expected." He then admonishes *physicians rather to acquiesce with resignation in the death of their patients*, than preserve them by impious means."[‡] And the part that "enlightened" Europe has acted in regard to witchcraft is only too notorious; thousands of unhappy wretches have suffered at the stake on this accusation, not always as a punishment for a presumed injury, or to gratify revengeful feelings, but in consequence of *cures effected by the simplest herbs* and through the aid of nature, after repeated failures of the faculty.

All this is melancholy enough; and a sad answer to those who talk of the dignity of human nature. But bad as it is, something worse remains behind, viz., that the clergy[§] of all

* Burton, "Anatomy Mel.," part ii. p. 220. edit. 1624.
† "Ils tournèrent même contre lui l'éclat de certaines cures, en l'accusant de les obtenir par des moyens magiques."—*Biographie Univer.*, art. "Galien."
‡ "Quanquam vero negari non possit Diabolum rerum medicarum notitiam peritam."—Sennert, tom. i. p. 234. De Peruoke.—See Moore's "History of Small Pox," p. 164.
§ In making this statement, I seek not the worthless distinction of liberality at the expense of my wiser and *her superior brethren*. But there are

H 3

persuasions have too generally led the van in these abominable persecutions.

Religion has been well termed, by one of our best living writers, "the medicine of the soul;"—"it is," he says, "the designed and appropriate remedy for the evils of our nature;"[*]—but this medicine, unhappily is not only easily polluted by the poison of superstition; but the dregs of human passion and human vanity too readily and too often mingle with the cup. The object, which the ministers of the gospel have in view, is of so momentous a nature, of an importance so above and beyond every other consideration, that it may seem, to zealous minds, almost to justify the adoption of any means towards its attainment. If the soul be but saved, what matter the process, says the carnal reasoning of the sophist. But, happily, we are forbidden by the highest authority to "do evil that good may come:" and even the salvation of sinners is not to be accomplished by unrighteous ways. Still, this golden rule of Scripture is too frequently forgotten by the young and by the ardent. Anxious to carry on the great work that is before him,—eager to enlarge the number of his proselytes, our enthusiastic teacher is not always sufficiently careful as to the quality of the argument he adopts in his persuasions. A little "pious fraud" he trusts may be very excusable. Not content with denouncing in words of gravest censure the ungodly and the vicious,—not satisfied with "reasoning on righteousness, and temperance, and judgment to come," he must needs travel a little aside into the region of the doubtful and the imaginative. And if he be a man of talent as well as of energy, he soon perceives the

points on which a well-known proverb must be brought to memory. Truth, especially gospel truth, ought to be dearer than factitious claims. And when religion is exposed to the scoff of the unbeliever, through the injudicious advocacy of its own supporters, it is necessary to show that the conduct which does the mischief is no part of the system, but the reprobated superaddings of a mistaken friend. This is essentially a scientific age; and the more needful is it to be understood that there is no other hostility between religion and science than what arises out of the grossest ignorance. God's works and words speak but the same language.

[*] Archbishop Whately, "Errors of Romanism traced to Human Nature," cap. i, p. 75., a book which every one that feels disposed to cast a stone at his brother-religionist, should read, not once, but once a year.

result. He sees his congregation perplexed, alarmed, and anxious. He finds out that fatal secret,—fatal I mean to the happiness of others,—the pleasure of wielding power. He learns the power of the strong mind over the weak,—of the crafty over the credulous,—of the fanatic leader over the bigoted follower. And this power, once tasted, is far too delicious to be laid down: it must now be maintained at any cost. One preacher promotes it by enforcing the most puerile and superstitious ceremonies; another by confounding things in themselves innocent and indifferent, and only blameable in their excess, with things positively sinful and forbidden in Scripture;—a third thunders forth his anathemas against the philosophic inquirer, and places on a level the man, who humbly searches into the wonders of Providence with one who is living without God in the world. And the more supple and complying that they find their people, the more exacting and progressive are they in their demands. This then is Priestcraft[*], be it exercised by what persuasion it may. It is that intolerable spiritual tyranny, that lording it over men's minds and consciences, which has done more injury to the pure evangelical faith,—which has more retarded the course of the everlasting Gospel, than all the writings of all the deists from Bolingbroke to Voltaire. It is in fact one of the very evils that have created deism. It belongs not in particular to one body of Christians more than to another, though the church of Rome has been taxed unjustly with an exclusive attachment to its use. Those, however, who look into the annals of the church, and analyse the springs of human action, will find it a feeling all but universal. Pope and Presbyter, Wesleyan and Baptist, have alike displayed it. The High Church movement at Oxford, and the Free Church schism at Edinburgh, are equally emanations of the same principle, though the accidents of their two systems may be widely opposite. Our evangelical party have, in their

[*] "Under the name priest," says Hartley Coleridge, "we comprehend all creatures, whether Catholic or Protestant, clerks or laymen, who either pretend to have discovered a bye-way to heaven, or give tickets to free the legal toll-gates, or set up toll gates of their own."—Biographia Borealis, p. 341.

own peculiar way, shown the warmest predilections for this power; no men have more domineered over the weak and ignorant than have they;—and the ministers of dissenting congregations, in spite of their loud professions to the contrary, have, where the occasion has been offered them, been as little free as any from the same hateful practice. And thus have they all succeeded in spoiling the simplicity of the Gospel through "vain deceit after the rudiments of the world, and not after Christ," and rendered its pure and blessed morality of none effect through their additions. But the strangest thing in the matter is the fondness of the people for wearing the yoke. Be the doctrine or discipline what it may, the laity seem always ready to receive the most monstrous statements, and to uphold the pretensions of the most ambitious, if the teachers themselves appear but in earnest. Affection for priestcraft would almost seem an inherent principle in the human heart. *Populus vult decipi:* or as the Prophet said of old, "*the people love to have it so*, and the priests bear rule by these means." Moderation never was and never will be popular. Bitterness, bigotry, extreme and extravagant opinions, these are the things that are palatable with the vulgar. And hence it has been that in all ages of Christianity, those who by their education and position ought to have taken the lead in promoting the claims of science, were the very parties that sought a reputation for sanctity by heading the outcry against it: and hence it is, that in the case of Mesmerism, in other towns of England besides that of Liverpool, some of the clergy have succeeded in tightening the chains with which they have enthralled the weakest members of their flock, by second-hand denunciations on the wickedness of the system, and by mourning over some of the most virtuous practisers of the art as the hopeless victims of satanic cruelty!*

---

* This is not asserted from a loose assumption. Those who disbelieve in Mesmerism, and have not given attention to its claims, have no conception of the strong language used on the subject, for the sanction of which appeal is made to the authority of Mr. M'Neile. Not many months since, I was staying a few days in one of our midland counties,—and on spending an evening with a friend, part of the family remained absent. I afterwards discovered that they refused to make their appearance, as a mesmeriser was in the room, and the conversation might turn on the practice. A short time

These things are matter of history; and it may be a useful, though humbling lesson to bring forward a few instances in proof. It may encourage a spirit of caution in those who teach; it may check the leaning towards credulity in those who hear. And without alluding to the well-known examples in the study of astronomy, of geology, and other branches of natural philosophy, I shall confine myself to a few remarkable cases taken from the practice of medicine, as bearing an affinity to the curative power of the mesmerist.

I begin, therefore, with witchcraft, for the charge of witchcraft, as was before stated, too commonly arose out of the medical success of the offender; and on this point, what a tale of horror has the conduct of the clergy to call up.

The persecutions for witchcraft did not commence in Europe till towards the close of the fifteenth century; that is, when what are called the dark or middle ages were rapidly passing away. In 1484, at the time of our Richard the Third, Pope Innocent VIII., in his conclave of cardinals, denounced death to all who should be convicted of witchcraft. The succeeding popes, Alexander VI., and even Pope Leo X., the polished and enlightened Leo, lent their aid in this fearful persecution. About 1515, just before Luther commenced his career, 500 witches were executed in Geneva: 1000 were executed in the Diocese of Como. In Lorraine 900 were burnt. In France the multitude of executions is called "incredible." In Germany, after the publication of the Pope's bull, the number of victims stated is so portentous, as to lead to the hope that there must be some mistake in the calculation; and we are told that the clergy went about preaching what were called "*Witch Sermons*," and inspiring the people with a fanatic ardour in the pursuit.*

---

previously to this visit, the clergyman of their parish had collected the most obedient members of his congregation together, and, addressing them in awful language, entreated their prayers for some lost brethren and sisters. These lost brethren were some benevolent and Christian people who had been devoting their days and nights to the relief of their suffering neighbours. And this in the 19th century!

* I have abridged the above facts and figures from Combe's admirable work on the "Constitution of Man," and rely on his accuracy for their correctness.

In England the executions were frightfully numerous, especially at the period when the Presbyterian and Independent clergy were in the ascendant. During the puritanic supremacy of the famous Long Parliament, 3000 victims suffered.

But it was in Scotland, after the Reformation, and more especially after the triumphant establishment of the Presbyterian Kirk, that some of the darkest scenes were enacted. The General Assembly passed an act for all ministers to take note of witches and charms, and over and over again pressed upon parliament a consideration of the subject. In following up the accusations, the clergy exhibited the most rancorous zeal, and were themselves often the parties who practised the worst cruelties. We may rail against Torquemada and his Dominicans, but it may be a question whether the Inquisition of Spain inflicted more real domestic misery than was endured under the galling bondage of John Knox and his platform. True, there was no *auto-da-fé*; but, in its stead, there was a system of *espionage*, of informations and visitations, which carried dismay and unhappiness to every household hearth. In fact, the spiritual tyranny of the Kirk of Scotland was often intolerable. Documents show that no habits of private life were left untouched by its meddling jurisdiction. And those in the present day, who are abetting the recent Free Church measures, should well consider what they are bringing upon themselves; for there can be little doubt, that the leaders of the secession, in spite of the apparently popular character of their proceedings, are aiming at a return to the old ecclesiastical domination, and to the prostration of the purses and persons of their people, under the iron rule of an ambitious presbytery.

Some curious books have been lately published which throw a valuable light on the old conduct of the Kirk. I allude to the Miscellanies of the Spalding Club. They ought to be well studied by the present admirers of spiritual discipline. In the first volume, there is a document published, called " Trials for Witchcraft," which contains no less than fifty papers relating to different trials before the kirk sessions for that offence. A second volume is called " Extracts from the Presbytery Book of Strathbogie," in which we may read how the clergy took fearful

cognizance of each action of private life, and accused and punished the " suspected " for their magical skill. A few samples may be instructive. There is a trial of poor Helen Fraser, who was convicted before the " presbeterie of Foverne," among other charges, for promising one " Johne Ramsey, who was sick of a consuming disease, to do quhat in hir lay for the recoverie of his health ; " but it was to be kept secret, for the " world was evil, and spake na gude of sic medicines." Janet Ingram had also sent for Helen to cure her.

There is a narrative of a meeting held at the kirk of Caldstane, and a poor victim is brought forward, who was accused of calling on George Rychie's mother, and promising to take off his sickness.

Mr. John Ross, the minister at Lumphanon, and the parson of Kincardine, O'Neil, send in documents to the sessions, accusing of witchcraft nine or ten persons.

At Belhelvie, one Janet Ross is accused of witchcraft, and denies it, but she confesses to prescribing to a patient, sick of fever, an egg with a little aqua-vitæ and pepper; she had used the same for herself in her own disease.

One George Seifright is summoned before the kirk, and rebuked for consulting about his wife's sickness, and bringing some poor woman to cure her.

Issobel Malcolme is accused of charming and curing a child's sore eye.

Isabel Haldone, of Perth, confesses upon accusation to having given drinks to cure bairns.

Three poor women are executed in 1623 at Perth for doctoring; and the kirk session called up and censured the parties who had sought cures at their hands.

In short, as the editor says in the preface, these charges were "generally connected with *cures wrought* or attempted for some *severe disease.*" The ignorant prosecutors could not explain what they saw: it was a paradox to them, how an old woman by the administration of simples could cure diseases, which had resisted the wisdom of the professor ; and so cutting the knot, which they could not untie, they trumped up a charge of sorcery as a salvo and excuse for their own folly.

William Perkins, a learned and pious divine of Marton, in Warwickshire, who died in 1602, wrote, amongst a number of other works, a "Discourse of the Damned Art of Witchcraft;" in which he says, that the healing or "good witch is the worser of the two."

"Of witches there are two sorts," he adds, "the *bad* witch, and the *good* witch. . . . The good witch is he or she that by consent in a league with the devil, doth use his help for doing good only. This cannot hurt, but only *heal and cure*. . . . Now, howsoever both those be evil, yet of the two, the *most horrible and detestable monster* is the *good* witch. . . . For in healing him, the good witch hath done him a thousand times more harm than the former. For the one did only hurt the body, but the devil by means of the other, hath laid fast of the soul, and by curing the body, hath killed the spirit." [*]

If the learned Mr. Perkins had been living in these days, what powerful "Discourses" he might have put forth against Ether and Mesmerism under a horror of their healing and pain-subduing virtues!"

Let us come to another instance. When, in 1649, the Jesuits imported into Europe the Peruvian bark, and for this act and for their philanthropic exertions in Paraguay made atonement to society for much of that conduct which has rendered their name a proverb, the most wonderful effects were produced in Rome by its use. Geoffroy, in his Materia Medica, states, that Cardinal de Lugo and his brethren distributed *gratis* a great quantity among the "religious," and the poor of the city. Agues and intermittent fevers were cured as if by enchantment. Geoffroy says that the cures were thought too rapid (trop prompt). And hence, as we learn elsewhere, not only did physicians interfere, but "ecclesiastics prohibited sick persons from using it, alleging that it possessed no virtue but what it derived from a compact made by the Indians with the devil." [†] And thus this useful, this invaluable drug was, on its first introduction, treated as Mesmerism is now, and ascribed to the invention of the father of all evil. And of course the spiritual guides of

[*] Perkins, W., Fol. vol. iii. p. 637.
[†] See Colquhoun's "Isis Revelata."

those days thought, with old Burton, that it was "better for the patient to die," than be cured of his ague by such a remedy!

When, in 1718, inoculation for small-pox was adopted in this country, the greatest uproar was stirred up against it. Not only was the whole medical world opposed to it, but farther, as Moore tells us in his amusing work on Inoculation, "some zealous churchmen, conceiving that it was repugnant to religion, thought it their duty to interfere. * * * They wrote and preached that *Inoculation was a daring attempt to interrupt the internal decrees of Providence.*" (p. 237.) Lord Wharncliffe, in his life of Lady Wortley Montagu, says, that the "clergy descanted from their pulpits on its impiety." Oh! if Mr. Paul and his Penny-Pulpit reporters had but been living in those days, what gems of reasoning and rhetoric might have been preserved to us! Fortunately a few *Folia Sybillina* are yet extant. A Mr. Massey preached in 1722 in St. Andrew's Church, Holborn, that "all who infused the variolous ferment were hellish sorcerers, and that inoculation was the diabolical invention of Satan." [*] And one of the rectors of Canterbury, the Reverend Theodore de la Faye[†], perhaps exceeded this in a sermon, preached in 1751, for he denounced with horror inoculation as the offspring of atheism, and drew a touching parallel between the virtue of resignation to the Divine will and its practice. Similar minds see similar objects under a similar view. And it is hardly necessary to observe the strong resemblance that exists between the arguments delivered in Holborn and Canterbury at the beginning of the last century to the expressions so recently uttered in the pulpit of St. Jude's at Liverpool.

But the zeal of Mr. De la Faye was not content with one explosion. In 1753, two years only after his first discourse, he published a second sermon, called, "Inoculation an Indefensible Practice,"—in which, if possible, he out-Heroded

[*] See a sermon by the Rev. Mr. Massey, against the sinful practice of Inoculation. July 8th, 1722.
[†] A Discourse against Inoculating; with a Parallel between the Scripture Notion of Divine Resignation and the Practice of Inoculation. 1751.

Herod, leaving all former declamations completely in the shade.*

The effect on the public mind † was so mischievously great, that, to counteract the evil, the sermon was answered by Mr. Bolaine, a surgeon at Canterbury, in a short and judicious "Letter."

This summoned our hero for a third time into the field ; and in a long Pamphlet, called "*A Vindication of the Sermon*," (which I have already referred to in the last Chapter,) he ransacked the regions of folly and intolerance in search of arguments to maintain his doctrine. The consideration of this melancholy invective is thus far useful, that it unfolds an instructive page in the history of the human mind, by the curious parallel it presents between the former horror of inoculation, and many of the present notions respecting Mesmerism. It is impossible not to smile at the strange coincidence between the respective reasonings. A few instances shall be given.

Mesmerism, we know, is constantly described as a quackery. Inoculation is here termed "an unsocial quackery,"—"an *irregular* practice, made to promise more than it can perform." (Pamphlet, p. 5.)

Mesmerism is called immoral. Inoculation is here represented as a "complicated immorality, exposing the soul to more important peril than what men dread from the disease," (p. 85.); —"a device so immoral," as to be utterly "inconsistent with the duty we owe our fellow creatures." (p. 61.)

Mesmerism is laughed at as ridiculous. Inoculation is here called "a practice *extremely absurd* in a physical view,"—"irrational" (p. 81.), and directly *contrary to the nature* of all physical means (192.).

Those who employ Mesmerism as a remedial agent, are said to exercise unlawful means for the benefit of their health. The

---

* Inoculation an Indefensible Practice, a Sermon preached at the United Parish Churches of St. Mildred's and All Saints, in the City of Canterbury, on the 3d and 24th of June, 1753. Second Edition.

† Mr. Cradock, in his gossiping "Memoirs," says, "At a very early age I was inoculated. At that time the prejudices ran so strong against such an innovation (presumption it was called) that my father could scarce in safety venture from his house for fear of the mob."—p. 6.

sermon calls inoculation "doing evil that good may come," (p. 8.)

Mesmerism is called satanic. Inoculation is described as "irreligious"—"a daring presumption against the Almighty," —"an *impious machination*," "which nature recoils at, reason opposes, and religion condemns," (p. 191.)—"a presumptuous exaltation of oneself into the high dignity of the supreme, all-knowing Creator," (p. 15.). *

On reading these monstrous paragraphs, and remembering that within a few years after their publication the practice of inoculation became generally prevalent, and prized indeed as a a divine "gift" most conducive to the welfare of man, one feels humiliated and shocked at the grovelling superstition of the Canterbury controversialist.

And yet our preacher might have been better instructed, had he condescended to look beyond the pale of his own miserable prejudices ; for good and pious men had not feared to lift up their voices on the other side, and to attempt to lessen, in some degree, the fanatical follies of their benighted people. Dr. Doddridge, the excellent and learned Doddridge, a short time before his death, took up his pen on the subject. A friend of his early years, the Rev. David Some, a Nonconformist divine of Harborough, had written in 1725 a tract called, "*The Case of receiving the Small Pox by Inoculation impartially considered, and especially in a Religious View.*" This pamphlet Dr. Doddridge published in 1750, with a Preface by himself. In this Preface he says, that "the *chief objections* against the practice were of a *religious nature;*"—and that it was to confute the mistaken application of Scripture to the remedy that the treatise was written.

The author mentions the usual objections, such as, that Inoculation "usurps the sacred prerogative of God, who wounds and heals as He pleases" (p. 18.) ; —that there "is a great deal of danger in it" (p. 20.) ; that it "came from the

---

* I have given these several quotations at length, from the feeling, that unless they were plainly placed before the eyes, the reader would not believe the lengths to which the anti-inoculation frenzy had reached. And what a lesson they also furnish to the anti-mesmeric crusader!

Turks,"—men "of a different religion" to ourselves (p. 87.); that "some learned divines are of opinion that the practice comes from the devil" (p. 87.); and that others consider the assaults of the evil spirit upon Job as an instance of satanic inoculation!

These objections Mr. Some answers successively, taking high and religious ground in defence of the practice.[*]

When vaccination made its appearance, the same hubbub arose. Again was the medical profession up in arms; again did the pulpits resound with denunciations. Some of the clergy discovered vaccination to be antichrist. Moore, in his History of Vaccination, says, that "the opposition to vaccination was much more violent in England than in other countries," (p. 115.). He says again, "the imaginations of *many females* were so much disturbed with tales of horror concerning it, that *they could not even listen to any proofs of their falsehood.*" (p. 122.). The learned author of the "Principles and Practice of Medicine" says, that when vaccination was introduced, "it was said, that it was taking the power out of God's hand; that *God gave us the small-pox, and that it was impious to interrupt it by the cow-pock.* When I was a boy, I heard people say that it was an irreligious practice, and that it was taking the power out of God's hand, forgetting that it is merely *using* that power which God has given us. *Sermons were preached against it;* and handbills were stuck about the streets. I recollect seeing it stated in a handbill, that a person who was inoculated for the cow-pock had horns growing in consequence of it," (p. 479.). These now are the annals of small-pox: and thus in a few years hence, when Mesmerism shall be firmly established,— and when it will be as much a matter of course for a neuralgic patient to apply to its influence for a cure, as it is now for a mother to have her infant vaccinated, the future historian will relate, among the curiosities of the subject, that two sermons were actually preached one Sunday in Liverpool, denouncing as impious and satanic the practice of so simple, so common, and so natural an act as the exercise of the mesmeric manipulations.

[*] This pamphlet is now scarce, I found it in the library of the Norwich Literary Institution.

Truly this satanic agency is a clever actor of all work! Numberless are the difficulties that are removed by it. "All the world's a stage;" and one and the same interpretation "plays in its time many parts." For,

Satanic agency first comes forward in the character of an old woman, curing the sore eyes of a boy by an infusion of dock-weed.

Satanic agency next appears in the character of a Jesuit, scowling darkly around, and curing a tertian ague by the Peruvian cinchona.

Satanic agency again appears in the character of Lady Wortley Montagu, importing inoculation from Turkey, and arresting the fearful ravages of small-pox!

Satanic agency again appears in the character of Doctor Jenner, convulsing the College of Physicians with his novelties, and saving myriads of infants by the process of vaccination!

Satanic agency lastly appears in the character of a modern Mesmerizer, healing, by his soothing power, some of the most distressing diseases, and expelling a whole train of neuralgic pains, which had defied the skill of the faculty!

And they, who utter these denunciations, think that they are doing God service!

Rather do they throw a serious discredit on religion; rather do they inflict on it material disservice. They make the infidel and barren spectator laugh, and the judicious and thinking Christian grieve. They overload the Gospel with a weight that does not belong to it. They affect the mind in the same way as the legends and false miracles of the church of Rome, "in leading captive" the silliest of women through a grovelling superstition, but disgusting men of sense by their absurdity, and converting the philosopher into half an infidel. Enjoined to believe *all* these statements, men end in believing *none.*[*] In this respect, then, these pious frauds are a mistake, if we may so speak. They do not accomplish the object aimed at. They do not increase, but rather lessen, the amount of real Christianity. But they are not merely a mistake,—they are far

[*] See the Life &c. of Mr. Blanco White, which strikingly confirms this observation.

worse,—they are positively immoral and sinful. In asserting this, we are far from singling out Mr. M'Neile as the object of our remarks. His views are but an indication of opinions that are afloat. He is but one out of many. We rather regret to see a man of his abilities lending the sanction of his name to such absurdities. He is a person of weight in the religious world; and therefore do we appeal to him, and ask,—if, in giving currency to these dogmata, he has well considered his responsibilities as a teacher. To speak of the bounties of Providence as the temptings of the evil one,—to treat a blessing as if it were a curse,—to condemn a benefit before it be examined,—as is the wont of the religious opponents of Mesmerism,—seems to me the conduct of a thoughtless unthankful spirit.* "If the Lord would make windows in heaven, might this thing be?" was the speech of the unbelieving Lord at the promised plenty to Samaria. (2 Kings, vii. 2.) "He doeth these wonders through Beelzebub, the chief of the devils," —was the answer of the hardened Jews to the works of our Divine Master; and what are the marvels of Mesmerism,—but equally the works of God,—equally flowing from the same heavenly fount as the miracles of the blessed Jesus,—the one indeed effected immediately at His word,—the other through those secondary agents of which He is the first and only source. We therefore say, that it is our DUTY AS CHRISTIANS TO SEE THE HAND OF GOD in the work,—that it is our duty to recognise so good, so merciful, so healing an influence, as a proof of the Almighty's care for his people. To do less than this argues a want of faith, and a lowering and an undervaluing of the Divine attributes. Our bodily frame may indeed be full of complicated and mysterious movements; but what is that to faith? a mystery is no mystery to the eye of faith. The Psalmist hath told us, that "we are fearfully and wonderfully made;" that it is God "who hath fashioned us behind and before,"—that it is "God who laid his hand upon us,"—and that "in his book all

* "Such notions are mere emanations of false pride and ignorant prejudice. He who conceives them, little reflects that they, in reality, involve the principle of a contempt for the works and ways of God."—Vestiges of Natural History of Creation, p. 335.

our members are written." To say therefore, that "the flesh of man's body cannot be placed in a Mesmeric state, except by supernatural means," is to show a forgetfulness of God. "Be ye sure that the Lord He is God; it is *He that hath made us, and not we ourselves;*"—we are but clay in the hands of the potter. The Divine Creator forms one vessel to honour, and another to dishonour;—he divides severally to each of us our separate qualities,—to some he gives spiritual gifts,—to others physical,—to others a union of both: "He will have mercy on whom He will have mercy, and whom He will He hardeneth," —but whether they be gifts of grace, or gifts of nature, they all flow from Him,—for "of Him, and through Him, and to Him are all things," and "by Him do all things consist."

Let not, then, the Christian misunderstand me. In thus opposing the main tenets of these anti-mesmeric pamphlets, do I make void the doctrine of satanic influence? Do I deny its truth? God forbid! yea, rather would I establish it. My own painful experience tells me, that in our religious warfare, we wrestle not with flesh and blood, but with the unseen powers and principalities of hell, with spiritual wickedness in high places. Firmly do I believe, with Holy Scripture, that the "devil goeth about like a roaring lion, seeking whom he may devour." Wherever is seduction or wickedness, there is Satan in the midst of us;—wherever is falsehood, imposture, and deceit, his kingdom reaches also;—wherever are unjust and railing accusations against the brethren,—wherever are "lying wonders," and claims to a false and pretended power, his presence may be known; and my daily prayer is, after the teaching of our blessed Master, to be delivered not only from evil,—but also from "the Evil One." This is a creed of which all the wisdom of this world will never make me ashamed;—I am only anxious to place this doctrine on a scriptural and legitimate footing. With the apostolic Heber, I believe that "no slavish fears, no trifling superstition can follow from these views, when regulated by reason and by Scripture." And while, with that lamented Bishop, I think that the "notions which God's word has taught us to entertain of evil spirits, are sufficient to discredit the ordinary tales of witchcraft," with

him also do I believe, that our tempters to sin are "mighty and numerous," and that the name of the great adversary is "Legion."[*]

But if no satisfactory reason can, after all, be advanced in maintenance of this charge of satanic agency, and if that position be abandoned as forlorn, our fanatical opponents shift their ground, in the next place, to an uncharitable imputation against the men themselves. The slavery of mind must be secured at any cost; and so the world is instructed, that the thing itself must be wrong, because the creed of its supporters is dangerous and unsound. The leading Mesmerists, they say, are deists, sceptics, materialists; and what good fruit, it is demanded, can grow or be gathered from such a stock? And who are they that thus join in the accusation against the persons and principles of the Mesmeric school? Many, who in their daily habits of domestic life are visited by practitioners, entertaining and avowing the very same views on religion to which they object. And to be consistent, therefore, they who make the charge should be careful that the rule applied to every other therapeutic novelty and invention in surgery. But granted, that their sweeping denunciation be correct, it were surely a new ordeal, wherewith to test the merits of a medical discovery. For, after all, the real question is, how can such a charge affect the truth of the science itself? If all geologists were atheists, the fact would still remain, that the imbedment of certain fossils in certain strata does determine the relative succession of the latter, and throw considerable light on the structure of our globe. If all phrenologists were materialists, the fact would still remain, that an habitual train of thought, of feeling, or of conduct does act through the brain on the external conformation of the skull, and furnish a faithful manifestation of the moral character. And so if all Mesmerisers were deists, the fact would still remain, that that Supreme Being, who formed man out of the dust of the earth, and breathed into his soul the breath of life, did impart in his organization a sym-

* See Heber's Sermon on the Existence and Influence of Evil Spirits; and a Sermon by Bishop Hurd on James iv. 7. : "Resist the devil, and he will flee from you."

pathetic susceptibility to magnetic action, and that through this process a curative influence may be evolved of the highest value to suffering humanity. And is it, then, the fact, that this healing, this merciful power is alone exercised or adopted by the scriptural unbeliever? Shame, then, on Christians who can so neglect it! Shame, then, on men who can thus arraign the bounties of Providence, and extract from the very gifts of creation the poisoned materials for their own uncharitable assumptions! But that the disciples of Mesmer belong so exclusively to the school of materialism, if we must not call it a libel, is at least a strange exaggeration of facts. That there may be some among them, is probable; for in what department of knowledge, where a consciousness of intellectual power leads men on, has not the light of revelation been too often overlooked and forgotten? Whether it be, as Bacon says in his Advancement of Learning, that "in the entrance of philosophy, when the *second causes*, which are next unto the senses, do offer themselves to the mind of man, if it dwell and stay there, it may induce some oblivion of the Highest Cause;" whether this be correct, I know not; but it is a common remark, that they, who by the habitual course of their studies, have been more accustomed than other men to look into the immediate causation of things, have been too generally found amongst the followers of Pyrrho and Epicurus; — but I have yet to learn, that the observation applies with greater force to the students of Mesmerism than to those of any other science. Many there are amongst them, whom no Christian community need blush to own; many, who by their faith and practice adorn the doctrine they profess; — some, with whom I have walked to the house of God in company; and all of them with whom I am acquainted, are less deficient in that most excellent gift of charity, the very bond of peace and of all virtues, than those of their impugners, by whom the wanton cry is raised of infidelity and materialism.

What, then, is the state of mind with which "wise, prudent, and Christian men should meet the present state of the question?"[*] I would not have them, from a disgust at the

* See M'Neile's sermon towards the close.

tendencies of this sermon, join the ranks of the infidel, and laugh to scorn the doctrine of Satanic agency, as the invention of men * — holy Scripture teaches it; experimental religion confirms it; but I would have them be cautious not to confound the ways of Providence † with the works of the Evil One; I would have them remember "how little a part" of God's wonders are yet laid bare to his creatures; I would have them look into the subject with a devotional spirit, anxious for truth, not rashly condemning that of which they are ignorant, lest haply, in their presumption, "they be found to be fighting against God."‡ "Christian men" need not fear to be present at scientific lectures or physiological experiments, if they go in a Christian spirit. Hard words are no argument. Accusations of "morbid curiosity," and "foolish novelties," and "devilish devices," carry no proofs of their truth to the *thinking* pious believer. If he goes, he goes with prayer — he goes with the Bible, if not in his hand, yet in his heart; he goes to study the book of God's works by the book of God's word; he goes with the full remembrance that "no science can save a soul," no natural knowledge bring us nearer to God. But if, on the other hand, it be sickness or bodily pain that hath entered into the Christian's dwelling, and that his knowledge of the healing properties of Mesmerism should lead him to make experiment of its power, what are the feelings with which he would commence a trial of this unknown and unseen remedy? He would

---

* "Whilst we endeavour to reduce divers ecstacies to natural causes, the ignorance of which causes we shall show to have been the cause of many evils, we would not be suspected to question the truth and reality of things supernatural, for which having the authority of the Holy Scriptures, no man can deny them, except he first deny the truth and reality of these as divine." — MERIC CASAUBON, *Treatise on Enthusiasm*, cap. 3. p. 60.

† Since the above was written, I have met with a clever paper, full of curious matter, called "Witchcraft and Mesmerism," in the London Polytechnic Magazine, No. 2, by Dr. T. Stone. The facts therein stated are very instructive.

‡ "Science, it is said, fills the soul with uneasiness and curiosity, and removes us from God. *As if there were any science without him*, as if the divine effulgence, reflected in science, had not a serene virtue, a power diffusing tranquillity in the human heart, and imparting that peace of eternal truths and imperishable love, which will exist in all their purity when worlds will be no more." — MICHELET, *Priests, Women, and Families*, p. 18.

"walk by faith and not by sight." He would regard it as only one out of many thousand gifts, bountifully bestowed upon us in this life by a merciful Creator; he would value it as a blessing sent to cheer and comfort him, when other and more customary means were failing to relieve him. He would turn to its use with prayer, with humble hope, with pious confidence; he would feel that the issue was yet with God, and the divine will would be his own. He would not, like the impious king recorded in Scripture, forget the Lord, and seek only physicians. No: the great Physician of the cross, the healer of our leprosies, bodily and spiritual, would, after all, be his main and only refuge. To Him would he look at morning, at noontide, and at the evening hour. Yea, he would feel that it was good to be afflicted, if his afflictions and their earthly remedies made him better acquainted with his own heart, and brought him to a closer and more abiding communion with his Saviour and his God!

All, however, that I have been saying in the above pages, has been so much more happily expressed in the following charming lines by that gifted poetess, Miss Anna Savage, that my readers cannot but thank me for introducing them to their notice.

ON HEARING MESMERISM CALLED IMPIOUS.

CALL not the gift unholy; 'tis a fair — a precious thing,
That God hath granted to our hands for gentlest minist'ring.
Did Mercy ever stoop to bless with dark unearthly spell?
Could impious power whisper peace the soul's deep throes to quell?
Would Evil seek to work but good, — to lull the burning brain,
And linger in some scene of woe, beside the bed of pain, —
To throw upon the o'erfraught heart the blessing of repose, —
Untiring watch the eye of care in healing slumber close, —
And as the agony of grief fell 'neath the Spirit's will,
O'er the wild billows of despair breathe tenderly — Be still!
Speak gently of the new-born gift, restrain the scoff and sneer,
And think how much we may not learn is yet around us here;
What paths there are where *Faith* must lead, that Knowledge cannot share,
Though still we tread the devious way, and feel that Truth is there.

Say, is the world so full of joy, — hath each so fair a lot,
That we should scorn one bounteous gift, and scorning, use it not,
Because the false thought of man grasps not its hidden source?
Do we reject the stream, because we cannot track its course?

I 3

Hath Nature, then, no mystic law we seek in vain to seem?
Can man, the master-piece of God, trace the unerring plan
That places o'er the restless sea the bounds it cannot pass;
That gives the fragrance to the flower, the "glory to the grass?"
Oh! Life with all its fitful gleams hath sorrow for its dower,
And with the wrong heart dwell the pang and many a weary hour;
Hail, then, with gladness what may soothe the aching brain to rest;
And call not impious that which brings a blessing and is blest.
The gladden'd soul re-echoes praise where'er this power hath been;
And what in mercy God doth give, O "call not thou unclean!" *

* "God hath shewed me that I should not call any man common or unclean." Acts, x. 28.

These lines have since appeared in a pleasing volume of poems by the
same authoress, called *Angels' Visits*. (Longman & Co.)

CHAP. III.

UNBELIEVERS IN MESMERISM.—AUTHOR'S OWN EXPERIENCE.—REMARK-
ABLE CASES.—MESMERISERS IN ENGLAND.—CURES AND OPERATIONS
IN ENGLAND.—PROGRESS IN SCOTLAND—IN GERMANY—IN FRANCE—
IN UNITED STATES.—MESMERISM PROVED TO BE A POWERFUL REMEDY
IN PAIN AND DISEASE.

BUT all this train of argument appears childish in the extreme
to a *second* class of opponents. It seems like fighting with the
wind. A medical friend, who for his ability and various attainments in science stands by common consent among the heads
of his profession, says in a letter, "It amuses me much to see
two grave clergymen making a serious debate on the subject of
Mesmerism." The editor of the Lancet says much the same
thing; "We cannot but smile at each theologian for seriously
attacking and seriously defending the practice." And a religious
periodical has made a few observations on the subject which require some little notice.

The Christian Observer * says, that they agree neither with
Mr. M'Neile nor with his opponent, for they believe Mesmerism
to be nothing else than the result of credulity or imposture. But
we will put the charge in their own language. "We believe
that the work is *strictly human*,—being in part imposture for
morbid vanity or *sordid gain*, and in part the irregular action
of an excited *imagination*, &c." Dr. Elliotson was "duped by
some *artful* patients, who *pretended* to respond to his magical
control. We calmly say, *duped*." He "exhibited his deluded
or *deluding* patients, suffering or *affecting to suffer*." * * * *
"In some instances the patients and exhibitors may be con-
federates; in others they may deceive the exhibitor; but that
there is *deception* upon the *part of one* or of *both*, we make no
question." Hard words these,—if not somewhat coarse and

* Christian Observer for September, 1843, in notice of "Mesmerism, the
gift of God."

unbecoming! It might have been expected that the editor of a religious publication would have known more of that evangelical virtue, which "believeth all things, and hopeth all things" favourably. "Charity never faileth." Charity always adopts the best interpretation. Such words as "dupe" and "imposture" are easily written, and save the writers unfortunately much laborious investigation. My original purpose was to treat of the religious aspect of Mesmerism,—or rather to show, that its practice was not so unhallowed as the timid Christian might deem. But in the position in which I have been placed,—and with the facts in my possession of which I have been a witness, such a narrow view of the subject appears to be inconsistent. And when a periodical of such deserved reputation as the Christian Observer can thus encourage its readers in their error by the most unjust aspersions; when the leaders of the medical profession (for the larger part of the junior members are happily an exception) can obstinately persevere in terming this valuable discovery a delusion and an absurdity; I should be wanting in my duty towards God, if I did not thankfully announce that which I have experienced; nay, I should be even wanting to my own character among my fellow-men, if I did not show that in thus advocating Mesmerism I had reasonable grounds for my conviction, and spoke but the words of truth and *soberness.*

It may be then desirable to state that I was an unbeliever in Mesmerism: perhaps it would be more correct to say, that I scarcely thought on the subject. A few years back I went to the Mesmeric exhibitions of the Baron Dupotet in Wigmore Street, and returned from them disgusted and incredulous; and from conversations that I subsequently held with medical men, I was led to resolve the whole appearances into "monotony," "imagination," and "nervousness." All this is stated, to show my previous state of mind. The change, then, that was wrought in me,—the change from scepticism or indifference to earnest conscientious conviction, was no sudden hasty impulse, but the result of cautious observation, and slow and gradual in its growth. I was placed in such circumstances, that in my own despite, I was compelled to be present and witness facts. I

watched them, however, with the most anxious jealousy. I trusted to my own eye-sight alone, and took nothing for granted. I have gone from case to case, and from one patient to another, and seen them all under different states of mind and body, and studied all the effects with the most unwearied diligence for months.* And if plain common sense, untrammelled by the jargon of science, may be allowed to give an opinion, my conclusion from the whole is, that there is no one fact in nature more unquestionable, than that in certain conditions, hitherto unascertained, of the human body, one person is capable of producing a powerful action on the physical system of another, and that through some medium perfectly independant of the imagination of the recipient: and this position I propose to prove in the following statements.

The patient, to whom I shall first refer, had been for many years in an anxious state of health. Palpitation of the heart, severe neuralgic pains, intense continuous headaches, had been a few of the more urgent symptoms; and though she had enjoyed the benefits of the very first advice both in London and the country, and often with advantage, yet still the constitution had at length become so enfeebled as to be little equal to meet an additional shock upon the system. Let it be sufficient to state, that the worst symptoms of her case were at length fearfully exasperated. The most agonizing pains succeeded. For seven long and tedious weeks, sleep, which is "often the last to come when wanted most," literally came not at all. Opiates not only failed to ease, but even tended to aggravate. Till at last, when a crisis was rapidly approaching; when the hopes of the patient's family were almost gone;—at that moment, when it was least expected, were their prayers heard;—a change was happily obtained; a new system of treatment was adopted;—and from that hour they saw the hand of God leading them on to health and to hope; they saw a gradual steady progressive improvement setting in, attended by circumstances of relief, which no language can express.

Mesmerism was that fresh treatment: but as a few facts

* I may now add, "for years."

will throw stronger light upon the action of this newly-discovered power, we will proceed to relate certain incidents in the case.

First let it be stated that this was not a case of confidence, or where faith in a fresh remedy brings about a realization of its own wishes. The very opposite was the fact. The patient's disbelief in Mesmerism amounted even to dislike: and when the medical friend, but too much alive to the necessity of a few minutes' sleep after such a fearful duration of wakefulness, caught at the idea of the Mesmeric action, and suggested its adoption, the proposition met with a peremptory repulse. And it was only through the firmness and intelligent explanations of the excellent friend that undertook the treatment, that this strong reluctance was at last overborne.

At the first séance, which lasted an hour, small apparent effect was produced; but on going to rest, the patient who had been in the habit of requiring the nightly aid of fomentations to lull the intolerable severity of her sufferings, lay perfectly still, and said that "the pain had been endurable." Sleep, indeed, did not visit the pillow: but much was thus far gained.

At the few next sittings sleep was obtained,—deeper too on each occasion,—and the effect of which continued after the patient retired to bed. And though this sleep was very short and much disturbed, still there was sleep; an effect, which for weeks "all the drowsy syrups of the world" had failed to procure. The patient soon declared that she had passed a refreshing night. All this was very encouraging, and called forth many expressions of gratitude; still nothing had hitherto occurred to convince me that the monotony of the passes was not the producing cause,—nothing, that is, of an extraordinary or unusual character; sleep with a gradual mitigation of pain were the blessed results; and we "thanked God and took courage,"—and only trusted that this simple treatment would not lose its effect, as we went on.

It was about the fourth evening, as I was sitting at a distant part of the room, silently watching the patient in her slumbers, that my attention was suddenly arrested, by observing her hand following the hand of the Mesmeriser, as by the force of

attraction.[*] Never shall I forget the feeling with which I started from my chair, ejaculating to myself, "*there is then something* in Mesmerism." A new light burst upon me. Here was a fact which no imagination could explain;—here was a case where no collusion was possible. The act was marked, clear, decisive. In what way, the unbeliever can account for this sympathetic movement, or into what solution it may be tortured, I know not. Common sense simply replies, that here is a plain evident action, in which the eye could not be deceived. This effect too, it may be as well to add, was not temporary, but was produced daily for weeks and weeks. The hand and the head invariably moved with the hand of the Mesmeriser; and certainly in witnessing this magnetic action, we could not avoid adopting the conclusion, that the term "Animal Magnetism" was not so inappropriate.

It is unnecessary to enter further into this case, though other phenomena might be mentioned, except to add, that the most essential benefits continued to be obtained; and that although with a patient of such an impaired constitution, a complete restoration to health was not to be expected, the action of Mesmerism has never on any occasion been employed on her behalf (and this is said after the experience of twelve months) without producing a relief and salutary effect, such as medicine fails in any measure to accomplish.

But my experience can give attestation to a very affecting case,—some of the events of which occurred under my own roof.

Anne Vials is the daughter of Samuel Vials, of the Abbey parish in St. Alban's, who formerly drove the mail cart from thence to Watford. For a short time this poor girl gained her livelihood by working in a silk factory; from the scrofulous habit of her constitution she was not always equal to full employment; but, in 1837, when she was only sixteen years of age, she was compelled to give up work altogether. For her mother fell sick, with a long and pining illness, under which, after much suffering, she finally sank; and during which she was confined

[*] See how this fact is confirmed in Reichenbach's "Researches," p. 12.

to her bed, and required the constant presence of a nurse. Poor Anne, therefore, left her calling at the factory,—took her place by her mother's couch, and was her unwearied attendant night and day. So feeble indeed was the patient, that she could scarcely be quitted for a moment; and for a long year, therefore, did this anxious and affectionate child sit by her parent's bed the whole night through. When death at length released the sufferer, a fatal discovery was made. The mother's disease had taken strong hold of the daughter, for the over-wrought exertions of a twelvemonth had now too clearly brought out the hereditary taint. Anne Vials in fact required a nurse herself; for not only was the general state of her health broken down, but the left arm, which for three or four years had been giving her much pain and uneasiness, became now in so diseased a condition, as totally to deprive her of its use. She was placed under the care of several medical men in succession; the best attendance in St. Alban's was provided for her; but the arm every day grew more and more painful. Through the kindness of some charitable friends, she was now admitted into different hospitals one after the other. She was first removed to Hemel Hempstead Infirmary,—thence to St. Bartholomew's Hospital in London, where she remained nine months,—thence to St. Thomas's in the Borough, and thence to Hemel Hempstead again, in none of which places did she obtain any effectual benefit. The state of her health at length became so serious, that to save her life some decisive measures were necessary; and she was taken up to London again to Guy's Hospital, where her arm was amputated by Mr. Morgan the 22d of March, 1841.

At the end of three months, when the wound was healed, she returned back to St. Alban's. After she had been at home some little time, a violent convulsive action commenced in the stump. This movement grew rapidly worse and worse. In fact, the stump moved up and down, night and day, unceasingly, —and much quicker, to use her own expression, than she herself could move the other arm. Her sufferings became intense, and her general health was affected in proportion. She was now removed backwards and forwards, as before, to the dif-

ferent hospitals, but without any relief. At the infirmary in Hemel Hempstead, they actually strapped the arm down with the hope of lessening the movement; but the confinement made it, if possible, worse, and they were compelled to unloose it. She was at length carried to St. George's Hospital; here she remained three months; her health gradually getting worse and worse, and the epileptic fits, from which she had been suffering for a twelvemonth, increasing in violence and duration; —when, with the only hope of saving her life, a proposition was mooted of taking the stump out of the socket. My readers may judge by this simple fact of the desperate state, to which this poor girl had now arrived; for with her shattered health, it could hardly be expected that she should survive even for a short time so serious an operation.

Fortunately for poor Anne, she had several benevolent friends, who, knowing all the circumstances of her history, had watched the fearful progress of her sufferings from the first; and by subscriptions and various little Christian kindnesses had done much towards lessening her load of sorrow: Mr. Basil Montagu, in particular,—that excellent man, whose long and useful life has been devoted to the benefit of his fellow-creatures, took the warmest interest in her fate;—she often went to his house; and there she received from Mrs. Montagu, that sympathy and consideration which woman alone is able to bestow. One day the thought struck both these kind friends, that if any thing could be of service to Anne in this extremity of misery, it might be Mesmerism. It was but the faintest hope, for they had but slight knowledge or belief of its power;—still they mentioned the case to their friend Mr. Atkinson, and suggested to him the idea of making a trial of what could be done.

Mr. Atkinson is not a member of the medical profession, but has devoted himself to philosophy and science. His acquirements are of the very highest order. He is well known among the advocates of Phrenology and Mesmerism; in the former science he has added much to our stock of knowledge; and in Mesmerism he is eminently successful. Whether in relieving deeply-seated pain, in arresting disease, or in subduing morbid

excitement, his power is equally strange and wondrous.[*] He is so calm, so gentle, and yet so firm, that it is a perfect study to watch him in the management of a case.—Hour after hour have I seen him with the most unwearied patience, devoting the whole energies of his powerful mind to the amelioration of suffering, watching the various symptoms as they arose, and undisturbed by any change that might occur. Never were philosophy and humanity more beautifully united. And in the instance before us, those who have the happiness of being ranked among his friends, require not to be told his answer to Mr. Montagu's suggestion. In spite of the feeling against Mesmerism, and the almost hopeless state of the patient, he at once on his own responsibility undertook the case; and seeing that it would require for months the most unremitting attention, he procured a nurse from St. George's Hospital, and had the poor girl removed to his own house.

It was in May, 1842, about fourteen months after the amputation, that Anne Vials quitted the hospital to make trial of Mesmerism; and this is Mr. Atkinson's description of the state in which he found her. " She had sometimes three or four fits in a day, of a most violent nature, which continued for more than an hour; the stump moved up and down without cessation, not a merely nervous twitching,—but violently up and down; she suffered continuous excruciating pain in the head and back,—and at the end of the stump too the pain was most excruciating;—she had pain too in all her limbs and joints, particularly in the elbow of the remaining arm, just as she had before amputation in the other. Masses of sores were constantly breaking out in different parts of the body; palpitations at the heart, pains in the chest, suspensions of the functions of nature, and a spitting of large quantities of blood accompanied by solid matter, were some of the other symptoms." In short,

* Among his other qualifications for the practice, Mr. A. possesses a peculiar sense of feeling, by which he detects the existence and locality of pain in the patient. This is occasionally the case with Mesmerisers. M. du Bruno, one of the earliest French Magnetisers, speaks of himself possessing this susceptibility. The passage will be found in Gauthier, " Traité Pratique," p. 235.

a more terrible complication of evils have seldom been united in one sufferer.

I shall leave it to Mr Atkinson at some future period to give to the public the interesting details of his success. Let it be sufficient to state, that the process was most painfully laborious, and occupying a large portion of his time, and that she remained in his house more than twelve months. At the first few sittings the epileptic fits were brought on, as if by the Mesmeric effect[*];—but this prevented their recurrence in her ordinary state. At the fourth or fifth *séance*, the deep sleep or trance was superinduced,—*when the action of the stump suddenly stopped*,—and from that moment it never moved in that way again;—the fits too ceased; the pains in the back of her head were almost immediately relieved;—and a gradual improvement in her general health set in. Upon the wonderful results of the Mesmeric treatment in this case, I shall make little comment; my readers can think for themselves;—they will see here a poor girl, carried to and fro from hospital to hospital, enduring the most exquisite torture, and her life placed in such a state of jeopardy, that the only hope of preserving it was recourse to a second and horrible operation. The arm was to be taken out of the socket! an effectual mode, in truth, for a prevention of its movement! But from this operation was she spared by the action of Mesmerism; and by its continued and regular application was a relapse prevented, and an improvement in her health obtained. Who does not see the goodness of Providence in vouchsafing such an agent? Who can deny that Mesmerism to her was the precious gift of God? The facts of her case,—of her sufferings,—of

* When a patient is treated by Mesmerism for epileptic fits, it is considered a favourable sign, if the manipulations bring on a paroxysm; and, from what I have seen, I am of that opinion. But to the inexperienced magnetiser, it has a formidable effect; he appears to be inducing the very disease which he wishes to cure. The case of Anne Vials is one in point; and Teste, in his practical treatise, having described a remarkable cure of epilepsy, says, " this case characterises the ordinary mode of action of magnetism in epilepsy. An *increase* in the number and severity of the fits constitutes almost always the *first* effect of the treatment. But these crises soon diminish in frequency and severity, and ultimately disappear altogether." —*Spillan's Translation of Teste*, p. 267. We shall recur to this subject in the last chapter.

the amputation,—of the movement of the stump, and of the other attendant evils, are known to numbers,—to medical men in St. Alban's,—and to the surgeons and nurses at the hospitals; and it is also known, that all the remedies suggested for her benefit were fruitless;—the best surgical advice was of no avail:—but the fifth day, after the application of Mesmerism, the stump ceased to move, and the other fearful symptoms of the case began to disappear!

But these are not all the marvels that accompanied the treatment. With the improvement of her health the most beautiful phenomena step by step developed themselves,—so beautiful indeed as to attract the admiration of a large number of inquiring spectators, who came to watch and study the case. She became what is called an ecstatic dreamer. Her nervous system had fallen into so peculiar and extremely excited a state, from the effects of this long and painful disease, that the Mesmeric action brought out an exaltation, and a great spiritual activity of the higher organs of the brain. And all these effects appeared spontaneously and unlooked for. Not only did she become a somnambulist,—*i. e.* not only were the common results of the *sleep-waking* state produced,—but an ecstasy,—a spirituality,—a rapt devotional feeling, such as appeared to draw a veil over the scenes of this lower world, regularly came on.* To make myself understood, I will describe the effects as they occurred on my first visit. A few minutes sufficed to throw her into the trance by the simple application of the hand held over the head without contact. First, would there come a slight nervous action of the stump, which was suddenly arrested,—a peculiar movement of the eyelids followed,—the eyes closed,—and she fell back in a deep stupor. From this state she could not be aroused by any application whatsoever; she appeared insensible to pain, and to the action of ammonia, or of lucifer matches burning under her nose. After the lapse of some minutes, she began to move uneasily,—when, on being

* "Not only have mesmerised persons been shown to reason with a perspicuity of which they were incapable at other times, but to display a grace and *freedom of gesture* wholly different from the constraint of their habitual deportment."—Townshend's *Facts*, p. 206. second edit.

addressed by her Mesmeriser, she answered, and sat up in a sort of *sleep-waking* state, conversing freely, though unaware of the presence of strangers. Suddenly she fell back again into the stupor. In this she remained a short time;—when slowly rising from the recumbent position, and gradually lifting up her arm, and pointing as it were to heaven, she opened her eyes, looking upwards with the most intense expression of adoration. The effect was truly sublime. It approached the character of what we may conceive of the devotional rapture of the seraph. Prayer,—veneration,—an admiration of the unseen world,—a contemplation of the divine and the celestial, seemed to absorb every faculty of her soul. Her features, which in her natural state are most homely, were lighted up with a spirituality almost angelic. Though she is nothing but an ignorant factory girl, and accustomed to the most menial occupations, her gestures in this state were beautiful in the extreme. In short, so striking,—so extraordinary was the whole appearance of this poor one-armed girl in her dream,—such a combination was it of the graceful and of the sublime,—that even a Siddons might have made her attitudes a study for the Drama, and Raphael himself not disdained to borrow many a hint for the highest flights of his pencil. Domenichino's Sybille in the Palazzo Borghese at Rome may give some idea of the elevated beauty of her devotions. In fact, I cannot describe the effect better than by adding, that one of the spectators, whose name on matters of taste is of the very highest authority, after witnessing the scene walked from the house down several streets preserving the most profound silence;—and upon his companion at length inquiring of what he was thinking,—"Thinking," he answered, "of what could I be thinking, than of what grovelling creatures we are,—while that poor girl seemed a being of another world!"

Of certain important conclusions*, to which this case gives confirmation, I shall speak by and by: at present my readers may doubt how far two or three visits to Mr. Atkinson's house entitle me to the character of a competent witness as to the

* See Seventh Chapter, with history of several ecstatic cases, and of presumed miraculous appearances.

reality of what I saw; I shall proceed, therefore, to describe some future circumstances in this history, in which I myself took part.

After a patience, an expense, and a labour of no small duration, and such as few men would be willing to bestow, Mr. Atkinson brought this suffering girl to a state of comparative health and comfort; all the formidable symptoms had completely disappeared; the nervous movement of the arm was cured; and there only remained at times a good deal of pain at the end of the stump, the effect probably of something that took place during the amputation. Anne Vials therefore returned home to her native town; and here we might have lost sight of her altogether. It so happened, however, that I passed last summer in Hertfordshire.* And so vivid was the impression that the touching scene I had witnessed left upon my mind, that in one of our earliest drives into St. Alban's we determined to find out our ecstatic dreamer. What, however, were our feelings on being directed to her dwelling! When last we had seen poor Anne,—she was the observed of all observers; —surrounded by the scientific and the curious, there she was secure from want and toil; and with all the freshness of restored health in daily communion with the seraphic beings of her ideal world! What a contrast met our eyes! We found her in a miserable lodging in a back lane, with all the usual accompaniments of poverty. Distress was marked on her countenance. She was neatly and cleanly dressed,—but everything else looked bare and miserable. Toil had done its usual work. A few weeks' necessary employment in seeking her daily food had brought back some old and forgotten symptoms. The stump was causing her great suffering, particularly at the extremity: the right arm was again beginning to be painful above the elbow; her health was giving way; and the expression of her features was indicative either of bodily or mental anxiety. For her father had lost his situation, and was unable to contribute to her support; her Union, which piques itself upon the strictness of its rules, refused any out-door relief; and desirous

* This was written in January, 1844.

of doing all that she could, and of keeping out of the workhouse, she strained her powers of exertion beyond what nature would allow. With but one arm, her choice of employment was limited; and so she carried about the town a basket with goods for sale, the weight of which pressed too heavily on her nerves, and was bringing back her pains in the diseased parts. Had it not been for the assistance of some charitable friends, her case would have been pitiable in the extreme. We took her at once to the house I was occupying; for I determined to try how far Mesmerism, with my inferior powers and experience, would be able to check the relapse with which she was threatened. My pleasure, then, was great on perceiving all the usual phenomena successively presenting themselves. There was the fluttering of the eyelids,—the stupor, the insensibility to pain, the strange and fanciful colloquy, the manifestations of the phrenological organism, and, lastly, the ecstatic dream, with all its varying appearances,—the rapture, the prayer, the uplifted eye, the extended arm, the bended knee, and all the usual signs of the profoundest adoration. The difference that existed between the effects produced by Mr. Atkinson and myself was this, that with him the dream was of a far more elevated and beatific character; with myself the cerebral responses to the touch were more pronounced and striking. However, the main thing to be noticed is, that the health of the patient improved under our management;—of course her freedom from daily toil was of no slight assistance; still she was benefited by her Mesmeric sleep; the pains in the head were removed, and those in the stump greatly lessened, and a countenance of health and serenity reappeared. She stayed with us, backwards and forwards, several weeks: we had the best opportunity of judging her character; and we found her an honest, well-conducted, right-principled girl; and this opinion was confirmed by many in the neighbourhood who had known her long. But we did more than this:—we determined to sift the case to the bottom; we determined to find out how much of truth there was in these startling phenomena. Undeniable as was the benefit to her bodily health by the action of Mesmerism, there were many who thought that the subsequent manifestations of the dream were

all assumed from some interested motive; and I will not conceal that some such suspicions did occasionally lurk in my own mind. But as Bacon says in one of his undying Essays, "*There is nothing makes a man suspect much, more than to know little; and therefore men should remedy suspicion by procuring to know more, and not to keep their suspicions in smother.*" We resolved, therefore, to probe the matter thoroughly. We had every facility for the work; leisure and retirement were not wanting; and we had no interest, moreover, in the decision one way or other. Fortunately our circle had been joined by a friend whose varied talents and acquirements rendered him a competent judge on any philosophic question. Mr. Mitford's [*] inquiring mind was determined to be satisfied as to the truth of our so-called science. He assisted us, therefore, daily at each séance. In fact, he often took the principal part. In conjunction with my wife and myself, he tested the case in every possible way. Experiments of the most opposite kinds were adopted by him. It would be tedious to relate them; it is enough to say, that we repeated them over and over again, and were satisfied at the conclusion as to the only inference to be drawn. And what then was that result? That not a shadow of a suspicion even for a moment could remain as to the reality and truthfulness of what we saw; that the poor girl was an honest unpretending person; that the phenomena produced were far beyond her powers of acting either to assume or to sustain; that the force of imagination could not explain them; —that the supposition of hysteria or nervousness was only solving one difficulty by another;—and that, in short, the whole scene, strange and pregnant with mighty truths as it appeared, was nothing else than the simple effect of this newly discovered agent, the effect of the nervous system of one human being acting on another. It is impossible to say how strong was the satisfaction we all felt at the close of our in-

---

[*] My accomplished friend, the Rev. John Mitford, the learned editor of Gray, and the author of many delightful and popular works, is the last man to sacrifice his judgment to the love of a new and startling theory. Let it be sufficient to say, that, originally a sceptic in Mesmerism, he is now a firm believer.

quiries into this most curious case. It was an opportunity for searching into truth that never might be offered to us a second time. And when the morning of our departure from the neighbourhood arrived, and poor Anne with tears in her eyes attended us to the carriage, we took leave of her with feelings of real regret, and drove away with many an anxious foreboding about her future fate. [*]

But I was also witness to a third case of Mesmerism, that occurred in my house during the summer we passed in Hertfordshire,—which is interesting, not only from the benefits that resulted to the party mesmerised, but also from the corroboration which it gives to the truth of a similar event, of which the newspapers have been lately full. I allude to the case of the sleeping boy at Deptford. James Cook [†] was there thrown

---

[*] It ought to be mentioned in explanation of the circumstances of distress under which we found Anne Vials, that her kind friends in London had gone to great expense on her behalf, as she was supported for some time through the benevolence of Mr. and Mrs. Basil Montagu, and subsequently by Mr. Atkinson, during her residence under his roof; and when she returned to St. Alban's, they entertained the hope that her former charitable neighbours in that place would not omit to renew their benevolent aid. But such was the strong opinion maintained by several in regard to the Satanic character of Mesmerism, that it produced an adverse feeling against the poor helpless girl. Others, too, disbelieving the powers of Mesmerism, were disposed to consider her in some measure an impostor, and assumed that her health, which had defied the skill of the ablest practitioners, had *come round of itself.* It was, therefore, to postpone to as late a day as possible her final reception into the workhouse, that the poor girl economised the alms which she had brought with her from London in as chary a way as possible. Among the friends, however, who remained firm to her, there is one who ought especially to be named. Mrs. Wilkins, of the Verulam Arms Hotel, has acted towards her with all the kindness of the good Samaritan. When staying in that neighbourhood, too, Mr. Mitford kindly set on foot a little subscription, which was most charitably responded to by some of the most influential families in the vicinity. I lately had a letter from Mrs. Wilkins (Feb. 22d, 1844), saying that the poor girl had been very ill again, but was now something better.

It ought to be added, however, that though she has often been subject to attacks of illness, and to great pain in her arm, the convulsive movement of the stump, and the violent epileptic fits, *have never returned.*

Since the above was written, Anne Vials has occasionally been seen in London at several private houses. Her health has varied, but she has always derived the greatest relief and benefit from Mesmerism. (1847.)

[†] This boy slept about three days. See a very interesting letter in No. xvii. of the "Zoist," from Mr. Smith of Deptford, giving an account.

into the mesmeric trance by his master's son, and remained in that state for so long a period, that one party collected round the house with fearful apprehensions at the dangerous condition into which he was plunged;—while a surgeon, from his apparent ignorance of physiology, deems the thing impossible, and writes a letter to the newspapers, pronouncing the whole a delusion. The sleep, as we have since learnt from the best authority, was neither assumed nor alarming; and I am able to confirm the probability of the narrative, from the almost similar circumstances that took place in my own household. A maid-servant of the age of eighteen, of a pallid complexion, and in delicate health, came to live with us in Hertfordshire, her mother being in hopes that country air might have a bracing effect on her constitution. But no such result was produced: she remained weak and languid, and unequal to any exertion. One day Anne Vials mesmerised her; and the next morning she expressed herself as much benefited by its effect. This in-duced a friend, who was staying with us, to repeat the experi-ment. And the result was so deep and prolonged a sleep*, that his endeavours to awaken her were for many hours un-successful; we tried every plan we had seen adopted in similar cases, and referred to different works on the subject,— but in vain. This state of somnambulism lasted for nineteen hours, at the end of which she awoke, and was perfectly ignorant of all that occurred during her sleep. It may be as well to state for the benefit of the sceptic, that this young girl was artless and inexperienced, and perfectly unequal to acting any part, or to resist the various plans pursued by ourselves and her fellow-servants to rouse her from her slumbers. It was an interesting

---

of this case, called, " Mesmerism not to be trifled with, though it kills nobody; or, James Cook alive and hearty."

* This prolongation of sleep is not so very uncommon, and is only alarming to the inexperienced. I was present when Martha Price, a patient of Mr. D. Hand's, awoke after a sleep of more than 48 hours. Dr. Sigmund published in the " Lancet " for 1837, a very curious case of heightened Mesmeric sleep (nearly 94 hours), when much unnecessary fear was experienced. The " Popular Record " contains a spontaneous case of prolonged coma, No. lvii. p. 200. I shall return to this subject in the last chapter.

sight, with which some anxiety was mingled, owing to her delicate constitution. But I have the satisfaction of stating that within a few days afterwards the beneficial results sur-passed all our expectations; the bloom of health returned to her cheeks,— the blood seemed to be circulating through her veins, her whole system was renovated, and she became lively and active. In short, so great was the alteration in her ap-pearance, that on her return to London a few weeks after-wards, her mother, surprised and delighted, exclaimed, "Ma-tilda, you are changed indeed,— I should not have known you!"

Since the above occurred (in 1843), my experience, of course, has very greatly increased. I have employed the treatment successfully with several of my parishioners, have often re-lieved severe pain, and made the science the subject of con-tinued practical study. Among the different cases, however, in which I have assisted, there are none that have given me more pleasure than two, which happened in 1844, from the remark-able refutation they afford to the favourite anti-mesmeric theory of imagination. I sent the account to Dr. Elliotson, who published it in the Zoist*, from the pages of which the following is extracted, and the reader, it is hoped, will not find the nar-rative uninteresting.

"H. B., aged 20 years, the daughter of a labourer in Flixton, was obliged to return from service last year on account of ill health, and early this spring was attacked with rheumatic in-flammation and swelling in one of the knee-joints. She is of a scrofulous habit, and the family are constitutionally subject to rheumatism. Her sufferings were intense, and the inflammation and the pain increased almost daily. The usual remedies, leeches, cupping, blisters, were in vain applied. Opiates were administered, but with no effect. I often went to read and pray with her; and in my whole ministerial experience, have never seen a human being enduring such frightful and con-tinued agony. The neighbours in the adjoining cottage were unable to sleep at night from the screams and cries of the poor

* Vol. ii. p. 200. Apr 1844.

girl. When she was moved in bed, her shrieks were as if she were stretched on the rack. Her miseries had now lasted for three or four weeks: she slept neither night nor day: and at last the able and kind surgeon who attended her began to think that amputation of the limb would be inevitable, to lessen the torture and save her life.

"One morning in April, I went to pay her my usual visit. As I drew near the garden gate I heard the fearful cries of the poor sufferer most audibly. A lodger who lived next door, said to me as I was walking in, 'Sir, this has been going on all night, and we have not been able to close our eyes.' I walked up stairs to the bed-side, and what a sight was before me! The miserable creature was writhing about under the intolerable agony, screaming and almost shrieking out, her face frightfully flushed by fever and distorted by the pain; and this, the mother said, had continued for several hours. Her daughter, she said, had not slept for a week; and the paroxysms of pain had been often as excruciating as what I was then witnessing. I attempted to address and comfort her, but of course fruitlessly. She was in too excruciating agony to heed what was said. I sat down by the bed-side in silent horror. The spectacle was oppressive. Here was a fellow-creature in a hopeless extremity of torture, and not a prospect of alleviation!

"Suddenly the thought struck me that I would try Mesmerism. I had never attempted it as yet beyond the walls of my own house, partly from having no great faith in my own power, partly from an unwillingness to perplex my parishioners with an unpopular novelty; but as I had known some cases of great success in its alleviation of severe pain, I thought I would make a quiet experiment. I said nothing, therefore, to the mother or the sufferer on the subject (they had never even heard of such a thing before); but standing up by the bed-side, and addressing and comforting the afflicted parent *all the time*, I moved my right-hand gently before the patient's face. I continued to speak to Mrs. B. during the process, for this reason, that as I had no great hopes of success, my wish was, that if I failed, they should not remark the action, but simply think that I was a little more emphatic and earnest than usual. This

is *the* noticeable point in the story; because the parties have both stated since, that when I began they were quite unconscious of any thing uncommon in what I was doing.

"At the end of about four minutes I was almost certain that there was an effect. The writhing on the bed seemed less violent, the cries had settled into groans, and there was somewhat more of composure in the face. I left off speaking,—begged the mother to be still,—and pointed the fingers of both hands steadily before the face. In less than ten minutes from the time that I first commenced, the poor suffering girl was in a deep sleep!

"Here, then, was a sudden change from the late horrible exhibition! Here was, indeed, a present mercy for which we had to bless God! The room was now silent; the groans had ceased, only an occasional moan being slightly heard; the limbs so lately tossed to and fro in anguish lay perfectly still; the face was gradually becoming less flushed and looking more tranquil, and the distracted mother, who had been wiping her tears and wringing her hands, stood looking at me speechless and amazed. I was thunderstruck at my own success. Much as I had known, and seen, and read of the healing virtues of Mesmerism, here was an actual living fact which appeared to equal them all.

"*Where was imagination here?* The poor ignorant mother and daughter, in their humble cottage, had never heard of Mesmerism.....It was in consequence of a sudden thought that I commenced the manipulations; and while I was proceeding with them, they did not even know what I was doing, or, in fact, that I was doing any thing; *and in less than four minutes there was a decided effect.*

"I continued the passes for about an hour. She now and then started, and cried out from a sudden pain, but she did not awake; the face had gradually become tranquil; the whole frame seemed comfortable, and I left her asleep. In about a quarter of an hour after my departure she awoke; and though the pain soon become again extremely severe and the fever high, yet there was a decided mitigation of suffering as com-

pared to what it had been; she no longer screamed out from the agony; her night was better, and she had a little sleep.

"The next day I put her into a deep sleep in five minutes: in less than a week, by the surgeon's own admission, she went to sleep in two minutes and a half; for he occasionally attended with me to watch the process (of which he had hitherto seen and known nothing); the severity of the pains also greatly abated, and she began to enjoy a refreshing night's rest. In fact, from the time of the first mesmeric visit, there commenced a gradual, though slow, amelioration; after each séance she was the stronger and better, and the idea of amputation was abandoned; but inasmuch as medical treatment was going on contemporaneously, I must not attribute the whole benefit to the magnetic power. But this fact is undeniable, that as I was often called from home at that period, at each interval of my absence the poor girl relapsed, and gave me great additional labour on my return. However, be the present far happier state of the patient owing to what it may, my medical friend most candidly admits that a great amount of suffering has been spared to her by this sleep,—that Mesmerism was so far an auxiliary to him, and that probably the improvement in her health has been greatly accelerated by its means. This is taking very low and inadequate ground; but even with this admission, what a blessing has Mesmerism proved to the unhappy sufferer!

"Though her general health has since very greatly advanced, and she is able to walk about on crutches, it is doubtful if she will ever recover the complete use of the limb, for it is feared that anchylosis, or union of the upper and lower surfaces of the bones forming the knee-joint may have supervened.*

"One point in the treatment is deserving of notice. She was generally mesmerised for half an hour, and would then continue to sleep about an hour longer. Occasionally, however, my time would be so limited, that I was only able to put her into the sleep and continue the passes for a short period, and

* The knee, as was feared, has become stiff-jointed; but she is able to walk without a stick; and though not equal to hard labour, is in the enjoyment of tolerable health.

she then awoke in about ten minutes after my departure. One might infer from this that the merely putting into a deep sleep in the first instance was not enough—that the battery required to be well charged—and that without a sufficient amount of power communicated, the effect would be but transitory. If this fact be observed in other cases, it would go far to confirm the theory of a fluid.

"I shall not weary you with the phenomena that were manifested in the case; such as the touch of gold causing a strong rigidity in the arms, the application of a sovereign on either side of the knee acting, like a galvanic battery, by moving the limb, and relaxing apparently the sinews and muscles: all these results are familiar to you. The important point in this case is, the *utter absence of all aid from the imagination*, as the party was not only in an extremity of agony, but absolutely unaware that any process was going on.

"And now, what do you suppose that our would-be philosophers reply to these facts? What is the class of objections with which the Suffolk sceptics meet this plain statement? They say that the patient is a woman! A poor, nervous, hysterical woman! And instead of praising Providence for placing within the reach of the sufferer such a merciful gift, they magisterially pronounce, that 'These girls are always up to such tricks, that there is no trusting them;' and then dismiss the subject as unworthy of enquiry! Come we, therefore, to the other sex; and let us learn how the everlasting 'hysteria' of the opponents is to explain the following fact:

"It was on Monday, the 26th of last August (1844), that I rode to inquire after the health of an old couple, whom I had missed the day before at their accustomed place in church. This is merely mentioned to show, that what occurred afterwards happened without design. On reaching the cottage I found the old people well, but one of their sons was very ill in bed, and had been suffering dreadfully for more than a week. I proceeded at once to the bed-side.

"James P., the patient, is a strong stout man, of the age of thirty-three, partly a fisherman and partly a farm labourer, and as little likely to be a subject for the imagination to play with,

as a president of the College of Surgeons himself. About twenty years ago, he had a sharp attack of rheumatic fever, which lasted more than four weeks and confined him to his bed still longer. About thirteen years back he had a second attack of similar duration; but his health since that period has been robust and vigorous, and he is a good specimen of a hardy English peasant. He was engaged in the mackarel fishery in the summer, and had returned to his village for the harvest; but during the first days of reaping had caught cold from the heavy rains that set in, and had returned to his father's cottage seriously ill.

"The poor fellow was now stretched on his pallet, in a severe state of suffering. It was an attack of his old complaint, acute rheumatic fever with a swelling of the joints. Large drops of perspiration were standing upon his face. He was evidently enduring great agony, hardly bearing the bed-clothes to touch him; and though he did his utmost to suppress what he suffered, the enemy was too strong for him, and he groaned out occasionally from the intolerable anguish. His mother said, that all the sleep that he had had for the last week, put together, scarcely amounted to an hour's length. He himself said, that the sleeping draughts that he had taken had done him more harm than good; for if he went to sleep for ten minutes from the effect, he awoke up afterwards feeling worse than before. It was a distressing scene; and had I not made a successful trial of my mesmeric powers with the other patient, I should have taken leave of poor P. after the usual conversation was over.

"As it was, I determined to make another experiment, and saying nothing whatever to the patient, I held my hand before his face, and in less than five minutes he was fast asleep! you shall not be wearied with an account of the mother's astonishment, or of my own gratification. Here was a sturdy unimaginative labourer, who a few minutes back had been in too great agony to converse, cast into a deep composing slumber, through the simple agency of our vituperated art! as the poet so beautifully expresses it, "that sweet sleep which medicines all pain," had steeped his senses in forgetfulness of this world's miseries. He was, comparatively speaking, in elysium,—and

all the work of a few minutes. I continued to make passes down his limbs for half an hour. Once he woke up suddenly, from pain; but instantly fell off to sleep again. After I left him, he slept the greater part of the afternoon, waking at times from a sudden pain, and then again dropping off; and he had the best night since his attack.

"When I called to see him the next day, he told me that though he was still very full of pain, the violent intolerable agony had quite subsided since that first sleep; and it may be as well to mention, that it has never returned since. He has had a good deal of suffering, of course, but different altogether in degree. In fact, the *acute* anguish of the rheumatic fever seemed to be *cut short* at once. I asked him now how he felt, as I was beginning, he said, 'It fared (seemed) as if something *cold* was walking over his brain.' He has described the same sensation several times in almost the same words. I then put him to sleep in three minutes, and when I pressed his forehead with my fingers, he *snored out*. I have since generally put him to sleep in a minute and a half; the last time he went off in half a minute. He says that when I begin, 'he cannot possibly keep awake.' It is unnecessary to add, that he never heard of Mesmerism.

"The touch of gold or silver seemed to give him pain, and he instantly awoke. The movement of my fingers near his hand would set his own fingers in a slight magnetic movement, causing a sort of twitching.

"As medical treatment has been going on at the same time, I do not place the whole abatement of the fever to Mesmerism. P. was greatly benefited by bleeding. But the surgeon, hitherto an unbeliever, in spite of what he had witnessed with our former patient, was astonished at the result, and admits that the way in which sleep was induced and pain overpowered, is something quite beyond the customary means of the Æsculapean art. To which of the two systems, the mesmeric or the medical, the main improvement be owing, I do not decide, though I have my opinion. I rather wish Mesmerism to be regarded, not as an isolated panacea, that holds no communion with other remedies,—but as adjunct, an

auxiliary; one out of many means, only simpler and less injurious than the usual narcotics. But the point in this case, as in that of H. B., is this, that *imagination could have no part in the matter: the patients were both ignorant of what was taking place, and their faith or fancy gave no assistance whatsoever.*

"How the learned of your profession will explain the above, I pretend not to guess. They must find some other theory than that of imagination. They have ridden that horse to death, and it will carry them no longer. Neither does the system of Mr. Braid meet the difficulty. The patients did not stare at me. They did not fix their eyes stedfastly at my fingers, and so drop off to sleep: they did not even look at me, —or know that anything was going on. I therefore send these two cases up to you, not as proofs of the curative influence of Mesmerism, (for of that there is already abundant evidence,) but as an unequivocal, undeniable illustration of the wondrous *sympathy that exists between man and man.* They prove that a sympathetic union does exist,—be the connecting chain either a fluid, or electricity, or any other undiscovered agent: and again I call upon our antagonist in your profession to enter upon the subject in a calm philosophic tone. Let them discard their vulgar jokes, and their affected silence, and meet the question openly like men. It is really sad to see the shifts and the interpretations that they employ; to see the rapture with which they pounce on a failure, and the smooth plausibility with which they forget a fact. It is melancholy to see this, and remember, that the inquiry is not about some unreal point in abstract science,—but whether there be a provision in nature's storehouse,—the soothing gift of a merciful Creator,—by which a vast amount of human suffering may be spared, and even the duration of human life occasionally prolonged."

Here then are a few remarkable cases. And what is the reply of the unbeliever? That the writer is a prejudiced, incredible witness? For I pass by as unworthy of notice the common charge of deception and "morbid vanity," with simply demanding, what reason I could have for upholding Mesmerism

except conviction of its truth? But I am an incompetent testimony,—it is meant; I have received no diploma from the College of Surgeons, and know nothing of the action of hysteria and of nervousness. There is a homely proverb which will admirably apply to these reasoners,—"An ounce of mother-wit is worth a pound of clergy." A little practical common sense is all that is necessary; and it is possible for an educated man, —even though he may not have received a medical degree,— to form a legitimate opinion of the appearances of Mesmerism, after a daily observation for several months. But setting all this aside,—and for the sake of argument admitting myself to be in error and the above a delusion, are these cases isolated ones? Is my experience a rare instance? Is nothing else producible? At this moment, hundreds and hundreds of cases, out of England alone, can be brought forward. A mass of evidence quite astonishing is in my possession. Cures and relief effected in an infinite diversity of diseases can be named. Not that it is pretended that Mesmerism is a universal specific. There are many disorders, which it does not seem to touch. There are many patients to whom it does not seem to be of use. Still a host of cases can be produced, in which a service, beyond all expression valuable, has been wrought; in which pain of the most intense agony has been removed; in which long chronic diseases have been subdued; in which sudden attacks have been mastered;—cases, too, in which medical men have been at fault, or which they had pronounced incurable and hopeless. In the metropolis alone a considerable number of Mesmerisers can be named. There is hardly a county in England, where it is not now practised. From York to the Isle of Wight,— from Dover to Plymouth, there can be produced a chain of evidence and a list of cures. Our Mesmerisers are not ignorant practitioners;—not hot-headed cracked-brained enthusiasts, but men whose standing in society is a guarantee for the correctness of their information,—temperate, slow-judging, careful thinkers, and as little likely to be led astray by a false light as their opponents themselves. Clergymen, military men, barristers, physicians, surgeons, ladies high in rank, and men of a distinguished position in the world could all be named: their

practice of the art is well known in their respective circles; and by many I have been favoured with information that is surprising and interesting in the highest degree. The details of their respective success are so copious that they would fill a thick volume. Of course, I am precluded by the brief nature of this little work from doing more than glancing at the leading points. If I selected a few cases for insertion, the choice would be most perplexing; and if I began, I should not know where to stop. They can only, therefore, be noticed in the most cursory manner. But even with this limited allusion, and with the addition of the names of some who have previously appeared before the public, but of whom many of my readers may not have heard, I shall be able to produce, what the lawyers would call such a mass of cumulative evidence, as nothing but the *scepticism of science* could prevent men from admitting to be at least a startling and important phenomenon.

Mr. Atkinson, then, of whom mention has been made before, has been eminently successful in his treatment of numerous diseases, some of which too generally defy all human skill. He has accomplished *three cures* in that most fearful of maladies, *tic doloreux*: one case was of *ten years' standing*; and the other two of several years' duration. He has cured several cases of fits, of hysteria and want of sleep, and of those determined nervous and sick headaches, which seldom yield to remedial action. He has been successful in various acute nervous pains and contractions of the limbs, in asthma, fever, long-standing cough, affections of the heart and spine, injured sight, and deafness, in melancholia, rheumatism, toothache, indigestion, and different functional obstructions. He has found Mesmerism efficacious to a most valuable extent in subduing cerebral excitement. He had a patient under his treatment, whose irritability of brain was becoming a source of much anxiety. By the application of Mesmerism every day for a fortnight all the formidable symptoms disappeared; the head became cool; the paroxysms ceased; and the functions of the brain were restored to a calm and healthy state. The efficacy of Mesmerism in maladies of this description is almost incredible. Its soothing influence has so speedy an effect. Mr.

Atkinson has indeed such copious and invaluable information to communicate, that the public have reason to hope that one day he may place the results of his experience before them.

Captain John James, of Dover, has great experience in the practice, and has contributed much towards its full appreciation. His patients have been numerous. He has found Mesmerism most efficacious in nervous disorders;—and in several other complaints, he has greatly alleviated the sufferings of his patients.

The late Mr. Chenevix, a well-known name in the literary world, the author of a beautiful article in the Edinburgh Review on "France and England," and a man of considerable scientific attainments, as his communications in the Philosophical Transactions show, was preparing a work to demonstrate the results of his experiments and observations on 442 persons, when an acute disease suddenly terminated his own existence. In the course of six months he once mesmerised 164 persons, of "whom 98 manifested undeniable effects. There was hardly one instance where disease existed, that relief was not procured." His efforts were immense; and his success proportionate. To mention a few instances,—he cured a case of epilepsy and spasmodic pain of six years' standing in twenty-one sittings. He succeeded completely in three other cases of the same disease, and procured immense relief in eight. He cured a man far advanced in a rapid consumption. He cured seven cases of worms; and produced a most powerful effect on *some men in the Coldstream Guards*. He was of service, also, to several inmates in Wakefield Lunatic Asylum. The reader is referred for further information respecting this lamented man to the first number of the Zoist.

The cases reported by the Reverend Chauncy Townshend in his philosophical work, called "Facts in Mesmerism," are remarkable from the answer they afford to the common opinion, that the effects of Mesmerism are limited to a few nervous and fanciful persons, chiefly of the weaker sex. While he has adopted Mesmerism extensively in cases of sickness, he mentions that when he first took it up, "out of *twenty-three* individuals, in whom he induced sleepwaking, more or less perfectly,

six only were women, one only a decided invalid." He gives the account of seven or eight young men "in perfect health,"—"in good and robust health," who were mesmerised by him. His description of his power over some sceptics at Cambridge is so curious and convincing, that it should be read by every candid inquirer. In respect to Mesmerism as a curative agent, he says himself, after much experience, "its capacity to serve, either as a calmant or a stimulant, according to the exigencies of the complaint, would alone give it the highest rank as a remedy. In this point of view, how valuable appear its offices, how unmatched by those of any substance in the Materia Medica." "Of all remedies, this alone pours its benefits direct upon the very springs of sensation." "In cases of deafness and blindness, which depend on nervous weakness, we possess a subtle means of acting efficiently upon the fountain-head of the calamity." Though "insulated cases of benefit," he adds, "might seem suspicious, benefits on so large a scale must finally vanquish distrust." And he concludes his notice to the second edition of his work, "with a deep regret that prejudice should yet stand in the way of so much alleviation of human suffering as it is calculated to afford, and with a humble hope that truth and time will lead to a discreet and grateful use of this wonderful gift to man."

Colonel Sir Thomas Willshire, commanding at Chatham, has practised Mesmerism extensively, and with great success. It is no new thing to see the gallant profession of arms lending the warmest aid to the cause of humanity: and many military men, with a zeal and benevolence that reflect the highest honour upon them, have taken up our science. To Sir Thomas Willshire, in particular, occupying as he does so distinguished a position, the highest admiration is due;—and while very many interesting particulars could be related by him, one is so striking that it cannot be too often laid before the public.

A nursery servant, who had been for a long time suffering pain in her upper jaw, of a most excruciating kind, was compelled to undergo a severe operation on its account. The pain was so intense, that she could scarcely bear a touch on the part affected. Sir T. Willshire put her into the Mesmeric trance,

and the surgeon commenced the operation. It lasted more than five minutes. She did not feel it the least. Not a muscle or nerve either twitched or moved. When Sir Thomas awoke her, she was not conscious of having gone through the operation.

It should be added that the sympathy of taste was developed in this case. When Sir Thomas took wine, the patient said she tasted it. The same experiment was tried with biscuit, and she "tasted biscuit." And though she felt not the pain of the operation, when Captain Valiant pinched Sir Thomas's hand, she immediately felt it, and said she did not like it.

Among other cases, Sir Thomas Willshire has cured a servant, named Catharine Cocks, of a pulmonary complaint, with which she had been very ill and affected for years. She is now perfectly restored to health and strength, and is "robust and well;" "though the medical gentleman, who had attended her for some years, had, previously to the Mesmeric operation, assured her parents that she could not survive the ensuing winter."

Earl Stanhope, whose philanthropy and Christian kindness are so universally known and admired, is a practiser of the science. This excellent nobleman is not deterred by popular prejudice, or by the ridicule which some newspapers have endeavoured to cast upon him for his zeal in the cause, from appearing as the advocate of truth. In a letter, of which he has permitted me to make use, the noble lord mentions several cases, in which he had been of signal service to some of his sick and poorer neighbours. In particular, he mentions the case of a young man, aged twenty-seven, who had been obliged to give up his place on account of a nervous affection, which produced syncope upon every trifling excitement. After being mesmerised a few times, he was perfectly cured. Another was the case of a young woman, aged twenty-two, the daughter of a day-labourer, who was afflicted with such violent epileptic fits, that she also was obliged to retire from service. After a treatment of a short duration, she was pronounced quite well, and returned to her situation with her former master. Other

rary interesting particulars could be added, if the limits of this work allowed it.*

Miss Wallace, a most benevolent lady in Cheltenham, whose exertions are unremitting in everything that can be of service to the cause of humanity, can give the strongest attestation to the truth of the Mesmeric power. She has had several most extraordinary cases under her management. She has cured two cases of decline,—the only two of the kind that she has attempted. She has cured sciatica,—the *most violent cramps,* epilepsy, head-aches, tooth-aches, ear-aches,—and some without sleep being induced. Several of her other cases are very remarkable; and I hardly know any one more able to give valuable evidence and information connected with the science, than this amiable and active-minded friend of truth.†

Several other ladies and gentlemen in Cheltenham and the neighbourhood have been for some time practising the art; and could speak in the strongest way of its beneficial effect with their patients.

Captain Valiant, of Chatham, who a short time ago was a "thorough sceptic," as he called himself, is now a most powerful and successful Mesmeriser. Numerous cases could be related in which he has relieved pain, reduced swellings, and obtained a complete cure. His power seems unusually great. He writes, "I have myself mesmerised *many persons of both sexes,* and have seen *others succeed with a great many more.* I have also, in many cases, without putting the patient to sleep, removed head-aches, tooth-aches, sore-throats, and several other pains, not only in women, but *strong men,* merely by manipulating the parts affected." Space is wanting for an insertion of some interesting facts connected with a few of his patients; but the attention of the reader is invited to the following: "In my practice of Mesmerism, I have met two curious cases which perhaps may be worth mentioning. In both of these my subjects were *powerful men,* brother captains in the army,

* The details of these cases have been since published in the "Zoist," vol. ii.

† See also "Zoist," vol. iv. p. 450, for report of many more cures by this excellent and kind friend.

whom I had repeatedly tried to mesmerise, but could only succeed in closing their eyes, without being able to put them to sleep, so that they could *not possibly open them,* till I demesmerised them. I could close their eyes in about two minutes, even by giving them a glass of magnetised water. I had also the power of catalepsing the limbs of one of them by making passes over them." Captain Valiant's testimony, like that of Mr. Townshend's, is a most valuable answer to those who think that Mesmerism applies only to patients that are "highly nervous and hysterical." *

Mr. Baldock of Chatham can bear most useful testimony to the curative powers of Mesmerism. "*Several cases,*" he says, "have presented themselves to him, in which relief has been given to the parties." In palpitations of the heart and severe head-aches, he has been very successful. One of his cures is so remarkable, that I shall give the particulars. It is that of Robert Flood, now residing at Caistor in Lincolnshire. Mr. Flood had for several years suffered most severely from disease in one of his kidneys. He had been under the care of different medical men,—and had been placed in a London hospital. His pains were so acute, that he could not leave his bed until the day was advanced;—and even then it was necessary for him to recline several times before retiring for the night. He had been in this state for several years. Mr. Baldock was the happy instrument of restoring him to health, after a Mesmeric treatment of three months. This poor fellow, great part of whose time was spent in bed from pain and weakness, "is now in such robust health that he can throw a quoit." Mr. Baldock has several other most valuable instances of cure and relief; and as he keeps a journal of his Mesmeric proceedings, we may hope that these interesting particulars will be placed more fully before us.†

Mr. Majendie, of Hedingham Castle, Essex, has practised Mesmerism with great advantage to the health of several

* Captain Valiant's statement is given more fully in "Zoist," vol. ii. p. 241.

† Since the above was written, Mr. Baldock has furnished several other cases to the Zoist.

persons. He says in a letter, "I have seen *much* of the curative effects of Mesmerism." Several of his cases are most instructive. Invalids, who had been incapable of any exertion or labour, through a deranged system, have been cured or restored to comparative health. One of the facts that he mentions, is so corroborative of the electrical theory of Animal-Magnetism, that it deserves to be recorded. "Without the slightest suggestion or prompting, the patient said she saw the sparks of fire pass from the points of my fingers into the water which I magnetised for her." This same phenomenon has been observed by other somnambulist patients. Mr. Majendie has given great attention to the subject of Mesmerism; and his opinion on all matters connected with it is of much value.

Mr. Topham, of the Temple, whose services in the well-known case of poor Wombell were so invaluable, and of whom, therefore, the Chirurgical Society seem to entertain a professional jealousy, has much experience in the practice. It may be useful to record one of his cases; that of a young man, aged 18, who, for four years and a half, had been subject to epileptic fits,—at least three a week, and each of two hours' duration. He suffered also from *incessant* pains in his head. Upon being mesmerised, *the pains immediately ceased altogether;* his natural sleep became sound and regular; and he had two fits only in the space of three months. The Mesmeric treatment was unavoidably discontinued in this case—before the cure became perfected; but the change in the young man's health is something quite remarkable.

Mr. Thompson, of Fairfield House, near York, is a very successful Mesmeriser. After much experience, he speaks in the strongest way of the utility of the science, and of the benefit that may be derived from it. He is often able to remove acute pain without producing sleep. He says, that he has tested this repeatedly "with almost invariable success; mitigating, and very often altogether removing, toothache, headache, rheumatic pains, and pains occasioned by contusions, burns, and any inflammation;"—and in some few cases, of a serous or acute character, he has been able to afford great relief.

One of his cases is such a beautiful illustration of the power

of Mesmerism, that I regret my inability, from want of space, to give the full particulars. It is that of John Bradley, a boy near York,—aged nine years, who had suffered for fifteen months from a diseased knee,—evidently of a scrofulous character. When Mr. Thompson first saw him, "the child had been suffering intense agony,—was unable to rest day or night, had a total want of appetite; there was great inflammation extending above the knee,—the knee was enormously enlarged, and it was evident that extensive suppuration had taken place in the inside of the knee." "The child was in a high state of fever, a deep hectic flush was on his cheeks, attended with quickness of breathing and a short cough." Mr. Thompson determined to try the "experiment of making passes over the knee for half an hour. Before the time had nearly expired, the child became calm and still, then began to smile, and said he felt a *warm heat come out of Mr. Thompson's fingers,* which had taken away the pain. He seemed a little drowsy, but no sleep was produced." After a certain period of treatment, the child's health rapidly improved,—the inflammation of the knee subsided, absorption of the matter took place, and in a month he was able to put his toe to the ground. After many other particulars, Mr. Thompson adds, "that it was in May that I commenced mesmerising him; by the latter end of August the recovery was as complete, as I thought it possible for a knee, so deformed from long-standing disease, could be." He has great use of the limb; is able to walk about very well,—suffers not the slightest pain or inconvenience,—and his health is very good. One fact is too curious to be omitted. "During the process of recovery, he *never but once went to sleep under the operation of Mesmerism.*"

Here is another valuable proof of the remedial power of Mesmerism in Mr. Thompson's hands. A gentleman who had been suffering for *nine consecutive days* from severe rheumatic fever, with acute pain in the shoulders, arms, hands, loins, legs, and knees; with the fever excessive; profuse night sweats caused by the agony of pain,—and loss of sleep and of appetite, placed himself under the management of Mr. Thompson. These are his own words: "In less than twenty minutes you had

nearly charmed away all the pain and restored warmth and
feeling to my feet. You then put me to sleep: the delightful
sensation of that sleep, after such extreme pain, I can scarcely
describe. When you awakened me, I felt like another person.
The fever was reduced: and the pain was gone. In four days
I was down stairs: every time you mesmerised me, I felt as it
were *new life*."

Mr. Thompson gives a description of three cures of severe
and long-standing neuralgic pains of the head. One of the
parties had been under the first medical advice in London;
"had a *great horror of Mesmerism* without *any faith in its
curing her.*" One day, when much worse than usual, *she asked
for its* application: in less than ten minutes she was relieved;
and awoke up entirely free from pain; and her general health
has been very good ever since."

Captain Anderson, of the Royal Marines, who is resident in
Chelmsford, is another very powerful Mesmeriser. His last
case is so very striking an instance of the merciful power of
Mesmerism that I shall give it somewhat in detail. Mrs.
Raymond, a lady residing at Chelmsford, had suffered for nine
years from a spinal complaint, being confined to her sofa, and unable to be moved day and night; she had also lost the use of her
voice. Her sufferings were dreadful. Blisters, caustic plasters,
leeches, setons, medicines of all descriptions, were tried in
succession, without any substantial good. These are her own
words: "During the nine years I was unable to be moved
from my sofa night or day; I was never free from pain; sometimes the agony was indescribable: the three last years I have
been entirely speechless. I had given up all hope of recovery,
and almost prayed for death." "At the very time that I had
resigned myself to my fate, and begged that my sufferings
might soon be ended, God in his great mercy made me acquainted with Captain Anderson, who offered to try the effect
of Mesmerism." "*I laughed at the idea*; but from his account
of the cures he had performed, I complied,—being anxious to

* Mr. Thompson, who is one of the most successful of Mesmerisers, has
sent a large number of cases to the Zoist. His power in willing, without
the manipulations, is most striking.

grasp at any thing which would do me good." Without following out the details, this is the result. "I am now able to
walk out daily, alone and unassisted. I am regaining my
speech;—and I am free from pain, sleep soundly, and take no
medicine, and am now seldom mesmerised." Well may this
excellent lady, when comparing "her past sufferings with her
present happiness," say, that she "feels thankful to God and
grateful to Captain Anderson." For here is a case, which
alone would be able to substantiate the healing virtues of this
blessed gift.*

Dr. Engledue of Southsea practises Mesmerism in his profession, and is a warm advocate in its cause. Whoever has
studied the fine intellectual forehead of Dr. Engledue, and
watched his clear eye, and calm, thoughtful countenance, must
acknowledge, that there stands a philosopher in the truest
acceptation of the word, and one little likely to be led astray
by the unreal fancies of a heated imagination.

Dr Sigmond, whose position in the scientific and literary
world gives the greatest value to his testimony, published in
the Lancet, for December, 1837, a most remarkable Mesmeric
case of his own.

Mr. Weekes, a surgeon at Sandwich, has "for two years
devoted a large portion of his time and attention to the great
remedial powers proceeding from the judicious application of
Mesmerism;"—and for this independent and noble-minded
conduct, he has been, of course, traduced by the ignorant and
the malevolent. He has, however, the satisfaction of knowing,
that the alleviation of pain, and the removal of disease, under
the Mesmeric treatment, and through his management, has
been considerable. His professional success has been great.
With him, Mesmerism has proved of use, "after the usual
modes of treatment, and, in some instances, abundance of
quackery to boot, had utterly failed; and rendered the case
more inveterate and distressing." Among the cases that he
mentions, are some of "dyspepsia, habitual and obstinate con-
stipation, paralysis, sluggish condition of the hepatic system,

* This case has been since published in the Zoist, vol. ii. p. 82.

and hypochondriasis, muscular contractions, stubborn and otherwise hopeless cases of chronic rheumatism, local pains, and several severe forms of neuralgia, cases of general languor and debility without manifest cause, as also a case of deafness,—the removal of two teeth without the knowledge of the patient, besides several affections of an anomalous character." Mr. Weekes is proceeding firmly and actively: his name ranks high with all parties; and he is reaping an abundant reward.

Mr. Gardiner of Portsmouth is a powerful supporter of the truth of Mesmerism. He gives a valuable account of the extraction of two teeth, attended by most painful circumstances, without the consciousness of the party. "During the whole of this trying operation not a groan or complaint escaped the patient." Other severe operations have been performed by him "without any manifestation of feeling" on the part of the patient.

Mr. Prideaux, of Southampton, is another great practical Mesmeriser. He reports three remarkable cases of the cure of St. Vitus's dance,—in which the "twitchings" diminished perceptibly from day to day, under Mesmeric treatment. From five different patients he has extracted teeth without their consciousness. His description of their demeanour under this usually painful operation is most curious. "The patient sat with the hands quietly folded in the lap,—the countenance was placid and serene,—and the whole attitude that of repose." "The insensibility was perfect" of the three other patients. The fifth "allowed me to operate for two hours with the most passive indifference." Mr. Prideaux, himself a medical man, says of one of his patients, "a case more conclusive of the power of Mesmerism as a remedial agent in the cure of disease, it would be difficult to conceive." "If imagination," says he again, "can work such wonders, she should be placed at the head of the Materia Medica." With many such enlightened practitioners as Mr. Prideaux, the well-attested facts of Mesmerism will soon force their way on the mind of the public.

Mr. Jeanson, of Pennsylvania Park, near Exeter, the President of the Exeter Literary and Philosophical Society, and a gentleman well known in that part of the world among scientific

men, is also a Mesmeriser, and can bear his valuable testimony to the therapeutic virtues of the science. He has been particularly successful in the treatment of tic-doloreux.[*]

Mr. Kiste, a most intelligent gentleman from Germany, and who has been resident some little time in Plymouth, has devoted much of his attention to the science. Among the cases in which he has found it efficacious, one alone can be particularly mentioned, which by itself would confirm the unspeakable value of Mesmerism. It was a severe case of spasmodic asthma. The patient had been subject to it for *twelve years*. She says herself, that such were her sufferings, that for "many days she was obliged to sit with a pillow on her lap to support her stomach." "The paroxysms were so violent that she was obliged to sit on the floor for four-and-twenty hours at a time." "To describe half my sufferings when the spasmodic breathing came on, is impossible." She had been attended by eight or nine medical men in succession, Cupping, blistering, hot baths, were tried, but without any important effect. In short, her own description of the periodical pains which returned every fortnight—of their severity, and of other attendant evils, is painful to read. A clergyman, well acquainted with the family, now writes to the Mesmeriser, and says, "It is now at this moment (Jan. 29.) nine weeks since she was subjected to the Mesmeric influence, and she has been *entirely free from asthma*, her general health is improved, and she is gaining flesh." I shall not enter into the further details of this very striking and interesting case; as we have reason to hope that Mr. Kiste will himself shortly bring them before the public.[†]

Mr. Holm, of Highgate, who, in a most philanthropic manner, devotes much of his time to the benefit of his fellow-creatures, has found Mesmerism a most efficacious remedy. He has obtained some very remarkable cures. He generally has a large number of Mesmeric patients under his management. He tells me that he has proved Mesmerism to be most valuable

* Zoist, vol. iv. p. 341.
† This case has since appeared in the Zoist, vol. ii. p. 415.

in epilepsy, rheumatism, brain fever, diarrhœa, headaches, and many neuralgic disorders. Mr. Holm has large experience in phrenology, and has tested with great success its connection with vital magnetism.

Mr. Charles Childs of Bungay "was *very much indisposed to receive the phenomena of Mesmerism as facts,*"—"but he was constrained to admit their reality, unless he would deny the evidence of his own senses." He says, "I have practised Mesmerism above four years; in this period, I *have proved its unquestionably beneficial results on several of the most afflictive maladies.*" In corroboration of the above, I can state, that I called on the mother of one of Mr. Childs's patients, and heard from her own mouth the details of a very remarkable cure of a child that had been frightened in a fearful manner. Every other remedy, but Mesmerism, seemed to fail in this case. Mr. Childs generally has about four patients at a time under his hands. Much attention has been awakened in his neighbourhood by the following operations. I quote from the very able letter which Mr. Webb, the operating surgeon, addressed to the editor of "The Medical Times." Mr. Webb says, that he does "not come forward to support the theory of any man. He desires only, as an unprejudiced observer, to record facts which he had himself tested." The cases are these: "Two young women, Mesmeric patients of Mr. Childs, who had suffered from toothache for some time past, consented to have their teeth extracted while in Mesmeric somnolency, but were not apprised of the time at which this was to be done. That they might have no reason to suspect what was about to take place, I was not sent for until Mr. Childs had put them into the Mesmeric condition, when I went and extracted for one a very troublesome stump, and for the other, a double tooth in the upper jaw. I am morally certain that no means were employed to produce this state of unconsciousness except the Mesmeric." * * * * "After a short time they were awakened, and were both wholly unconscious of all that had taken place."

"Nor was this all; for neither at the time when they were awakened, nor on the following day, did they experience either

pain in the jaw or tenderness in the gum."* Evidence, like this, coming from the surgeon himself, has a twofold strength.

A similar operation took place at Hinckley in Leicestershire, last June, upon a young man, named Paul. The tooth was extracted during the Mesmeric sleep, without consciousness. Paul told a correspondent of mine, that "he did not feel any pain whatever."

Mr. Nicholles, of Bruton Street, has extracted two or three teeth from patients in the Mesmeric sleep, *without their knowledge.* In this last case, he says, "The pulse was 108 under the Mesmeric influence, and rose a little during the operation. On being awakened, she expressed the most lively gratitude and delight at having lost her troublesome companion."

Another striking case of this kind was the extraction of a tooth from W. Gill, at Edinburgh, without pain, on May 1. 1843, by Mr. Nasmyth, Surgeon-Dentist to the Queen. Several medical gentlemen were present. Mr. Craig was the Mesmeriser. Gill had no feeling, when the tooth was being extracted,—but after he was awakened, he felt a soreness and pain in the gums.†

Mr. Carstairs, of Sheffield, who practises Mesmerism, has extracted teeth from parties who were not aware of the operation. He has also performed several minor operations, such as opening an abscess and dressing the wound; cutting a large wart from a patient's hand;—inserting a seton, without the parties feeling the slightest pain or suffering any inconvenience. —Other medical men in Sheffield have employed Mesmerism as a medical auxiliary, and could bear testimony to its usefulness.

Mr. Chandler, a surgeon of Rotherhithe, has much experience of the beneficial effects of Mesmerism. Among other cases, he has had one of insanity, in which his Mesmeric power was invaluable. He "produced a cure, rapid and perfect, when

* Mr. Charles Childs has had some still more interesting cases, which I have enjoyed the opportunity of witnessing, the account of which is published in the Zoist, vol. iii. p. 36.

† See Introductory Chapter, for the report of extraction of teeth by different dentists.

bleeding and powerful medicines, and medicines given powerfully and perseveringly, had all been unavailing."*

Mr. Purland, of Mortimer Street, Cavendish Square, offers an honourable instance of the triumph of truth over prejudice and preconceived opinions. I met Mr. Purland last July at the house of a friend: his opinions against the existence of Mesmerism as a fact were most decisive; I had much conversation with him,—but did not shake him in the least. He consented, however, to witness some Mesmeric experiments;—and after giving them a due and patient investigation, he became a convert, and is now a valuable ally,—and has practised the art with great success. He has cured his father in a dreadful and most distressing malady, in a case where no relief was procured from medicine. He has cured cases of asthma, hysteria, lameness, and deafness. At various times he has relieved patients of headache, toothache, pains in the chest, &c. He calls Mesmerism, in a letter I lately received from him, " a science of much importance;" and this from a gentleman, who a few months back was a determined sceptic! Such, however, is the force of truth, where straightforward and honourable intentions go hand in hand with the inquiry.†

Mr. Boyton, a surgeon of Watlington, in Oxfordshire, is another honourable example of a manly independence of mind. His acknowledged reputation in his profession gives value to what he states. He has cured a severe case of fits; and another serious case of injury, accompanied by much pain, and general ill health. He says, "I do not mean to recommend the indiscriminate use of this agent in every case, nor substitute it for acknowledged remedies. But in some cases I should not hesitate to employ it; it *strengthens the nervous system, improves the digestion, and tranquillizes the mind.*" This is most important testimony.

Dr. Wilson, of the Middlesex Hospital, is so well known by

* A large number of most interesting cases, under the treatment of this able and indefatigable Mesmeriser, has appeared in the later numbers of the Zoist.

† The produce has already recorded the large number of teeth which Mr. Purland has extracted in the Mesmeric state.

his publications on the subject, to be a firm supporter of the truths of Mesmerism, that it is only needful to allude to his name. Some readers may, however, be interested in learning that Dr. Wilson has cured a case of insanity, or intense melancholy, by the aid of Mesmerism.

Dr. Ashburner, of Grosvenor Street, and lately physician to the Middlesex Hospital, is a most energetic friend to Mesmerism. As was also the lamented Dr. Buxton, of Brownlow Street.

Dr. Storer, of Bristol, has published a valuable little treatise, recommending the practice.

Dr. Simpson, of York, has been one of the earliest friends to the science.

Dr. Arnott, of Edinburgh, is another advocate.

The names of several other medical men can be added. Mr. Symes, of Grosvenor Street. Mr. J. Hands, of Duke Street, Grosvenor Square. Mr. Decimus Hands, of Thayer Street, Manchester Square, a most successful and benevolent promoter of the good cause. Mr. Morgan, of Bedford Row. Mr. Flintoff, of Great Titchfield Street. Mr. Clarke, of Kingsland Road. Mr. Case, of Fareham. Mr. Adams, of Lymington. Mr. Chater, of Norwich. Mr. Weddal, of Scarborough. Mr. Nixon, of Wigton, Cumberland. Mr. J. B. Parker, of Exeter. Mr. Sargent, of Reigate, Surrey, &c. Most of these gentleman have sent papers to the Zoist.

Mr. Johnston, Surgeon, 22 Saville Row, bears honourable testimony to the efficacy of Mesmerism in a remarkable case, recorded in the second volume of the Zoist, p. 42.

Mr. Newnham, Surgeon, of Farnham, the well-known author of "Human Magnetism," has proved himself a valuable and unexpected ally. He was requested to "write a paper against Mesmerism, and furnished with materials" for the purpose: but the very inquiry convinced him of its truth. The result has been as honourable to Mr. Newnham, as it must have been mortifying to his sceptical prompter!—

" For 'tis the sport, to have the engineer
Hoist with his own petard."

Mr. Laxmore, of Alphington, Exeter; and Mr. Hollings of

Leicester, are amongst our most unwearied friends. Mr. Vivian, of Woodfield, Torquay, is another supporter.

The readers of the Zoist must also have noticed the benevolent exertions of Mr. Briggs, of Nottingham Place. (No. 14. p. 226.)

Mr. Mulholland, of Walsall, is a most earnest and successful Mesmerist. He has reduced a wen of eleven years' standing, and of the size of a goose's egg, so completely, that it requires acute observation to detect it.

Mr. Stenson, of Northampton, is another valuable supporter of the cause. He has cured cases of fits, melancholia, &c. &c. He says that he looks forward with well-grounded hope to Mesmerism being more generally applied as a curative means.

Mr. Summers, of Chatham, has acted successfully upon a case of obstinate hernia by Mesmerism.

Dr. Cryer, of Bradford, states a case where a young girl, named Louisa Taylor, who had lost the use of her arm and leg by paralysis, was materially benefited by the Mesmeric treatment of Mr. Prest of that town.

Mr. Brindley, of Stourbridge, has cured various diseases by this power: an affection of the heart, of seven years' standing; a case of general debility of the nervous system; and several cases of fits and rheumatic pains, &c. &c.

Mr. Tubbs, of Upwell Isle, in Cambridgeshire, has proved the reality and efficacy of Mesmerism in the treatment of many diseases. Delirium from grief, muscular pain, chronic rheumatism, and several other cases could be named, where he found the Mesmeric treatment most successful. This earnest friend to the cause of humanity has found Mesmerism most efficacious in several operations,—in the extraction of teeth, &c.:—Mr. Tubbs has had some most interesting patients under his care.*

Mr. Donovan, the able phrenologist, can give very valuable testimony as to the powers and virtues of our science.

In Wolverhampton, Mesmerism is making vast strides in popular estimation. Dr. Owens, of Stourbridge, a medical

* A number of other cases, by Mr. Tubbs, have since appeared in the Zoist. He is a most steady and able practitioner.

gentleman, lately made many converts, by the following operation: "A young woman, suffering dreadfully from toothache, was thrown into the Mesmeric sleep, for the purpose of having the tooth extracted. A sceptical dentist happened to be present and undertook the operation. There was much difficulty in the case. The key slipped from the tooth twice; and a splinter, nearly an inch and a half in length, was broken from the alveolar portion of the jaw. Still there was not the slightest manifestation of pain; and the patient, on being brought to herself, had not the slightest idea that the operation had been performed." The dentist said, that "there was no more movement than there *would have been in a corpse.*" About eighty persons were present.

Mr. Gibbon Wakefield, who is so well known in the political world, and was such a staunch unbeliever in the science, is now "satisfied of its truth, and has since mesmerised many hundred persons."

The names of several clergymen could be given; in fact, they would furnish a long list. Mr. Pyne, incumbent of Hook, Surrey, has published a most useful little book (Vital Magnetism), in which he has communicated the results of his experience. The Rev. John Edwards, of Prestbury, Cheltenham; and the Rev. L. Lewis, of Gateacre, Liverpool, have both sent papers to the Zoist.

Mr. Spencer Hall, the original magnetiser in Miss Martineau's case, and the author of "Mesmeric Experiences," is a most successful practiser of the art, and well entitled to the confidence he has so invariably received. Some of his patients have exhibited very interesting phenomena.

A long catalogue of non-professional advocates yet remains to be mentioned. Among them are Mr. Fradelle, of Percy Street; Mr. Holland, of New Cross; Mrs. Jones, of Salisbury; Mr. Davey, of Devonshire; Mr. Edmund Fry, of Plymouth; Mr. Parsons, Marine Library, Brighton; Mr. Reynoldson, Renshaw Street, Liverpool; Mr. Brown, Low Leyton, Essex; Mr. S. Selfe, Bridgwater; Mr. Hayman, of Sidmouth; Mr. Vernon, the promoter of the Mesmeric Institute; Mr. C. Caillard, of Leicester; Mr. Hicks, the well-known and able

Lecturer; Mr. Saunders, of Ivy Cottage, Bath; Mr. W. Warenne, of Hull; Mr. H. Hudson, of Liverpool; Mr. Alexander Walker, Bainsford, N. B.; Mr. Bailey, &c.

In Scotland Mesmerism has taken a firm root. Its remedial power has been tested over and over again. And Mr. Lang's useful little work on " Mesmerism, with a Report of Cases developed in Scotland," should be read by every person solicitous of the truth.

Dr. Elliotson's eminent success in the practice is too well known to require notice. All, who really seek for valuable information on this head, should consult his Papers in the Zoist. They will there see the cases reported in detail,—and enriched by medical observations of the highest value. Let it be sufficient to state that he has cured cases of insanity,—cases of St. Vitus's dance, of palsy, of loss of voice,—of deafness and dumbness, of epileptic and other fits; cases where every other medical treatment had utterly failed. The increasing circulation of the Zoist has placed these wonderful facts so completely within the reach of the medical student, that this brief allusion to them is no otherwise necessary than to make our list of leading Mesmerisers complete.

Here, then, is a train of witnesses in favour of our science! Here is a succession of evidence from men of ability, of education, of honourable standing in society, from whose report alone, the existence of Mesmerism as a fact in nature might be confidently predicated![*] And this list might have been swelled to any extent! What an amount, moreover, have we here of happiness conferred! What a mass of pain, of sickness, of sorrow, lightened or removed! Here at length are a few pleasing pages in the long sad chapter of human life! Here, at last, is a delightful study for the philanthropist and the Christian! And all these blessings communicated by means of a power that is derided, or dreaded, or disbelieved! We have confined our testimony to what has occurred in this country alone and within the last few years,—but what a pile of narratives could have been added to it, if the limits of a

humble work like this would have allowed it. It might have been added, that on the Continent Mesmerism has been received as a fact (un fait accompli) for years: that in Germany it is studied and practised to a considerable extent[*]; that in Prussia many physicians make use of it under the authority of government; and that in Berlin in particular the greatest success has attended its use;—that in Stockholm degrees are granted in the university by an examination on its laws; that in Russia, the Emperor appointed a commission of medical men to inquire into it, and that this commission pronounced it " a very important agent,"—that the first physician of the emperor, and many others at Petersburgh, speak in favour of its utility; and that at Moscow a systematic course of treatment under the highest auspices has been employed for years. In Denmark, physicians practise it under a royal ordinance, and by a decree of the College of Health. In Holland, some of the first men take it up. In France, the extent to which it is practised is considerable indeed.[†] A commission of the Royal Academy of Medicine there recommended that Mesmerism should be allowed a place within the circle of the medical sciences (comme moyen thérapeutique devrait trouver sa place dans le cadre des connaissances médicales). Some of the first physicians in Paris, affixed their signatures to this report. I might mention the cases related by Foissac in his report[‡]: I might give extracts without number on the subject from different French and German works. I might quote from De Leuze, Puysegur, Wienholt, Treviranus, Brandis of Copenhagen, &c. usque ad nauseam. The great name of Hufeland, of Berlin, is a host in itself.

I have a curious little French work by me, called " La Vérité du Magnétisme prouvée par les Faits," in which the list of cures effected by a lady in Paris is quite marvellous.

---

[*] See Miss Martineau's Preface on this point, p. 6.

[*] The famous Jean Paul Richter practised Mesmerism for the sake of his friends, when they were ill.—See his Life, vol. ii. p. 150.

[†] See " Exposé des Cures operées en France depuis Mesmer jusqu'à nos Jours" 1826), with attestations by more than two hundred medical men.

[‡] Rapports sur les Magnétisme Animal, par M. P. Foissac, Docteur en Médicine.

M 3

In the United States the same mighty progress has been made. Mr. Buckingham, the distinguished traveller, told me, that it is there practised to a very great extent. In his amusing work on that country he mentions several curious Mesmeric cases and phenomena that he witnessed in Philadelphia, at the Asylum for the Deaf and Dumb, tried upon children in the presence of several physicians and legal gentlemen, when it appeared proved beyond suspicion, to the satisfaction of all present, that "there was a complete suspension of the susceptibility of pain during the state" of Mesmerism. Dr. Mitchell, an eminent physician of Philadelphia, mentioned an operation performed by him in the extraction of a tooth under most painful circumstances, when no feeling was experienced,—and no recollection of the fact existed afterwards.* And who and what are the men that have thus advocated Mesmerism? I shall answer in the words of the celebrated French physiologist, Dr. Georget,—who says,—"It is a very astonishing thing that animal magnetism is not even known by name among the ignorant classes: *it is among the enlightened ranks that it finds support.* It is men who have received some education who have taken its cause in hand: it is partly *learned men, naturalists, physicians, philosophers*, who have composed the numerous volumes in its favour."† And what is the reply of our opponents to this pyramid of facts? That they are all cases of delusion? Granted, for the sake of argument, that very many might be so,—that in several instances the ablest men might be deceived: what then? still, even with the largest deduction under this head, what an accumulation of evidence would yet remain! As Mr. Colquhoun observes, "Upon what evidence are we permitted to believe any series of facts? What amount of proof is required?" The host of competent and highly qualified men who have narrated their experience, forbid the supposition of a universal delusion. Some other theory must be adopted. Mesmerism is a science of facts. To facts we appeal: and we do not believe, as has

* Buckingham's "America," vol. ii. p. 119—125.
† Apud "Isis Revelata," vol. ii. p. 45.

been well observed, that "any science rests upon experiments more numerous, more positive, or more easily ascertained." *

To facts, then, it is repeated, do we appeal. What the nature of those facts is, it is superfluous to mention. I presume that most of my readers have a general notion respecting them; that they are aware, how that after certain manipulations a deep sleep comes on;—how that this is followed by the phenomena of attraction, of sympathy, of insensibility, of phrenomagnetism, and other singular manifestations, all varying with various sleepers; and how, that when the patient is awakened, a sanative or soothing effect is generally experienced. To the higher order of phenomena, such as *clairvoyance*, internal vision, and so forth, I have made little allusion. Not that I disbelieve, or have not witnessed something of them. But this work aims strictly at a practical character. I have no wish to astonish or amuse. Those wondrous facts of *clairvoyance*†, which cause the faith of so many to hesitate, have no necessary bearing on the therapeutic qualities of Mesmerism. They might all be false, and yet the healing virtues of the magnetic slumber remain unquestioned. At the same time, it may not be useless to mention, that there is not one single phenomenon of the higher order of Mesmerism, which has not been found to exist in a natural state, and spontaneously, in some recorded cases of extremely-diseased individuals. The annals of natural somnambulism are full of them. Mesmerism simply brings out in the process of cure, and by artificial means, what nature throws forth in the action

* "Il a été établi en France, et dans presque tous les pays du nord, des traitemens magnétiques, où des milliers des malades ont trouvé la santé. La relation détaillée d'un grand nombre de guérisons a été publiée, soit par les particuliers, soit par les sociétés de l'harmonie."— Foissac, Rapports, p. 500.
This was said by Foissac, a medical man himself, more than ten years ago,—in 1833, before the practice of Mesmerism was much known in England. If Foissac could say in 1833 that there were thousands of sick persons who had received benefit from the art, what might he not state now? This, let it be remembered, is the main question; that the number of successful cases proves the power.
† One of the most successful cases of clairvoyance occurred at Plymouth, in the house of Mr. E. Fry, with a patient of Mr. Lendle, the well-known lecturer.—See the report in Zoist, vol. iv. p. 82.

x 3

of disease. Take the staggering fact of reading with the eyes closed, through, what I believe, an electric communication. This has occurred in a natural state.* The report is to be found in the 88th volume of the French Encyclopædia, on the authority of the then Archbishop of Bordeaux. It was the case of a young ecclesiastic, who walked in his sleep, took pen, ink, and paper, and composed and wrote his sermons, and read, with his eyes closed. To test him, the archbishop held a piece of pasteboard before his face to prevent his seeing, — but he appeared to see equally well. Now, we repeat, that this case had no connection with Mesmerism, — that it is quite independent of it, — that it occurred spontaneously and in a natural state, and is established on as high authority as any single fact in science. It was simply the effect of a morbid action on the nervous system of the young man. And so of all the other strange phenomena of Mesmerism; there is not one of them but has its parallel in some instance of common somnambulism: and I know no study that would so well prepare the mind of the student for a due apprehension of this question, as a perusal of the marvellous facts that have been recorded in the histories of many natural sleepwalkers. However, a further allusion to these singular manifestations is foreign to our purpose. My object is wholly utilitarian. And my endeavour has been to prove by a copious body of statistics, that there is a state into which the human frame can be placed, from whence the most powerfully remedial results may be obtained, even in cases of extremest suffering.

* See Appendix for several instances.

CHAP. IV.

ARGUMENTS AGAINST TRUTH OF MESMERISM. — MONOTONY. — HYSTERIA. — IMITATION. — FAITH. — IMAGINATION. — "MESMERISE ME, AND I WILL BELIEVE YOU." — FIRST FRENCH REPORT. — SECOND FRENCH REPORT OF MEDICAL MEN ALONE. — MR. WAKLEY. — LONDON UNIVERSITY. — ROYAL MEDICAL AND CHIRURGICAL SOCIETY. — BRITISH ASSOCIATION AND MR. BRAID. — BRITISH ASSOCIATION AND PHRENOLOGY. — BRITISH ASSOCIATION AND ETHER AND MESMERISM. — GREAT NAMES AMONG BELIEVERS IN MESMERISM.

AND what is the reply of certain medical men, who presume *ex cathedrâ* to give an opinion on the subject without condescending to look into it, — what, we demand, is their reply to the representation of this state? Simply, that it is impossible; the thing, they say, is in itself impossible; — and consequently that no farther investigation is requisite for the student. To say that facts are extraordinary, — are difficult to conceive, — are contrary to previous experience, is but the duty of a philosopher, who should suspend his belief till every reasonable doubt be done away.* But to begin with asserting, that a thing is *impossible*, — and that it is contrary to the laws of nature, because it differs from our early opinions, is irrational in the extreme, and eminently absurd in days like our own, when every year we see things accomplished, which in our youth were deemed impracticable. The real question is, — *what are the laws of nature?* Are they all known and established? But inasmuch as to set limits in this way to the operations of nature, and call a thing which is occurring every hour "impossible,"

* Wienholt in his Lectures says, " Philosophers, when they have once deduced a number of general principles from a certain range of experience, are not easily brought to admit of exceptions from these general laws, when once established to their satisfaction. *They endeavour to reduce all subsequently supervening facts, however anomalous, under subjection to these laws.* They twist them in all directions, until they get them — *nolentes volentes* — accommodated to their theory; and if they do not succeed, they consider this circumstance as a perfectly good ground for throwing them aside; and, accordingly, they are at once struck out of the category of facts."—Colquhoun's *Wienholt*, p. 41.

is not quite satisfactory to the philosophic inquirer, a few ingenious theories are propounded by the faculty to silence the
unreasonable questionings of the "impertinently curious."

One gentleman will tell you, that "Monotony" is the secret.
The constant movement of the hands before the face [*], — a continued friction by passes down the arm, has, they say, such a
dull, deadening effect, that the mere monotony of the action
induces somnolency. All this is granted: many a restless
invalid has been lulled into slumber by some such soothing
process. The tickling of a feather, or the reading of a dull
book in a drowsy tone for a prolonged period, will often per-
suade to sleep. But this explanation will not meet the difficulty.
It applies but to a few isolated instances. And first we ask,
how many times would this experiment answer in the case of a
feverish patient? For days? for weeks? for months? A
daily repetition of the trial would, I fear, soon break the charm.
Not so with Mesmerism. The mesmeric sleep is obtained only
the more easily and more quickly at each renewal of the process.
But with some patients, these monotonous movements, made by
parties unskilled in Mesmerism, not only do not soothe, but
have even an irritating effect; — to whom, however, the mesmeric action, applied in a judicious way, succeeds at once. I
can speak to this point from my own experience. But this is
not all. Many Mesmerisers scarcely use monotonous movements
at all. The mutual contact of the thumbs, the application of
the points of the fingers near the eyes, the pressure of the hand
upon the crown of the head, are the plans that I have seen most
usually adopted, and which I have found most successful myself.
Often and often have I seen patients in a state of cerebral excitement put to sleep in two, in three, in four minutes, by the
contact of the balls of the thumb. A lady has told me that
ofttimes from the moment her thumb touched the thumb of the
Mesmeriser, a leaden weight has settled on her eyelids, making
resistance to sleep impossible, — and this in a case where every
other soporific method had been worse than idle. No: mono-

[*] "To the *waving motion of the hands*, in what are termed the "*passes*," I
attribute all the phenomena which animal magnetism is said to induce in
patients who submit to this mummery." — *Unity of Disease*, by Dr. Dickson,
p. 22.

tony will not explain the difficulty. In fact, so little has monotony to do with the effect, that none but those who have seen
little or nothing of mesmeric action could invent this theory for
its solution.

Driven from this post, our opponents next establish themselves behind the entrenchments of "*Hysteria*." This is the
explanation, that is for ever being advanced in anti-mesmeric
works and lectures at the hospitals; and I think it more especially worthy of answer, as I have heard it made by some
able and enlightened friends. The patient, they say, is "highly
nervous and excitable; it is simply an hysteric action, — nothing
else." Now there is much plausibility in this representation.
Its vagueness catches the ear. The undefined character of the
word "nervousness" includes almost every thing in common
parlance. Merely say that a patient is nervous, and all difficulties are removed. But we must pin our philosophic friends
down to something more specific. These loose generalities carry
no meaning in them. And first we would observe, that it is
not nervous patients who are always the most susceptible to
mesmeric action. The idea is convenient; but the fact is often
the reverse. Stout, strong-minded men have been mesmerised;
and I have seen patients who were termed "highly nervous"
resist the influence altogether.[*] But let us analyse this explanation more closely. *What is Hysteria?* Is it hysteria,
when a pin is forced into a delicate female's hand, far enough
to draw blood, and she feels no pain, and exhibits no change of
expression? Is it hysteria, when a brute strikes a sleeping
boy a violent blow with a walking-stick, and no movement or
consciousness results from it? Is it hysteria, where excitement and strong cerebral irritation are soothed and calmed
down into tranquillity and repose? Is it hysteria, when intolerable heat and throbbing in the head are carried off and leave
not a vestige? Is it hysteria, when racking, torturing pain is
relieved or completely taken away? And all these effects not
happening once and accidentally, but over and over, and over

[*] Teste says, "I would almost venture to say there might exist an obtuse-
ness to commonsensation in excessive sensibility." (p. 41.) My experience quite confirms
this view, in opposition to what is vulgarly entertained.

again? According to common experience, these effects would rather result from hysteric action than be removed by it; and certainly it is a novel doctrine, when we are taught, that an abatement in feverish or cerebral irritability is the product of hysteria. However,—it is now said, that all these states are the effect of hysteria. Hysteria includes every thing. Whatever may be the condition of the human body,—be it unusual repose or unusual excitement,—be it exquisite sensibility to pain, or an utter unconsciousness of its presence, hysteria is the cause. Be it so. And how much nearer are we now towards resolving the difficulty? For again I ask, *what is hysteria?* Do the medical men know themselves? Can they explain it? Can they say what are its causes, proximate or remote? Are they not confessedly in the dark on the subject? To explain Mesmerism, therefore, by hysteria, is but to exchange one difficulty for another. It is but a shifting of position, not an approximation towards the truth. It is a moving of the feet, not a marching forwards. With far greater judgment did one of the most superior and rising members of the profession observe to me, that "Mesmerism, if true, rather threw a light on hysteria, than hysteria on Mesmerism." It would rather lead them, he said, to a solution of their very difficulties on that question. But be this as it may, to explain one difficulty by another is a most unphilosophical proceeding,—and one through which no approach whatever is made to an illustration of the truth. But on the other hand, if Mesmeric action be nothing but hysteria[*], —as perhaps it is,—then we assert, that hysteria, when produced artificially and intentionally, ceases to be a disease,—but becomes a condition full of medicinal and healing virtue; as the inexhaustible catalogue of cures accomplished by its power incontrovertibly proves.

"IMITATION"[†] is a favourite explanation with others;—and certainly imitation is a key which interprets many facts

[*] See a cure of Hysteria, by Mr. Spencer Hall, and some very judicious observations.—" Mesmeric Experiences," p. 35.

[†] Imitation is one of the explanations given in the *Dictionnaire des Sciences de Médicine*, t. vi., p. 594.; and also by M. Virey in his article on Animal Magnetism.

in the science. Imitation is one of the most powerful agents for working on the human mind;—much that is good or wicked in human conduct is the result of imitation alone;—and it may be a curious study for the physiologist to trace the secret springs of imitation to their native source. But though imitation may explain many parts in the conduct of a Mesmeric patient,—it goes but a small way. How can we explain this fact, that young and artless girls, — the deaf, — the dumb, — the blind, — patients who had never heard of Mesmerism[*], — who knew not what process was going to take place, have all equally exhibited the same class of phenomena? Imitation is often used, too, for a synonym of *Imposture.* But when employed in this sense, it assumes that the capabilities of the human mind are great indeed, and that the histrionic talent is far more common than is suspected. The lovers of the drama complain that the days of tragic and comic excellence are departed, and that not an actor remains to tread the stage. Unfounded regret! If the charges of our opponents be correct, and imitation (or imposture) be the clue to Mesmerism, then indeed actors and actresses of the highest talent abound in every district, — artists, before whom the genius of a Garrick would grow pale, are making the circuit of the country in every direction, — and the art of Roscius is now at its zenith. I have seen ignorant, uneducated, simple persons transformed by the touch of the Mesmeriser into the most finished performers. Yes, — if imitation (or imposture) be the solution, then is a greater wonder established than the supposed discoveries of Mesmer, —and the histrionic powers of the human mind proved to be something beyond the range of old experience. Either way, "the laws of nature" must be remodelled;—old systems are not sufficient; for mentally or physically, a new and wondrous power has been detected, which henceforward must find a place amidst the schemes and divisions of the philosopher and metaphysician.[†]

[*] See Spencer Hall, p. 6.

[†] See Wienholt, i. ii. p. 57., on the fact of the somnambulist, "conducting himself as perfectly in his first sleep as in his tenth." Practice does not make more perfect.

FAITH *or confidence in the power*, and a *desire to be healed* by the process of Mesmerism, are again suggested by others as a cause to which we may ascribe some of the cures of which we have spoken. On this theory, how are we to explain those instances, where the patient had a positive aversion to the practice; where, so far from the existence of faith, disgust and disbelief were the strong predominant feelings;—and where the remedy was adopted almost by compulsion, and yet the cure and the benefits have been most marked and unequivocal? Here I can again come forward with my testimony.[*]

Again, therefore, is a fresh interpretation needed, and all is resolved by another party into the large, the comprehensive phrase of "Imagination." Truly has it been observed, that this reference of all these difficulties to the influence of imagination is but "a cloak to cover ignorance." That imagination has a most powerful effect on the habit of the body, we all know. Numerous striking events can be clearly traced to it. Several wonderful cures have been produced by it. It is a valuable, a useful auxiliary. None but an idiot would deny its power. Still, imagination, with all its vehement effects, has a limit. There is a time when its influence wears off. An invalid often "imagines" that a new medical adviser has been of service,—that a change of medicine has done good,—that a different treatment has been beneficial; and repeatedly has a healthier action been brought about by this power of the mind upon the nervous system. But much too generally the spell is dissolved at an early day. Before the tedious week shall have run its round, a relapse has occurred, and the benefit is forgotten. Not so, again we say, with Mesmerism. The longer it is tried, the more powerful is the hold. A patient may be sent to sleep by imagination two or three days in succession; but would the same method succeed day after day for several months? Here is a point on which I can speak with confidence.

---

[*] So far from "Faith" being an active cause, it sometimes has worked prejudicially by over-exciting the patient through the expectation of benefit. "From my excessive nervousness, and being *full of faith*, I expected soon to find myself spell-bound, and subject to its sleepy influence," writes a patient in Zoist, No. 19, p. 317. But days and weeks passed over without an apparent effect. "It seemed to banish sleep," he says.

The process, which was comparatively feeble in its effect upon a patient in my family during the first week is now, at nearly the expiration of a year, more efficacious than ever. Look again to its influence on pain. We hear at times of pain disappearing suddenly through some operation of the mind. An individual, suffering from a raging toothache, has been known to walk to a dentist's door, when the simple ringing of the bell has so wrought on his system as to stop the pain and change the condition of his body. But who believes that this power of the mind would be continuous? Who supposes that the daily experiment of a walk to the operator's house would suspend the agony, if the pain recurred every morning? The unlucky tooth would in the end require extraction. Not so with Mesmerism. Pain is removed only the more speedily by a repetition of the manipulations. The oftener they are tried, the quicker are their effects. This notion of "imagination" will not therefore get rid of the difficulty. It is a convenient mode of explanation, and a courteous; when, in reality, the insolent charge of fraud is really meant, and is the only alternative. Either certain facts are true, or they are false; for the mind has nothing to do with them.[*] Is it imagination, when the hand of the sleeper follows the hand of the mesmeriser? Is it imagination, when the touch of any one but the mesmeriser throws the sleeper into extreme and convulsive agitation? Is it imagination, when the sleeper hears no other voice but that of the mesmeriser? Is it imagination, when what the mesmeriser tastes is recognised by the sleeper, be it bitter or sweet, or water or wine? These questions might be multiplied indefinitely; but here are sufficient: and what is the answer? We reply, that there is a physical impossibility that the mind, according to what we understand by that term, should have any thing to do with such effects. The *sleeper is fast asleep, and knows nothing of them.* Either they are the result of some newly discovered power on the nervous system, or patients, as honourable and virtuous as the opponents themselves, are as-

---

[*] See two Mesmeric cases of my own, recorded in 2d cap. p. 154. 155, where the theories of "mesmery," and of "imagination," are at once upset by the facts.

suming an appearance for which they have no earthly induce-
ment. "Imagination," in the usual acceptation of the word,
can afford no explanation to these phenomena in any way
whatever.

A few other facts may be stated on this point. Children
are often easily magnetised. Foissac mentions the case of a
child, aged twenty-eight months, that he placed in somnambulism. Deaf and dumb persons, and some that were blind[*],
have been thrown into this sleep, without being aware at the
time of what was intended or what was going on. Animals
have been powerfully affected. Dr. Wilson's experiments on
the brute creation are most conclusive.[†] Several sceptics, and
those men of powerful intellect, have been mesmerised. Mr.
Townshend, in his "Facts," gives some remarkable instances
of what took place at Cambridge with some unbelieving adversaries.[‡] Professor Agassiz, of Neufchâtel, in Switzerland,
was put to sleep by Mr. Townshend, according to his own
statement, after he had done every thing in his power to resist
the influence. But there is one point more decisive than any
which we have just mentioned,—and which, as Colquhoun
states, is well known to all practical mesmerisers,—viz. "that
if we attempt to manipulate in contrary directions, the usual
effects will not be produced, whilst others of a totally different
nature will be manifested."[§] In short, of all the explanations
that have been offered, the least tenable is that of "imagination."
Still, what is in a name? If the phrase be more acceptable
than that of Mesmerism, let it be adopted. All we ask and
want is, that the system itself be not neglected. "If imagination," says Mr. Chenevix, "can cure diseases, then cure by

---

[*] See the very interesting case of Captain Peach, "a gentleman perfectly
blind for eleven years," recorded in 5th volume of Zoist.

[†] See "Wilson's *Trials of Animal Magnetism on the Brute Creation*." (Baillière.) Dr. Wilson is physician to the Middlesex Hospital.

[‡] See Townshend's "Facts," book ii. sec. 2., for these interesting cases.

[§] Teste, p. 156. mentions the bad effects of magnetising upwards. Gauthier, p. 12. of his "Traité Pratique," gives a strong caution against it, and
quotes D'Eslon, who says, "la tête du malade s'embarrasserait, et on pour-
rait lui donner une commotion funeste au cerveau ; peut-être une apoplexie."
But if it be nothing but imagination, how could there be a disturbing
effect by ascending passes?

---

imagination, and the sick will bless you."[*] We have no wish
to supersede the labours of the faculty in their important department: what is rather desired is, that the treatment of the
mesmeric process should be under their direction and control,
—as is the case in many countries on the Continent. In
Russia, in Denmark, in Prussia, none but medical men, or those
under their superintendence, are permitted to exercise the art.
Let, then, the profession take the practice up, and we will
sacrifice the name. Let "Imagination" be placed on the pharmacopœia; let "Imagination" be written on their prescriptions;
let the students at the hospitals be instructed how to exert
the ideal faculty: only, as Dugald Stewart so sensibly observes,
let them not "scruple to copy whatever processes are necessary
for subjecting diseases to their command." Let them not culpa-
bly refuse to increase the resources of their art; and I, for one,
would gladly consent that the management of this mighty
agent should be left mainly in their hands, and that the name
of Mesmerism should be discarded and forgotten![†]

But our concessions and explanations fall unheeded on the
ear. The grand *coup de théâtre* yet remains; "Mesmerise
me, and I will believe you." Often have I heard the most
conclusive answers presented to these objectors; every misconception has been disposed of by argument, by facts, by
analogy, when the unbeliever suddenly escapes from the controversy by a demand that the experiment be tried upon himself. And if, as is almost certain, the experiment fail, the
question he considers as finally settled. I was attending a mes-

---

[*] Mesmer said from the beginning, that medical men were alone com-
petent to superintend the treatment. (See Gauthier, Traité, p. 697. See
Elliotson, Zoist, vol. iv. p. 377.) We have entered on this point in the
Introductory Chapter.

[†] Let us note what M. Bertrand, a physician himself, says :—"Il est de
toute évidence que si les savans et les médecins veulent guider et faire tourner
au profit de l'humanité et des sciences la nouvelle découverte qu'on leur
annonce, il faut qu'ils commencent par s'en emparer. A quel titre voudront-
ils la juger, s'ils sont convaincus de ne pas la connaître ? Et n'est-ce pas
une chose honteuse pour ceux qui s'occupent de l'art de guérir, de voir les
supérieurs le plus ignorans se montrer plus instruits qu'eux sur un grand
nombre de phénomènes qui appartient à la connaissance de l'homme malade?"
—BERTRAND, Traité du Somnambulisme, p. 431.

meric lecture one day, when a gentleman present sat down on the chair, and requested the lecturer to try his skill upon him. The usual manipulations went on for a certain period; much interest was felt by the spectators; when after a given time our unsusceptible gentleman rose up,—looked round the room with a triumphant smirk of self-satisfaction, declaring that he "felt nothing," and then left the company with the air of a philosopher who had refuted the claims of Mesmerism once and for ever!* and this is called experiment! as if certain *conditions* were not indispensable. What *all* those conditions are, we are not prepared to show; but common sense might teach us, that *some* conditions were at least required. In chemical experiments on impassive material substances certain conditions are demanded; how much more so, on the delicate human frame, where the mind can in addition offer a resistance, and the party himself strain his utmost to reject the sleep? Those who have been present at lectures on Galvanism or Chemistry must have observed how slight a cause will disturb the simplest experiment. A change of atmosphere will affect the machinery and spoil the electric action in a moment. If a conductor be *overcharged*, a result different from the one expected will be evolved. If a body be *saturated* with any ingredient that it holds in solution, the effect will not be the same, as when the substances are united in more congenial proportions. In some experiments, the *presence* of a small quantity of water appears always necessary to develop certain acid properties. And thus we might go on *ad infinitum.* And why are not similar laws equally applicable in the practice of Mesmerism? And why is it that the parties, who, more than any others, know the necessity of such conditions in regard to natural philosophy, are the very men who dispense with their presence in the analogous experiments on the human frame. My own opinion on the subject, after much observation, is, that sick and delicate persons are more susceptible of the

* Dr. Esdaile says truly, "a person in health resisting the influence is no proof that he will remain insusceptible to it in an altered state of the body, when there may be a craving from the nervous system for this sustenance from without."—*Mesmerism in India,* p. 13.

magnetic influence than those in robust health. Not but what cases can be produced, where the healthiest individuals have been readily mesmerised, and the delicate invalid remained unaffected: but these are the exceptions rather than the rule.* Where there is any unequal action,—any irregularity in the system, any improper or feeble circulation,—any extreme or overwrought activity of the cerebral or nervous temperament, there the Mesmeric influence seems to produce an effect. Its tendency appears to be to *restore the equilibrium of a disturbed or irregular distribution* of the nervous power.† Such an irregularity may exist, unknown and unsuspected, in the system of a robust man, and explain his readier susceptibility to the equalising power; while a more delicate patient, from the absence of some other condition, which is equally necessary, may resist the influence altogether, although the general state of his organisation and temperament might, but for this one and unknown circumstance, have rendered him peculiarly alive to the magnetic force. However, all this is but conjecture—and touches not the truthfulness of the facts recorded.—It ought, moreover, to be added, that sleep is not the only or a necessary symptom. Great effects may result,—and no sleep take place.

* If mesmeric influence be, as I believe, a means of communicating energy, or of equalising the circulation in an impaired system, one must expect, *primâ facie*, that a person in health could not be affected. It seems, therefore, absurd to make the attempt. Yet occasionally it succeeds. Mr. Townshend has mesmerised eight young men in robust health. Mr. Atkinson has mesmerised several. Mr. Kiste has done the same. I saw a lady put a gentleman in the full vigour of manhood into a deep sleep in less than ten minutes. Captain James "found a stout recruit in his late regiment more susceptible than any female that he had ever seen." *I never make the trial myself, believing it to be a foolish and improper waste of time and strength.* Reichenbach, speaking of his experiments with crystals, says that the "sensitiveness of healthy subjects is so limited as not to be sufficient for the investigation." p. 20.

† Mr. Newnham says, "It may be remarked as a general rule, that the constitution with the highest order of intelligence and in the best health, is the least susceptible of magnetic influence,—while the feebler nervous systems, and those in inferior health, are the most susceptible; and that is perfectly consistent with our supposition, that magnetism is the *medicine of nature,* and consists in imparting the exuberant life of the healthy to relieve the feeble life of the disordered:—while the strong and healthy, not requiring the agency of such medicine, are not susceptible to its impression."—*Human Magnetism,* p. 62.

Sleep is only one out of many symptoms, though of course the most general and intelligible. Among the other conditions, a physical sympathy between the parties seems the first requisite; what that sympathy may be is a difficult question; but it is a known fact, that a patient yields to the influence of one Mesmeriser rather than another.[*] A superior state of health, or of muscular energy, or of mental power, on the part of the Mesmeriser over the patient, seems another condition;—and yet this is by no means invariable or without exceptions. Again, it should be borne in mind, that an apparent external effect is not always to be expected at the first sitting. Sleep may not be produced for a week, for a month,—for three months; but it may come at last, and a cure be effected. In the case of individuals in good health it is especially less probable that somnolency should come on at the first trial; and in fact, few things are more ridiculous or misplaced than the exhibition of a vigorous muscular man offering himself to the manipulations of the Mesmeriser. Would the loss of the same quantity of blood,—or the administration of the same amount of medicine,—have the same or equal effect on two opposite constitutions or habits of body? The abstraction of ten ounces

---

[*] The best practical writer on this subject is Deleuze: his experience has been great. I refer my readers to what he says on this point — as to a safe authority : — " Tous les hommes ne sont pas sensibles à l'action magnétique, et les mêmes le sont plus ou moins, selon les dispositions momentanées dans lesquelles il se trouvent. Ordinairement le magnétisme n'exerce aucune action sur les personnes qui jouissent d'une santé parfaite. Le même homme qui était insensible au magnétisme dans l'état de santé, en éprouvera des effets lorsqu'il sera malade. Il est telle maladie dans laquelle l'action du magnétisme ne se fait point apercevoir ; telle autre sur laquelle cette action est évidente. On n'en sait pas encore assez pour déterminer la cause de ces anomalies, ni pour prononcer à l'avance si le magnétisme agira ou n'agira pas ; on a seulement quelques probabilités à cet égard ; mais cela ne saurait motiver une objection contre la réalité du magnétisme, attendu que les trois quarts des malades en moins en ressentent les effets.

" La nature a établi un rapport ou une sympathie physique entre quelques individus ; c'est par cette raison que plusieurs magnétiseurs agissent beaucoup plus promptement et plus efficacement sur certains malades que sur d'autres, et que le même magnétiseur ne convient pas également à tous les malades. Il y a même des magnétiseurs qui sont plus propres à guérir certaines maladies. Plusieurs personnes se croient insensibles à l'action du magnétisme, parce qu'elles n'ont pas rencontré le magnétiseur qui leur convient."—DELEUZE, *Instruction Pratique*, cap. i. sect. 21, 22.

---

of blood might hardly be felt by a strong athletic yeoman, while the depletion would be far too reducing for his feeble attenuated daughter. One man has been known to swallow with impunity more than twenty of Morison's drastic pills; while two of the same precious preparation have induced a distressing and painful result upon his apparently healthier and more enduring brother. And why is there this difference? simply,—*because men's constitutions are different*. And is Mesmerism to be an exception to this general rule? Be the party mesmerised delicate or robust, the same Mesmeriser only throws off a certain amount of Mesmeric influence (whether through the medium of some electric fluid we know not),—and why therefore should the same effect be expected in those opposite conditions within the same period of time? However, upon this point we are as yet in the dark. The above observations are rather meant as suggestions for consideration, than the exposition of actual knowledge. And though the question is not one quarter exhausted, enough has been said to show the unreasonableness and absurdity of those who demand an immediate effect on themselves as a test of this power.[*] What I always reply to medical men, who request to be placed under the process,—is,—" Do not ask to be mesmerised yourself; go and mesmerise your patients,—and depend upon it, that you will not only accomplish much benefit, but you will soon have a proof of the truth of my words." But far better would it be to quote the language of Bacon in his Essay on Seeming Wise. " It is a ridiculous thing," says he, "and fit for a satire of judgment, to see what shifts men have. . . . . . Some think to bear it by speaking a great word, and being peremptory, and go on and take by admittance that which they cannot make good. Some, whatever is *beyond their reach will seem to despise*, or make light of it, as impertinent or curious, and so would have their *ignorance seem judgment*."

Here, then, is the position on which I take my stand, and to which I respectfully invite the consideration of the scientific

---

[*] Teste thinks that " all men may become by turns, and according to the physical or moral conditions in which they may be placed, magnetisers and magnetised."—Cap. iii. p. 56.

world,—that be the exciting or immediate cause, imitation, monotony, hysteria, imagination, or so forth, this accumulation of evidence, out of Germany, out of France, out of England, and many other countries, proves beyond a doubt, that a strong curative effect in a certain class of diseases can be produced by what is called Mesmerism,—so strong, indeed, that the physician and the philanthropist are alike bound, for the sake of humanity alone, to give the subject the fullest and fairest trial.

But, says the "Christian Observer," all farther investigation is needless,—for the French commissioners have long ago decided the question. "Their report," it adds, "was full, candid, elaborate, and satisfactory." And the "commissioners proved that no magnetic influence was evolved,"—and that "Mesmer stood convicted of being a conscious impostor."

Often as this statement has been rebutted, it is still necessary to go over the ground again. For not only must such a representation have its effect, but there is, moreover, a general impression afloat, that the decision of the French *savans* has been adverse to our system.

The Reviewer says,—"We are not aware whether the report of the commissioners has been reprinted, since the revival of these follies."[*] And from the manner in which he treats the question, it may be doubted, whether he has read the report himself, and has not taken his opinion, second-hand, from some careless or prejudiced writers. At any rate, I have read the report, or rather reports. Before I ventured to express an opinion, I went to the British Museum, and read them carefully and analytically through. And the attention of my readers is requested, not only to the real representation as to how far the reports go,—but also to the important resolutions of a second and far more valuable Commission.

It may, perhaps, be desirable that this statement be preceded by a slight sketch of Mesmer and of the proceedings of his opponents.

Animal magnetism, it is generally supposed, has been always

[*] The report is reprinted in Bertrand's "Magnétisme Animal."

more or less practised by a select class, who, through some means or other, had arrived at the discovery. Many names could be mentioned under this head. But be this as it may, it was about 1776, that Anthony Mesmer, a native of Switzerland, and a physician and resident of Vienna, who had been for some time making use of the common magnet in his medical practice[*], perceived that he was able to produce a variety of phenomena of a very peculiar character without the magnet at all, and by the influence of some power proceeding from his own body. Repeated experiments confirmed him in this opinion: he applied this new treatment extensively among the sick; great success attended him; and his name became notorious. He now removed to Paris, as to a wider theatre for his labours. After a time considerable progress was made by him there in the dissemination of his views; patients of all ranks flocked to his house; he began to accumulate a large fortune; and the French government even offered a very handsome pecuniary remuneration for the communication of his secret.

Not satisfied with his success, Mesmer must needs put forth a 'theory.[†] He contended that there was a *subtle fluid* pervading the whole universe, which was capable of being put into motion, and through which the most powerful effects could be obtained. He went at great length into an examination of this theory, on which it is now needless to dwell. But it is important to add that this theory was an essential part of his system,—that he pressed it strongly upon the attention of the learned;—and that this assumed subtle matter he designated by the name of the *magnetic fluid*, and his treatment of his patients he called *animal magnetism*.

But this was not all. His enemies say that Mesmer was not

[*] Reichenbach's Researches go far to prove the use of the magnet, and, as Professor Gregory observes, to "restore to the statements of the early magnetisers the credit of which they had been unjustly deprived."—Preface.
[†] Colquhoun, in his introduction to Wienholt, says, "Whether the theories, by means of which Mesmer and others attempted to explain the fact, be accounted satisfactory or not, is a matter altogether of inferior importance; the fact itself remains, and stands quite independent of our theory," p. 13. I have already quoted Dr. Jenner and Bishop Thirlwall in justification of those who prematurely put forth their theories.

a really philosophic inquirer. Truth, for its own sake, and for the good of his species, was not his single aim. According to their statement, he invested his practice with a dramatic and unreal character;—he assumed a mysterious demeanour,—clothed his experiments with a magical obscurity,—assumed a masquerading costume, and was as much of the *charlatan* as of the scientific discoverer. All this, however, is as strongly denied by his partisans and followers.[*]

These proceedings, however, attracted the attention of the wits at Paris. His medical brethren were in an uproar; the public journals attacked him; the philosophers were disgusted; and few besides the sick were on his side. Yet Mesmer grew bolder and bolder: he asserted that "there is but *one health, one disease,* and *one remedy;*" and this remedy, he said, was alone to be obtained through his *magnetic subtle fluid.*

Government at length took the subject up. The amiable and unfortunate Louis the Sixteenth issued a mandate in 1784, requiring a commission to investigate the matter. The commissioners appointed were some of them members of the Academy of Sciences, some of the medical faculty, and others of the Society of Physicians, and contained in their number a few remarkable names. Among them were Lavoisier, who might almost be called the father of modern chemistry; Bailly, whose subsequent fate in the French Revolution was so memorable and melancholy; Guillotin, who in the same revolution obtained such an unfortunate distinction from his recommendation of that slaughterous engine which was called after his name; Jussieu, the illustrious botanist; and, lastly, that great statesman-philosopher of the other hemisphere, to whom has been so happily applied the line of the poet,—

"*Eripuit cœlo fulmen, sceptrumque tyrannis.*"

[*] The cautious and conscientious Deleuze said of Mesmer, "that it is impossible not to recognise in him a distinguished metaphysician and a *profound observer.*" (Histoire Critique, tom. ii. p. 90.) Bruno spoke of him as "a genius entitled to the gratitude of the human race, as one to whose memory every honest and virtuous man owed a tribute of veneration and respect." (Discours Préliminaire, p. 9.) Those who wish to see a candid statement respecting the character and conduct of Mesmer may turn to the Abbé J. B. L., chapters 6. and 7. See also the *Isis Revelata.*

Of course, to men like these, to say nothing of the other able names that were included in the commission, the profoundest deference is due. Though authority cannot overthrow facts, yet still authority is to be heard with grave attention in a report on those facts;—and here the question is, how far these commissioners have decided, or *intended to decide,* against the facts of Mesmerism,—and how far their opinion goes in subverting the reality of the cures effected by its power.

The answer is, that they decided nothing on the subject: the facts they have left untouched; the cures in great measure undenied; their main drift and aim was *against the theory.*

It has been said,—in opposition to one of the statements of the "Christian Observer" in regard to the "candid" manner of their inquiries,—that the commissioners behaved most unfairly,—that their examination was incomplete and superficial,—and that they took but small trouble to observe. All this I cannot bring myself to believe; their names are a guarantee against any such imputations. Men like Bailly and his colleagues *must* have intended all that was fair and candid. But that their examination was "full or satisfactory," I deny. That they entered upon the subject with strongly-formed prejudices is well known. Their experiments were not continuous enough,—were not followed up closely by the same parties, and were not conducted in compliance with the rules required for their success; and with Lavoisier, the great chemical philosopher at their head, their object was to detect the presence of Mesmer's subtle fluid, and failing in that, they considered the real labours of the commission virtually at an end.

The idea of "utility" was not lost upon them; and one might have thought that such a view of the question would have interested Franklin, and secured a careful investigation. "Le Magnétisme Animal," says the Report, "peut bien exister sans être utile, mais il ne peut être utile, s'il n'existe pas." But the fact is, Franklin was not in good health at the time; and from the language of the Report, it would appear almost certain that he was not present at Paris during any of the experiments. The commissioners all went one day to his house

at Passy; there a few experiments were made; there he himself was magnetised, and *felt no sensation*; and this imperfect examination and personal trial seems to have satisfied him. He signed the report; and his name therefore is always quoted as an authority on the subject [*]; but the world must judge how far the opinion of a man, whose energies and bodily activity were at that time in abeyance, can legitimately be claimed as decisive, especially after so brief and unsatisfactory an inquiry.

But the other commissioners, though, doubtless, all in good faith, omitted, in their experiments, many conditions, which they were told were indispensable. They were not steady in their attendance; and the experiments, moreover, were not conducted in the presence or under the superintendence of Mesmer himself, — but of one of his pupils (D'Eslon), who afterwards protested against their reports [†] (for there was more than one) as incorrect and unsatisfactory.

And what did these reports at length declare? Did they deny the facts? Rather they established their reality. They speak of "a great power influencing the sick."[‡] They say that, having ascertained that an animal fluid cannot be perceived by any of our senses (*les commissaires ayant reconnu que ce fluide magnétique animal ne peut être aperçu par aucun de nos sens*), they come to the conclusion that nothing proves the existence of this magnetic animal fluid;—that, therefore, not being in

existence, it cannot be useful;—(*que rien ne prouve l'existence du fluide magnétique animal; que ce fluide, sans existence, est par conséquent sans utilité, &c.*); and, consequently, they decided that some other theory must be brought forward to account for the facts (*les effets*).

The existence of many of these facts they acknowledge; they describe some of the most important phenomena; they mention many singular convulsions, involuntary movements, and *sympathies* (*rien n'est plus étonnant que le spectacle de ces convulsions ... des sympathies qui s'établissent.*—Rapport de Bailly): but Mesmer's theory they consider null and void;—and declare that the reality of the fluid could only be proved by its *curative effects*; as if these curative effects were not, after all, the most essential point towards which the commissioners could look (*son existence ne peut être démontrée que par les effets curatifs dans le traitement des maladies*).

And what is the theory they offer in opposition? "Imagination," "Imitation," and "Touch;"—these they asserted were the causes of all that occurred. (*De ces expériences, les commissaires ont conclu que l'imagination fait tout, que le magnétisme est nul. Imagination, imitation, attouchement, telles sont les vraies causes des effets attribués au Magnétisme Animal*).

It is unnecessary to enter upon a refutation of their hypothesis;—all the commissioners attempted was to pull down one theory, and build up another;—and this their Report, inconclusive, unsatisfactory,—and, if we may so speak of such men, unphilosophical in the extreme,—is declared by the "Christian Observer," and other writers, to be decisive of the question, and as having convicted Mesmer of being a conscious impostor.

We next come to the Report of their colleagues, the medical commissioners, who equally attack the existence of a fluid, and the theory of Mesmer, but scarcely utter an opinion as to the unreality of the facts alleged; and they sum up the result of their labours with two resolutions.

"There exists no evidence," they say, "of the existence of an agent or fluid, that is supposed to be the principle of

---

[*] I met lately at Paris in the *Bibliothèque Royale* a characteristic *billet* from Dr. Franklin to Madame Helvetius, which is here copied for the amusement of the reader. "M. Franklin n'oublie jamais aucune partie où Me Helvetius doit être. Il croit même, que s'il était engagé d'aller à Paradis ce matin, il ferait supplication d'être permis de rester sur terre jusqu'à une heure et demi, pour recevoir l'embrassade qu'elle a bienvoulu lui promettre en le rencontrant chez M. Turgot."

[†] There were four reports altogether. The first, signed by Bailly, Lavoisier, Franklin, &c. 2. The medical one, signed by Poissonnier, Caille, Mauduyt, and Andry. 3. Jussieu's, who had belonged to the medical section, but did not sign with them. 4. The Secret Report, signed by all together (excepting Jussieu), relating to "danger as to morals,"—not denying facts, but doubting the utility as to medical treatment. The three first are in the British Museum; all four, however, are to be found reprinted in Bertrand's "Magnétisme Animal," which is now becoming a scarce book.

[‡] "On ne peut s'empêcher de reconnaître, à ces effets constans, une grande puissance qui agite les malades, les maîtrise," &c. p. 7.

Animal Magnetism (p. 23);" this is their [first and grand conclusion:—" the theory is altogether wanting in proof."

Their second resolution relates to the utility of the discovery, as a curative means, which they pronounce to be valueless, except in certain very peculiar cases.[*]

The process, however, by which they arrived at these conclusions, is so amusing in itself,—so naïvely told,—and so indicative of the feeling with which they entered on the inquiry, that it ought not to be forgotten. " We have not thought it necessary," they say, " to fix our attention on rare, unusual, or extraordinary cases which appear to contradict the laws of nature!"[†] Can anything equal the absurdity of this conduct unless it be the sweet simplicity of the confession? As if the whole subject had not been "extraordinary!" They were actually appointed commissioners, because it was "extraordinary," and yet they decline to investigate its most "extraordinary" part! Verily, these commissioners would have been fitting associates of the Medico-Chirurgical Society on that memorable night when the latter refused to examine into the amputation of Wombell's leg, from the absurd pretensions of the man to an "extraordinary" insensibility to pain.

As to all that the Medical Commissioners next remark about the dangers of magnetism (pp. 36—40); about its action on the brain, and its being the source of great evils of a physical and moral nature (p. 46); the whole may be dismissed without consideration. Their original bias peeps out in every paragraph.

If a body of turnpike-trustees had been converted into railway commissioners, and required to send in a report on the practicability of the new system of transport, we should naturally have expected resolutions as to the dangers and injustice of the proposed novelty: but even these gentlemen would scarcely have declined to witness an experimental ex-

cursion of a few miles, on the grounds of the "unusual and extraordinary" nature of the conveyance!

The case is precisely in point.

Be this, however, as it may, the reader should know, that the Medical Report, like the one from Bailly and Franklin, did not conclude the question as to the unrealities of magnetism,—but confined itself to objections against the theories of Mesmer, and the assumed utilities of his system; and it is to be hoped, that, after this full exposition of their proceedings, we shall hear no more of the decisive report of the French Commissioners.

But, inconclusive even as this Report was, there is yet a more noticeable shortcoming. One great name is wanting to the signatures. The virtuous and intelligent Jussieu,—he who in the study of botany is an authority of the first rank,—paid the closest attention to the proceedings; and, "notwithstanding the pressing solicitation of his colleagues, and the menaces of the minister, the Baron de Breteuil," refused to subscribe his name, and actually drew up a special Report of his own. In that Report he states that the "experiments he has himself made, and those of which he has been ° witness, convince him that man produces upon man a decided action by friction (frottement), by contact, and, more rarely, by an approximation at a little distance;—that this action seems to belong to some animal warmth existing in the body;—and that judged by its effects, it occasionally partakes of a tonic and salutary result;—but that a more extended acquaintance with this 'agent' will make us better understand its real action and utility."[*]

---

[*] " Nous pensons en conséquence, 1er, que la théorie est un système absolument dénué de preuves; 2de, que ce prétendu moyen de guérir réduit, &c. &c.—est au moins inutile pour ceux dans lesquels il ne s'ensuit," &c.

[†] "Sur des cas rares, insolites, extraordinaires, qui paraissent contredire toutes les lois de la physique."—p. 25.

---

[*] " Que les expériences qu'il a faites, et dont il a été témoin, prouvent que l'homme produit sur son semblable une action sensible par le frottement, par le contact, et plus rarement par un simple rapprochement à quelque distance; que cette action, attribuée à une fluide universelle non démontrée, lui semble appartenir à la chaleur animale existante dans les corps; que cette chaleur émane d'eux continuellement, se porte assez loin, et peut passer d'un corps dans un autre; qu'elle est développée, augmentée, ou diminuée dans un corps par des causes morales et par des causes physiques; que, jugée par des effets, elle participe de la propriété des remèdes toniques, et produit comme eux des effets salutaires ou nuisibles, selon la quantité de chaleur communiquée, et selon les circonstances où elle est employée; qu'enfin un

Jussieu further says, "I have frequented the apartments of M. Deslon;—to avoid mistakes, I have been anxious to see much and operate often myself;—and I have given considerable time to the experiments." (p. 10.)

Having thus examined very many cases himself, he divides his facts into *four* orders; and admits that a large proportion of them may be explained away by "Imagination," &c., without the assistance of any external agent.

At last he comes to his *fourth* section, and here he asserts, that he has a different class of occurrences now to record.

"These facts," he says, "are small in number, and with little variety,—*because I was anxious only to enumerate those that were well established, and on which I had not the smallest doubt.* They are, however, sufficient to make us admit the possibility or existence of a fluid or *agent*, which is communicated from one man to another,—and sometimes exercises on the latter a sensible action." (p. 87.)

A large part of Jussieu's Report is full of "Reflections" (as he calls them), and attempted explanations and reasons of his "Facts." Perhaps these "explanations" weakened the effect of his statement with the public. He comes, however, to the conclusion at last, that warmth (*chaleur animale*) is the principal source of the magnetic treatment and success. (p. 78.)

Jussieu blames the course adopted by Mesmer and his followers, in aiming so much at the promulgation of a theory,—before the facts themselves have been fully established:—but he shows the utility of the system as a remedy.

Upon the whole, the Report is a very cautious, well-considered document,—not asserting or predicting too much —nor running wild with enthusiastic approbation. It is the evident production of a safe and sober man.

Here, then, is a significant fact in the history of this science, which ought to have arrested the conclusions of the faculty. But Jussieu's counterstatements were laughed at and set aside.

usage plus fecodes et plus riddeshi de cet agent fers mieux connoitre so veritable action et son degré d'utilité."—p. 80.

It was everywhere reported that the commissioners had put the matter to rest; and that large body of the public who never think for themselves, or care to distinguish, assumed that the refutation of the theory was a refutation of the facts; and so Animal Magnetism was considered as extinguished and buried for ever. While the stirring scenes of the approaching Revolution, and its sad and tragical horrors, and still more the wonders of Napoleon's reign*, so diverted men's minds from the subject, that to the great mass of the French people the existence of Mesmerism was a forgotten fact in history.

But truth is eternal, and the triumph of its enemies but short-lived and inglorious. Though a passing cloud may overshadow it, and appear to darken the prospect hopelessly, it is only that it may shine forth with greater brightness than ever. As one of our most glowing writers says of certain favourite principles, "Though they fall, it is but to rebound;—though they recede, it is but to spring forward with greater elasticity; though they perish, there are the seeds of vitality in their very decay;"—and so it is with truth and with the facts of Mesmerism. This exploded science "lived on,"—"brokenly," indeed, as the poet says,—and "showing no visible sign" of existence;—still it "lived on,"—and after a time gradually began to increase, and then to flourish, and at last to lift up its head only higher than before. The "crushing report" of the commissioners had not killed it.† Numbers of able and learned men still adhered pertinaciously to its cause. Schools were formed,—societies established for its promotion. The Marquis de Puysegur, a gallant soldier, devoted his whole soul and time to the treatment.

* See Seobardi.—Preface, p. t.
† Great facts in nature or art are not so easily got rid of by one crushing article, though their course may be somewhat retarded. Many of us remember the appearance of the "Excursion." The Ettrick Shepherd wrote to Southey: "I suppose you have heard what a crushing review in the Edinburgh Jeffrey has given Wordsworth." "He crush the Excursion! Tell him he might as easily crush Skiddaw!" was the Laureate's answer to Hogg. And so with Mesmerism. The article in the Quarterly, which is well-known to have proceeded from the pen of Sir B. B., was reported everywhere to have settled the question: but Mesmerism, it is well remarked, "is like the polypus; the knife may mutilate it, but it spreads again stronger than ever."—*Rapport Confid.* 4.

His success was immense. The cures performed by him were numerous. In Germany, in France, more especially at Strasburg and Paris, the subject was taken up with as great zeal as previously; and what is more to the purpose, with a judgment and sober consideration, and an utter absence of all *charlatanerie* and mystery.[*]

So signal was the progress, that a decided sensation was now made on the medical world. A young physician at Paris, the amiable and learned Foissac, made a stirring appeal to his brethren in its behalf. In 1825, he addressed a memorial to the members of the Royal Academy of Medicine, pointing out the necessity of a fresh and more satisfactory inquiry. Without entering upon the details, let it be sufficient to state, that a SECOND COMMISSION was appointed; that this commission consisted exclusively of medical men, some of them of very high standing in their profession; — that a most careful and scientific investigation took place; — and that in 1831 a Report on their Magnetic Experiments was laid before the Academy. And what was the nature of this Report? Was it evasive, cold, neutral, condemnatory? It was satisfactory and decisive in the highest degree. After having given a most interesting and circumstantial account of their proceedings, they finish with a series of conclusions, to which they had arrived: they are thirty in number, and ought to be read, as well as the Report itself, by every one interested in the subject; space can only be afforded for a few extracts, but these are decisive enough. They say:—

[*] " *Magnetism is a bêtise that is dead and buried,*" said M. Renauldin, a member of the Academy of Medicine, in 1825. "In one sense, our honoured colleague is right," observes the preface to the *Rapport Confidentiel.* " Magnetism was condemned *first,* then tried in the year 1784 by the scientific and the doctors; but it is notorious, that, since that epoch, the said magnetism, far from regarding itself as dead, has not ceased to spread itself in a deplorable manner in France, in Germany, in Prussia, &c., to the great satisfaction of the sick, and the great disappointment of the faculty, who know not what to make of these sort of *resurrections!*" (p. 2.) I am indebted to Mr. Newnham's work for my acquaintance with this very clever production, which professes to be a translation from Scobardi, an Italian Jesuit, in his report to the Grand Master of the Society of Jesus. The richest vein of irony runs through every page. All who love Mesmerism and sarcasm should read it.

8. A certain number of the effects observed appeared to us to depend upon *Magnetism alone,* and *were never produced without its application.* These are well established physiological and therapeutic phenomena.

29. Considered as a cause of certain physiological phenomena, or as a therapeutic remedy, *Magnetism ought to be allowed a place within the circle of the medical sciences;* and consequently, physicians only should practise it, or superintend its use, as is the case in the northern countries.[*]

And they conclude with saying,—" We dare not flatter ourselves with the hope of making you participate entirely in our conviction of the reality of the phenomena, which we have observed, and which you have neither seen, nor followed, nor studied along with us. We do not, therefore, demand of you a blind belief of all that we have reported. We conceive that a great proportion of these facts are of a nature so extraordinary that you cannot accord them such a credence....We only request that you would judge us as we should judge you,— that is to say, that you be completely convinced, that neither the love of the marvellous, nor the desire of celebrity, nor any views of interest whatever, influenced us during our labours."

This Report was signed by nine physicians. The two who did not sign did not consider themselves entitled to do so, from not having assisted at the experiments. The Report was laid before the Academy, who resolved that manuscript copies should be taken of it (*faire autographier le Rapport*). To this no objection was made: and the adversaries of Mesmerism resigned themselves, as far as the Academy was concerned, to an absolute silence on the subject. And from that hour, Mesmerism has been gaining ground in France, with such an im-

[*] 8. Un certain nombre des effets observés nous ont parus dépendre du magnétisme seul, et ne se sont pas reproduit sans lui. Ce sont des phénomènes physiologiques et thérapeutiques bien constatés.

29. Considéré comme agent de phénomènes physiologiques, ou comme moyen thérapeutique, le magnétisme devrait trouver sa place dans le cadre des connaissances médicales; et par conséquent les médecins seuls devraient en faire ou en surveiller l'emploi, ainsi que cela se pratique dans les pays du nord.— FOISSAC, *Rapports,* p. 205.

petns, that, as I have heard, a fourth of the medical men in Paris are stanch upholders of the science.*

"But," says the "Christian Observer," with a pertinacity worthy of a better cause, "if the French Commissioners have not decided the question, Mr. Wakley has." "Mr. Wakley laid bare some of the impositions to the conviction of unprejudiced observers."† "The wary coroner quietly slipped the wonder-working talisman (a piece of nickel) into a friend's hand, and substituted for it a piece of Queen Victoria's vulgar copper coin." "It was impossible that the hopeful young lady,"—as the writer unbecomingly terms as respectable a person as himself,—"could have exhibited such characteristic indications of Mesmeric influence if she had not been duly nickelised." And the editor of the "Lancet" is for ever referring his readers to those identical proceedings, and assuming that there is no appeal from his infallible tribunal. It is a new sight to behold Mr. Wakley and the "Christian Observer" yoked together in the same car of "compact alliance." Misery, they say, makes us acquainted with strange companions; and a bad cause appears to have much the same result. Not that Mr. Wakley's opinions are undeserving of attention. Mr. Wakley has "done the state some service." His first establishment of the "Lancet" was a useful act; it emancipated the minds of the junior members of his profession from a sluggish deference to official authority; and it often threw considerable light on some more than questionable proceedings within the different hospitals. In fact, it furnished an abundance of valuable information for all classes. Mr. Wakley's conduct in

* In 1837, there was a *third* investigation in Paris, composed almost entirely of the members of the Medical Academy, who were most hostile to Magnetism, and who of course returned an unfriendly report. It related only to two female somnambulists who had manifested some phenomena, and did not bear on the curative question. This report is notorious for its flagrant dishonesty in one or two points, and for its *suppressio veri*. The particulars will be found in the preface to the third edition of the *Isis Revelata*,—in Mr. Newnham's Human Magnetism,—and the recent French works. As the Abbé J. B. L. observes, "though the commission only made half a dozen experiments on two somnambulists, they have embraced the *whole* of magnetism in their conclusions." (p. 397.) This report was completely refuted by M. Husson, and M. Berna in their replies.

† In the article for September, 1843.

Parliament, in spite of his political ultraism, has been often marked by an honest detestation and exposure of abuse. And as a coroner, though occasionally officious and meddling, he has brought the reluctant authorities to a better knowledge of their duty. Still Mr. Wakley is not oracular on *every* subject. Clever as he is, he may, like other men, occasionally be mistaken, especially on points which he has little studied, and to which he comes for a novel and first experiment. He has so often enlightened the world with a description of what he tried in the cases of two of Dr. Elliotson's patients, that it is needless to repeat the story. It may be as well, however, to state, that it was in a set of experiments with nickel and lead, and which, he says, most egregiously failed, and proved the falsehood and imposition of the pretended sleepers. Those who have read Mr. Wakley's strictures should know that every charge has been again and again successfully answered. Dr. Elliotson, in the Letter to his Pupils on resigning his chair in University College, has entered fully into every part of the subject. Those who adopt the accusation should, at least, look into the reply. They will there find it stated, that some part of the proceedings were "entirely suppressed." They will there see how necessary it is in an experiment with metals on the human frame to proceed with the greatest caution and observation. They will there learn what slight disturbing effects change the nervous condition of the patient, and alter and affect the result of the experiment. "He acted," says Dr. Elliotson, "as though Mesmeric susceptibility is always present, and *always the same*; whereas the reverse is the fact; and experiments with water and metals frequently repeated so derange the susceptibility that we are often obliged to desist." Many a school-boy has made the trial of tasting, with his eyes bandaged, alternate glasses of white and red wine, till at last his palate has become so disordered, that he has been unable to detect the difference, and know the one from the other. In Mesmeric experiments, whether in phreno-magnetism or with metals, it is indispensable with most patients that the action of the first experiment be removed, or wear off, before a second and different one be attempted. They will otherwise clash and injure each other.

Time and the greatest nicety are requisite. The slightest circumstance may upset and disturb the patient, and so produce a *real failure* in the experiment, and a *seeming imposture* on the part of the sleeper.* With some somnambulists the trial with metals is complete; with others it is most uncertain. This is mentioned as a caution to those who quit a public lecture with their scepticism only the more strengthened, because the mesmerised metals have not obtained the promised effect.† But waving all this for a moment, let us suppose that these two most respectable patients of Dr. Elliotson,—patients with whom the editor of a religious periodical might not be ashamed to be acquainted,—let us suppose that these two patients were "deluding," and "affecting to suffer," and, for "sordid gain," "pretending to respond to the magical control" of the magnetist. What then? does the cause of Mesmerism depend upon the truthfulness of one or two cases? Granted that they were false, it would be rather a strong inference to assume that every thing else were a mistake. What yet becomes of the thousand-and-one cases that could easily be counted up, if a careful statistical body of evidence were collected from all quarters? It is to facts without number that we appeal; to facts confirmed by experiment and observation; and a hundred failures, or a hundred cases of imposture, would detract but a small amount from the actual heap:

> "Suave est ex magno tollere acervo."

But we must inform these cruel and thoughtless writers, who, for the sake of a pungent sentence, care not what libels they scatter against amiable and unoffending women, that these two sister-patients of Dr. Elliotson were *not* impostors. One

* "People are not very acute in distinguishing the causes of *failure*," says a clever article in the Examiner newspaper, "and the tide of fashion runs indiscriminately against a scheme," which appears to miscarry.—July 5th 1845.

† To shew how necessary it is to proceed most leisurely, and with intervals between experiments of every kind, the reader is referred to Zoist, No. 13, p. 244, for the interesting case of Mrs. Shewing. I was myself present on the day mentioned by Dr. E. p. 242, when the Archbishop of Dublin and Mr. Scarlett assisted in the experiments, and can bear testimony to the accuracy of the doctor's statement.

of them is most respectably married; and both have secured the good opinion of all who know them. But as one test of sincerity is better than fifty assertions, let us state an actual fact, and see how far it will serve as a set-off to Mr. Wakley's charges. Mr. Gibbon Wakefield, "as hard-headed and little credulous a man as exists," had often excused himself, when invited, from going to University College Hospital to witness the Mesmeric phenomena in the cases of these two sisters. At last he went, and was astonished; but still would not make up his mind to believe what he saw. "When the experiments were over, and he was passing through some part of the hospital to leave it, he accidentally noticed one of the sisters with her back to him, hanging over the balusters carelessly, and looking down, still in the Mesmeric delirium, and therefore highly susceptible. He thought this a favourable opportunity to test her, because he was satisfied that she could not see anything that he did. He made a pass behind her back at some distance with his hand directed to her, and she instantly was fixed and rigid, and perfectly senseless. He had sense enough to believe his senses,—and was now satisfied of the reality of all he had beheld."* This was a convincing fact; and might satisfy the brother-editors of the "Lancet" and of the "Christian Observer" of the truthfulness and honesty of the calumniated sleeper. A similar thing occurred to a friend of mine, as clear-headed and strong-minded a man as any of my acquaintance. He made a pass behind the patient's back (one of the sisters Okey), at Dr. Elliotson's house, when she was occupied in conversation with some one else, and was unconscious of his presence and intention. In truth, he was hardly conscious of the intention himself; for it was the thought and act of a moment. But the poor girl was instantly seized, and fell back in a state of torpor. The gentleman who told me this is no believer in Mesmerism: he merely mentioned it as a circumstance that occurred within his experience. Facts, however, such as these will receive the attention of the candid and the impartial; they refute the imputation of deception;—and it is by

* Zoist, No. I. p. 44.

o 2

such plain statements that we reply to the ungenerous slanders of Mr. Wakley and his new ally, the "Christian Observer."

But if Mr. Wakley did not succeed in disproving the honesty of two excellent sisters, there was one thing in which he was eminently fortunate. The thunders of the "Lancet" had their intended effect on his medical brethren. Though anything but a favourite with them before, he henceforward became their pet authority. And strange to say he also became their terror. Fearful of being hitched into a line of the next week's "Lancet," as believers in the so-called absurdity, some gentlemen straightway swallowed their rising convictions with wry faces and reluctant hearts;—while the remainder, almost to a man, refused for the future to be present at any Mesmeric demonstration whatsoever. Like Mr. M'Neile at Liverpool, they carefully retreated from the evidence of their own senses, but from a different reason altogether. My clerical brother judged that there was something supernatural in these cases;—he regretted that he had not faith to play the part of exorciser and bid the devil depart*, and from want of this faith would "*see nothing of it.*" But the fears of the liberal profession were of a different order. It was not of an evil spirit that *they stood in awe*; it was of Mr. Wakley,—of the evil genius of the "Lancet,"—of the gibes and jeerings of a substantial, corporeal editor, before whom they shrank rebuked. This was the demon whom they dreaded: and though we might have expected better things from such a body of men, it is a fact, that mainly through an apprehension of having their names brought forward before the public in the pages of a clever periodical, very many gentlemen turned their backs on the subject, and from that hour declined all invitations to visit and examine the phenomena for themselves. And thus it went on for a few years. The progress of Mesmerism was seemingly suspended in this country. It appeared stifled in its birth, an unlucky abortion, of which nothing more would be heard. But silently and steadily was it making way. A change was gradually coming on. Day by day fresh accessions were

* See Sermon, p. 147.

counted in its train. The leaven was fermenting; and even from the ranks of the faculty a few adherents occasionally dropped in. I hope that I may now say confidently that a better spirit has decidedly sprung up among them. In that noble profession, which is alike distinguished for its humanity, its ability, its love of science, its love of truth, its large and comprehensive philosophy, I believe that the far greater number would be ready to give, even to the hateful study of Mesmerism, the benefit of a faithful and dispassionate inquiry. I am sure that there are many who would cheerfully admit that the field of usefulness is enlarged by it, and the means of lessening human ills considerably extended. I know that there are several, who, at the risk of damaging their worldly prospects, do not hesitate to step forward fearlessly and manfully, as believers in, and practisers of, the calumniated science. More especially from among the *younger* members of the profession, there are to be found many zealous and talented men, taking a high and independent position, anxiously devoting their attention to the study, gathering facts as they arise, and prepared to employ the aid of this new power among the means of cure at their disposal. *O si sic omnes!* For there are others, and particularly among the leaders* in more than one metropolis, who, to judge from their conduct and their language, would seem to have the same horror at being witnesses of Mesmeric phenomena, as *the bat has at the approach of light.* They sneer or smile when the subject is brought forward, according to their own turn of mind, or rather according to the temper of those with whom they argue. But *to be present,—to*

* Apropos of leaders in a profession: Hume says that "Harvey is entitled to the glory of having made, by reasoning alone, without any mixture of accident, a capital discovery in one of the most important branches of science. He had also the happiness of establishing at once his theory on the most solid and convincing proofs; and society has added little to the arguments suggested by his industry and ingenuity. . . . It was remarked that no physician in Europe, who had reached forty years of age, ever to the end of his life, adopted Harvey's doctrine of the circulation of the blood, and that his practice in London diminished extremely, from the reproach drawn upon him by that great and signal discovery. So slow is the progress of truth in every science, even when not opposed by factious or superstitious prejudices! He died in 1657, aged 79."— *Hume's History of England, cap. 62.*

have their names bruited about as testimonies of a fact,—
to be unable to resist their own convictions,—to be unable to remain in the bliss of ignorance,—this is a position
from which they fall back with a secret dread of approaching
danger. They can be sharp-sighted enough in detecting
narrowness of spirit in any other quarter,—advocates for
freedom of conscience in theology,—ameliorators of our criminal code in matters of jurisprudence,—liberal, tolerant, and
haters of abuse;—but the moment that Mesmeric influence is
proposed as an auxiliary to their practice, that instant they are
as sensitive, as angry, as staunch adherents of what is old,—
as stout opponents of what is new,—as though the charter and
privileges of their order were being jeopardied for ever! *
Doubtless, in all experiments of a strange and novel character,
the public do expect from the medical profession the most
cautious, slow, and deliberate frame of mind. They expect
from their closer cognisance of subjects of this nature the most
searching, scrutinizing, hesitating conduct. Nay, they would
not even be displeased to see an inquiry carried on in a sceptical,
unbelieving spirit. But still they *do* expect inquiry of some
kind.† They do not expect to see a subject of this important

* Miss Martineau observes, "The systematic disingenuousness of some
medical journals on this subject, and the far-fetched calumnies and offensive assumptions with which it is the regular practice of the faculty to assail
every case of cure or relief by Mesmerism, looked very much *as if they were in
conflict with powerful truth, and as if they knew it.*"—Preface, p. 7.

† It would be unjust not to acknowledge, that many medical men, and
some with whom I have the pleasure of being acquainted, have made a
most fair and straightforward inquiry into the subject. But we too often
meet with much of a contrary character. A letter was read to me from the
West of England, saying, "We have had a lecturer on Mesmerism here; all
our medical men were present, and behaved in the most brutal and outrageous way." A lady, where I was on a visit lately, said, "We have had a
Mesmeric lecturer in our town: Mr.——, a surgeon, behaved in the most
bullying manner, and did all he could to intimidate the parties." In Norwich a Mesmerist was recently giving a lecture. A most intelligent
inhabitant of that city told me that many of the medical men "were furious"
on the occasion. One of them, who was present, suddenly took out a lancet
and ran it deeply into the patient's finger *under the nail into the quick*; a part
most exquisitely sensitive, as we all know: no expression of pain was evident at the time; but the poor boy suffered a good deal after he was
awakened. I neither know nor wish to learn the name of the party who
was guilty of this unmanly outrage. A strong feeling, I understand, has

nature treated with the vulgarest vituperation and ridicule;
its supporters stigmatised as credulous, its operators defamed
as fraudulent, its patients mocked at as impostors. They do
not expect to see the heads of a profession which piques itself
pre-eminently on its liberality, exhibiting the bigotry of the
priest, and the special pleading of the lawyer. Look, for
instance, at what took place a few years back at the London
University through the instigation and promptings of certain
members of the faculty. Often is the world invited to sneer
at the blind prejudices that disfigure the banks of the Isis;—
often have the venerable doctors of Oxford been satirised for
their love of the useless and the obsolete to the prejudice of
some nobler branches of knowledge; but in spite of all the
faults of Alma Mater,—in spite of all her past and present
absurdities, I would contrast her conduct on a memorable
occasion in academic history, with the intolerance and hatred
of novelty that recently marked the more modern institution.
Are the circumstances, for instance, under which Locke was
expelled from Christ Church one whit more disgraceful in
themselves, than the treatment which induced Dr. Elliotson to
withdraw his name from the Professorship in the University of
London? Was the temple of science more liberal than the
hall of logic? was the new foundation more friendly to
enlightened investigations than the old? What, in short,
were the respective circumstances of the two cases? In the
ancient seat of learning, the timidity or servility of a dean and
chapter expunged the name of the philosopher from the books

been entertained respecting him. But these are the ways in which an
inquiry is conducted,—if conducted at all, rather than with a calm, patient,
philosophic temper, solicitous of truth. A most acute observer, though no
believer in Mesmerism, lately remarked to me:—" From what I read in
different provincial papers, and from what I have heard from other quarters,
it seems to me, that medical men attend these meetings, not with the humane
desire of discovering a valuable auxiliary, but solely with the hope of detecting imposture." It is too nearly the truth. I have also read some curious
accounts of what took place lately at Bedford and at Exeter. The conduct
of certain parties to Mr. Vernon at Greenwich must be fresh in every one's
memory. See also in Miss Martineau's lecture another "brutal assault," by
a surgeon, who "violently seized the sleeper's arm, and shouted out that the
house was on fire," p. 25. The whole story is worth reading.

o 4

of his college at the mandate of an arbitrary sovereign; James the Second was the real cause of the expulsion of Locke, though the University of Oxford had long endured a most unjust opprobrium on the subject, till Lord Grenville cleared the matter up[*]: while in the model institution, the vacancy in the Professor's chair was the result of an opposition to physiological experiments on the part of *soi-disant* friends to scientific inquiry,—an opposition that was set on foot by Dr. Elliotson's own colleagues, and carried out to its completion by the despotic members of a liberal council!

But this subject will bear a little further examination.

The University of London, or, as it has since been designated, University College, was originally formed on the most liberal principles. No tests,—no subscriptions were admissible;—but to promote the largest amount of knowledge amongst the largest number of students, was the projected theory of its friends and founders. The *stare super antiquas vias*,—the clinging to old usages,—the rejection of new truths,—this was the favourite charge against the elder Institutions; but with the rival establishment in Gower Street, an order of things was to arise which would lead men forward to fresh fields of knowledge. Nay, so liberal were they, that the very name of Religion was not to pass their threshold; each man was to do what seemed right in his own eyes; and worship his Creator (or not) after the fashion he liked best. "But," says a clever article in the Spectator Newspaper, "there are few, even among the most liberal, who apply their liberalism to every point. Some are liberal on commercial, some on theological, some on political, and some on juridical questions;—but beyond the pale of their own peculiar subject, they are often *as intolerant as ignorance can make them.*"[†] And thus, in the University of London, though every one was to be his own theologian, the same latitude was not granted in the matter of medicine. Here all was by precedent and prescription; here the conventional customs of the faculty were deemed sacred as the Thirty-nine

[*] See "Locke and Oxford," by Lord Grenville.
[†] Spectator, Nov. 11th, 1843.

Articles elsewhere; here, whatever was not stamped with the orthodox seal of the College of Surgeons, was shunned as a heresy, to be burnt by the hands of the common hangman. As for the spiritual state of the students,—for their immortal and better part, no matter what was the result, these young men might become Budhists, Mahometans, Atheists, or Muggletonians;—any thing they pleased, so long as their freedom of choice was not interfered with;—but for the perishing bodies of the sick, all must be done *selon les régles*; cure or relief was unimportant, so that the prejudices of the practitioner were not offended. Accordingly, when Mesmerism was introduced into the Hospital by their most distinguished Physician,—though the patients themselves were willing recipients,—though the most signal benefits were being daily experienced,—though the academies at Paris and Berlin had not thought the question beneath their notice,—this new,—this liberal,—this consistent University stepped forward to aim a blow at a science in its birth. The *free-thinking* Council met and passed the following Resolution:—

"Resolved,—That the Hospital Committee be instructed to take such steps as they shall deem most advisable to prevent the practice of Mesmerism, or Animal Magnetism, in future within the Hospital."

No sooner was this Resolution passed, than Dr. Elliotson *sent in his resignation*. It ought, however, to be made known that four Members of the Council, true to their own principles and to the great cause of humanity, constituted an honourable minority in a vote on a proposition that Dr. Elliotson should be invited back to resume his chair. These four were Lord Brougham, Sir L. Goldsmid, Mr. Tooke, and Mr. Bishop. But the Council rejected the proposition.

And so much for the liberal University of London!

Turn again, for a second example, to the proceedings of the Royal Medical and Chirurgical Society on a late occasion.[*] See the alarmed and almost frantic feelings with which certain

[*] See "Numerous Cases of Surgical Operations without Pain," &c., by Dr. Elliotson. (Baillière.)

parties discussed the remarkable report of the amputation of a man's thigh during the Mesmeric state.[*] See how anxious they were to put the matter down, and bury the fact in oblivion. A Bible thrown into an old Spanish convent could not have more convulsed its inmates, than did this unfortune treatise that learned assembly. Mr. Topham has much to answer for. The conscience of Mr. Ward must be weighed down with bitter self-reproach. True, these gentlemen established a great fact in physiology: true, they assisted an unhappy sufferer with unexampled relief during a formidable operation;—but they cannot be otherwise than painfully mindful of the bile and bad blood they engendered amongst the members of the society on that unlucky evening. Poor Wombell, indeed, enjoyed a composing sleep during the horrors of amputation; but contrast that with the sleepless feverish nights of the angry opponents, and then what has humanity gained in the matter? The thing was "irrational,"—was "ridiculous,"—was "impossible," and so what need was there for the Society to discuss the subject? Like a country bench of double-barrelled squires assembled to convict a suspected offender against the game laws, this philosophical audience arrived at a "foregone conclusion," before the merits of the case had even been opened. The Mesmeriser and the poacher must both be silenced:—the one has no licence to kill, nor the other to cure; and so defence or explanation are alike inadmissible. One gentleman declared that he would not believe the facts had he witnessed them himself.[†] Another expressed his perfect satisfaction with the condemnatory reports made by others, and *par conséquent*, the needlessness that he should be *present and examine them himself!* Really, in passing through the account of this debate,—in noting the anxiety of certain members to expunge all record of the proceedings from their minute-book, I could have fancied that I was reading the discussions of a knot of mendicant friars

* See "Account of a Case of successful Amputation of the Thigh during the Mesmeric State, without the Knowledge of the Patient." Read to the Royal Medical and Chirurgical Society, November, 1842, by W. Topham, Esq., and W. S. Ward, Esq. (Baillière, Regent Street.)

† Etherisation has since proved the truthfulness of these facts in Mesmerism.

terrified at the dawn of the Reformation;—I felt myself transplanted, as it were, into the Vatican, where was a letter from Luther, frightening the holy conclave from its propriety. All the time that I was reading the speeches of certain opponents, there kept involuntarily rising up in my mind the outcry of Demetrius, the Ephesian silversmith, "Our craft is in danger to be set at nought: and, Sirs, ye know that by this craft we have our wealth." (Acts, xix. v. 25. 27.) One would suppose that these gentlemen would remember the treatment of Harvey, the *circulator*, as he was termed;—the averted eye that at first was turned on Jenner; and the disbelief with which many great and mighty discoveries have been received, and be more cautious and circumspect for the future. Oh! if a love of ancient usages,—if a hatred of new and unpalatable truths is to bear away the bell, Oxford may now hide her diminished head,—Salamanca "pale her uneffectual fires,"—the doctors of the Sorbonne part with their old pre-eminence, for competitors are stepping in from the "liberal professions," able and willing to take the lead. And yet we are all aware of the sarcasms with which "the faculty" and the "philosophers" treat the "learned ignorance" of the clergy, and their presumed dislike to scientific inquiry; and perhaps we are too often a fair subject for such animadversion, more especially if many such sermons as the one preached at Liverpool are delivered by us: but I can tell "the profession," in return, that I should often have more hope of bringing home a new and important truth to the minds of a simple ignorant peasantry than of combating successfully the bigotry of the philosopher, and the prejudices of an educated and scientific assembly.[*] Yes: save me from the credulity of the sceptic,—from the intolerance of the tolerant,—from the tyranny of the ultra-liberal! Experience has shown us some of the bitterest opponents of real freedom of conscience amongst the stanchest sticklers for religious liberty; we daily see men, who will *believe nothing*, even upon the strongest testimony, in contradiction to their preconceived systems, *believing everything*

* " Rarement un savant, qui a recueilli, comparé beaucoup d'idées trouvées avant lui, peut et veut comprendre un ordre de vérités nouvelles." — Magnétisme devant le Cour de Rome, 45.

against the veracity and competency of the most credible witnesses[*];—and here we have had a free-thinking council opposed to freedom of inquiry,—and a body of gentlemen, whose
whole professional career is based on experimental evidence, on
one occasion declining to witness facts, and upon another,
thrown into a confusion, worse than that in King Agramont's
camp[†], from the recital of a case, which, even if attended by a
few erroneous conclusions, was at least deserving of a candid
investigation.

Look, for another instance, to what occurred not long ago
in Manchester. When the British Association, in one of its
erratic flights, was preparing to visit that city, and by aid of
railway excursions in the morning, and concerts and conver-
saziones in the evening "cram" its money-making population
with the *areana* of science, Mr. Braid[‡], a surgeon of that
place, who had long devoted his attention to Mesmerism, offered
a paper on the subject to the medical Section, and proposed
"*to produce as many of his patients as possible in proof* of
the curative agency" of his particular system. He thought
that "gentlemen of scientific attainments might thus have an

---

[*] "I would rather believe," said a surgeon to a friend of mine, "that all
Mesmerisers and their patients were impostors, than give credit to one of
their facts, however well authenticated." "You must rather believe," said
an anti-mesmeric lecturer, "that all your wives and sisters and children are
false, than think any of these cases true."

[†] The wild and fanciful poet describes Discord as hastening with her
bellows to blow up the strife:—

> "La Discordia . . .
> Corre a pigliare *i mantici* di botto,
> Ed agli accesi fochi ossa aggiungendo,
> Ed accendendone altri, fa salire
> De mali cori un alto incendio d'ira."
>
> *Orlando Fur.*, canto xxvii. 39.

From all accounts there were no bellows wanted that evening in Berners
Street. The fire was kindled before the match was applied.—Gibbon sneers
about the "Monks of Magdalen," and the "port and prejudice" they im-
bibed. The monks of Magdalen, with their venerable president, may now
turn the tables against their liberal scoffers.—What is the favourite beverage
of the Chirurgical Society, I know not. A friend, more witty than wise
suggests that, to judge from the temper of the meeting, the potations that
night must have been gin and bitters.

[‡] See Braid's "Neurypnology, considered in relation with Animal Magnetism: illustrated by numerous cases of relief and cure of disease."

---

opportunity of investigating the subject, unbiassed by local or
personal prejudice." He himself "hoped to *learn something
from others*, on points which were mysterious to him, as to the
cause of the phenomena." And when we know the character
of some of his alleged cures,—when we learn that many successful cures in paralysis,—in tic-douloureux, and in rheumatism,
and of improvement in sight, where amongst them, the public
might naturally conclude that these *savans* would gladly accept
the offer, and bring their scientific knowledge to bear upon
the subject. Here was a concentration of talent and philosophy met together; and now was a golden time for going into
the question, and of putting down for ever a ridiculous pretension, or of satisfying their own minds as to the truth of the
practice. But no: "The committee of the medical section
declined entertaining the subject." As the professor at Padua
refused to *look through* Galileo's telescope at the moon;—so
these gentlemen at Manchester were unwilling to *look at* Mr.
Braid's patients, for reasons that can only be known to themselves. Either they had some secret misgivings, some fears
touching their own conversion, some dread of having to *unlearn*
much of their former acquirements, or the rules of the Association would not permit the arrangement, or their time, perhaps, at this important juncture was not quite at their disposal.
As a committee of the British Association for the Advancement
of Science could scarcely be afraid of meeting facts,—let us
see how the matter stood with them in respect to time. On
turning, then, to a record of their proceedings[*], we find, that
the "section was thinly attended,"—that several tedious papers
were read, most of which could have been studied more pro-
fitably at home,—and that out of the six days on which the
Sections met, there were two on which no business at all was
transacted before the one for medicine, some part of which
time might at least have been surrendered to Mr. Braid and
his experiments, even if the rules of the society forbade a more
formal lecture. These "learned Thebans" had flitted from
their homes and travelled many a long and weary mile, and

---

[*] See Literary Gazette and Athenæum for 1842.

what was their object? Was it not the detection of error, the discovery of truth, and the good of human kind? and might not Mesmerism or Neurypnology fall under one of these classes? Oh! let us not be too severely critical:—the visit to Manchester was not wholly without fruit. While one party was listening to a learned treatise on the "*Palpi of Spiders*," by which the arachnologist "would be prevented from falling into the *too common error of mistaking young spiders for old ones*[*]," another Section was instructed by certain "microscopic researches in fibre," and on the "therapeutic application of air-tight fabrics." Released from these arduous duties, and this strain on their cerebral functions, our professors could only find repose by a promenade through the adjoining gardens; here where Flora and Pomona vied with their most tempting gifts, and the eyes of beauty smiled reward on the learned labours of the lecturer[†], who could expect even an anchorite to tear himself away, and find leisure for Mesmerism with all its cares? And then came the banquet with its venison and its wines;—and then the self-applauding speeches, where one Section bepraised the other; and then followed music and the charm of song, till at length wearied out with this train of endless occupations, "Section E" could only recline their heads upon the pillow, with the self-satisfied assurance that they had not, like Titus, lost a day! To be serious, there is something melancholy in the state of mind here exhibited. These papers have their uses, and are valuable. But after all, the "proper study of mankind is man;"—the palpi of spiders are not so interesting as the nervous system of a patient; and when a subject like Mesmerism professes to mitigate the maddening throes of pain,—to give relief to thousands,—and to effect a cure, where a cure had been pronounced impracticable, to see men of education like those at Manchester pass over to the other side with offended dignity rather than be spectators of the fact, is a scene both painful and humiliating. The question ran counter to all their previous views,—and so with sullen

[*] See the reports in the Athenæum.

[†] See Times Newspaper and Literary Gazette.

silence they declined to witness an art which promises to multiply their remedial resources to an extent, at this moment, beyond calculation.

Though Section E, however, declined to countenance Mr. Braid by their medical presence, a large body of visitors did not think his curious experiments beneath their notice, and his lectures were attended by a numerous and scientific audience.[*]

The above, however, is not the only occasion, on which the British Association has flinched from free investigation. *Nitor is adversum* is evidently *not* its motto. It loves the popular and the fashionable, and to run along the smooth road of acknowledged and prevalent studies. *Primâ facie*, one would ignorantly assume that an association for the promotion of science would seek truth wherever it could be found, and love facts in nature at all price, and from any source. *Primâ facie*, one would assume, that the object of such an institution would be to extend the frontiers of knowledge in every direction of physics, with the feeling that the atmosphere of examination and opposition was one that it must often expect to breathe. But no : such assumptions argue a rustic unacquaintance with erudite corporations. The subject must first be scientifically orthodox, approved of in high places and academic bowers, and then the views of its promoters may be pushed to any extravagance and any length. "The bounded reign of existence" is then too narrow for our soaring and enlightened lecturer, who has "exhausted old worlds" with his theories, and must now "imagine new" ones for the edification of his auditory. All this is legitimate and pleasant enough. But why need the very same man be blind to facts, in a different province of nature, that lie within his arm's length? Why does he not examine truths that are accessible to his very touch? Why

[*] These searching Sectionists had a narrow escape from extinction at the Cambridge meeting in 1845. Their utility was actually called in question by their more active brethren! But a means termless was discovered, which has saved and, it is hoped, will enlarge their services. A new name was given them! Section E is no longer the "medical" but the "physiological" *Mæsto novd virtute. Novo nomine.*

does he spurn the easiest of all information, the evidence of his own senses? the

> "quæ sunt oculis subjecta fidelibus, et quæ
> Ipse sibi tradat spectator?"

Alas for philosophy! The study, perchance, is full of thorns, not yet admitted within the circle of inquiry,—unpalatable in leading quarters,—"opposed to the philosophy of ages," and apt to involve its advocate in unpopularity and rebuke. The advancement of *heretical* truths in science might be damaging and difficult; the advancement of the views of a friendly confederated majority is a far more pleasing and easy occupation.

The respective fates of Mesmerism and of Ether, of Geology and of Phrenology, within the halls of the British Association for the advancement of science, may furnish a commentary on the above observations.

Geology, not many years back, occupied the same position in the intellectual world that Mesmerism does now. It was the pursuit of an unpopular minority. Those who adopted its more extreme doctrines were regarded with coldness from the assumed danger of their theories,—if not frowned down upon as atheists and impugners of revelation. The tables are now turned. Geology is a favourite study; and to quote "Lyell" and "Murchison," and dilate on rocks "primitive" and "tertiary," an indispensable part of a finished education. Accordingly, when in 1844 the Association assembled at York, and a "Cathedral Doctor" (to use Ben Jonson's phrase) fulminated his feeble notions against certain views in the science, a splendid castigation was inflicted on the spot, for, in a reply that "annihilated both space and time" from the extent and liberality of its opinions, the great Cambridge Professor championed forth the claims of his beloved study against the assaults of an obsolete bigotry, and Geology shone out, amidst an applauding crowd, enthroned upon a free and fearless philosophy![*]

---

[*] Some persons thought that the reply, able as it was, showed more tartness than was necessary, that it smacked of the wormwood that occasionally is

"Look here upon this picture, and on this!"

Mr. Hewett Watson tells us in his useful work on Phrenology[*], that when "the British Association held its annual meeting in Edinburgh, about a week previous to their assembling, Mr. Combe addressed a letter to Mr. Robison, one of the secretaries, offering to give a demonstration on the national skulls in the collection belonging to the Phrenological Society. Mr. Robison forwarded the letter of Mr. Combe to the committee, and the gentlemanly courtesies of the persons *officially* concerned will be apparent from the following notice of the matter, borrowed from the ninth volume of the "Phrenological Journal:" 'Mr. Combe was duly admitted a member of the Association, and attended meetings of several of the Sections; but he *was not honoured with any reply whatever to his communication.* From Mr. Robison he received the most polite attention; and the reason of the silence of the committee became apparent at the first meeting. Mr. Sedgwick, the president for last year, before resigning his office, addressed the Association in a speech, in which he urged most strenuously the necessity of keeping in mind the objects of its institution, and of confining their researches into *dead matter*, without entering into any speculations on the relations of intellectual beings; and he would brand as a traitor that person who would *dare* to overstep the *prescribed boundaries* of the Institution.'" Strong language this for a philosopher and investigator, if it be rightly reported! "*Dare* to overstep the prescribed boundaries!" What boldness in one science! what caution in another! The uninitiated mind of Mr. Combe (a true philosopher himself, and a genuine lover of truth), assuming in its ignorance that a collection of crania came under the category of "*dead matter*," offered to give a public demonstration: but he was soon disabused of his error. However,

---

found in articles of the great "Northern Review," when a popular author, and original and inconvenient theories, are to be got rid of and silenced. Upon this I am not competent to offer an opinion.

[*] *Statistics of Phrenology,* p. 42. Mr. H. Watson has the credit, in some quarters, of being the author of a recent popular and scientific work, which has already passed through several editions. Is this the case? "Vestiges" of his opinions, it is thought, may be clearly traced in it.

as Mr. Watson remarks, "it is of small importance to any one wishing to instruct others, that he should be '*branded as a traitor*,' in return for his good wishes. But we apprehend that a demonstration of the peculiarities of national skulls was completely within the 'boundaries' of the institution. * * * Besides, part of the time of the Association was occupied with subjects of very trifling importance, when compared to this one, the description of fossil fishes, the colour of chamelions, and the circulation of tortoises; and surely the anatomy of the human head was a matter of as much consequence to mankind as 'such questions.'" But the explanation is easy. There are popes in science, as well as in theology; and the articles of "prescribed" belief are as carefully guarded in the one school as in the other. Canon law rules elsewhere than at Rome.*

Again, when the British Association assembled this year at Oxford, the same exclusiveness and self-induced ophthalmia appeared in their proceedings. "None are so blind as those that will not see." And Sir Robert Inglis, the president, addressing our friends of Section E, rejoicing then under their new appellation of the "Physiological," spoke most appropriately of the great blessings of Etherisation, and of the well-recorded instances of operations under its influences, "as a subject eminently deserving the attention of that division" of the philosophers. Nothing could be more just and becoming than every syllable that fell from the lips of the amiable speaker: but to read what he said, the ignorant would scarcely suspect that an insensibility of the same nature had ever been before attainable, or that upwards of 300† *operations under the Mesmeric influence* had been previously registered in chi-

---

* See also in Zoist, No. 16., a letter from Mr. Prideaux, with an account of the proceedings of the B. A. on another occasion before the *Ethnological* Section, when, on certain developments in the foreheads of some old skulls being pointed out, the chairman called to order, as "Phrenology was a prohibited study." What truth-loving philosophers!—to prohibit the study of the brain in an examination of the diversities between different peoples! The omission of the "character of Hamlet," as in the Irish play-bill, seems no longer an invention.

† See Summary, given in Introductory Chapter.

rurgical annals. But luck is every thing in this world; and Mesmerism has not *yet* been fortunate enough to secure the sanction of scientific magnates. In the words of the favourite ballad, "Oh, no, they never mention it; its name is never heard" within their committee-rooms and dining-halls; and so they hope, that, by appearing themselves thus ignorant of its influence, the knowledge of its very existence may escape the recollection of their audience. But "Leviathan is not so tamed," nor so readily disposed of. The absence of all allusion to the topic shows the *animus* of those who gave the cue to the discourse: for prejudice itself must admit, that when the subject-matter of an oration is insensibility to pain during the operations of surgery, to pass over a cognate condition of the human body, under which more than three hundred cases of a similar character had actually been recorded, marks an intentional omission in the argument more significant in its silence than a thousand bold allusions.*

In observing the cold-blooded indifference to human welfare with which science could thus "*remember to forget*" a fact in nature, because it happened to contradict a preconception, I am almost tempted to exclaim in the indignant language of Festus,—

> "Thank God! I am a man,
> Not a philosopher!"†

It is, indeed, a common remark, that no great reform or improvement in a profession has ever proceeded from its own members. One or two may have originated the idea;—but

---

* Every one knows, that on this occasion the good-natured member for the University of Oxford was confessedly the mouth-piece of a learned professor, an early and unforgiving opponent of Mesmerism. But surely the "prescribed boundaries of the institution were overstepped" when the professor "dared" to prompt an allusion, in the president's speech to the "effects of ether on the nervous system" (if we decide according to the speech of a former president, before quoted). The subjects for a surgical operation are not yet "*dead matter*," the strict line for investigation drawn at Edinburgh, although if ether be injudiciously applied, they would be very apt to become so. We must leave the two professors to decide between them, as to who ought to be "*branded as a traitor* to science," the man who intentionally omits, or the man who interdicts, or the man who introduces, a subject for investigation.

† Festus, p. 84.

the adoption of the plan has generally been forced on them from "without." This is eminently true in regard to ecclesiastical matters. They were not the clergy but the laity that led on the movement in Church reform. The same may be said in regard to law. The illustrious Romilly commenced his parliamentary career with propositions for an amendment of our criminal code; but it is notorious how unpopular in Westminster Hall were his suggestions; and it was public opinion alone that carried out his views. Again, may the same remark be applied to the medical body. Men of a certain standing in the profession are unwilling to depart from the old routine; they are afraid of losing *caste*; they care not to *unlearn* their early teaching, and to begin with some fresh laws of nature, of which they were unaware; and so, sooner than sacrifice themselves, they sacrifice truth. It is thus in the instance of Mesmerism. It was a medical man that first discovered it; but they were not medical men that took it up; —and their attention,—must we say their unwilling attention, was at last obtained, only through the firm attitude that their own patients often displayed on the question. And yet, even if Mesmerism had been an unreal phantom,—there were reasons why they need not have felt such shame in looking it impartially in the face. Great names could be numbered amongst its adherents. Some of the first men of our day,— the first in science and philosophy, have not blushed to express their strong convictions of its truth. That can be no common delusion upon a subject, on which La Place, the most profound and exact of mathematicians, could state, that " on his own principles he could not withhold his assent to it;"—and on which he could write, that " it would be unphilosophical to deny the existence of the phenomena, because, in the present state of our knowledge, their operations are yet inexplicable to us."[*] That can be no weak fancy, when Cuvier, by common

* Mr. Chenevix states, in the London Medical and Physical Journal, that he had more than one conversation with La Place upon Mesmerism, about 1816 and 1817, and that the expression of that great philosopher constantly was, "that the testimony in favour of the truth of Mesmerism, coming with such uniformity from enlightened men of many nations, who had no interest to deceive, and possessed no possible means of collusion, was

consent the first of modern naturalists, could say, that " the effects produced by Mesmerism no longer permit it to be doubted, that the proximity of two living bodies in certain positions and with certain actions, has a real result, independent of all participation of the imagination."[*] That can be no vague notion, of which a Hufeland,—if not the first, in the very first rank of German physicians, has expressed himself a firm and conscientious supporter. The catalogue of able and superior men that could be found among the friends of the science would run on to " the crack of doom."[†] From my own experience, I assert that those of my acquaintance who are its known and confessed believers, are as clear-headed, as strong-minded, as sober-thinking, as free from that wild enthusiastic feeling which prompts men to catch at the newest fancy, as any individuals in the kingdom. All of them, I think without exception, were strong unbelievers, if not op-

such that, applying to it his own principles and formulas respecting human evidence, he *could not withhold his assent to what was so strongly supported.*" The following are his own words, in his Essay on Probabilities: " Les phénomènes singuliers qui résultent de l'extrême sensibilité des nerfs dans quelques individus, ont donné naissance à diverses opinions sur l'existence d'un nouvel agent, que l'on a nommé magnétisme animal : * * * Il est naturel de penser que l'action de ces causes est très-faible, et qu'elle peut être facilement troublée par des circonstances accidentelles; ainsi, parceque dans quelques cas, elle ne s'est point manifestée, on ne doit pas rejeter son existence. Nous sommes si loin de connaitre tous les agens de la nature, et leurs divers modes d'action, qu'il serait peu philosophique de nier les phénomènes, uniquement parcequ'ils sont inexplicable dans l'état actuel de nos connaissances." — LA PLACE, *Essai Philosophique sur les Probabilités.* Paris. 4th edition, p. 191.

* This is Cuvier's own language : " Cependant les effets obtenus sur des personnes déjà sans connaissance avant que l'operation commençat,—ceux qui ont lieu sur les autres personnes après que l'operation même leur a fait perdre connaissance, et ceux que présentent les animaux, ne permettent guères de douter, que la proximité de deux corps animés dans certaines positions et avec certains mouvemens, n'ait un effet réel, indépendant de toute participation de l'imagination d'une des deux. Il paroît assez clairement aussi que ces effets sont dus à une communication quelconque qui s'établit entre leurs système nerveux."— CUVIER, *Anatomie Comparée,* tom. ii. p. 117. " Du Système nerveux considéré en action."

† I have already mentioned Coleridge and Arnold in the preface, and quoted some passages from the "Letters" of the latter. Here is an additional extract from one of his sermons: " In our own times the phenomena of animal magnetism have lately received an attestation, which, *in my judgment,* establishes the *facts beyond question.*"— Sermon, vol iii. p. 245.

ponents, till they practically and experimentally looked into
the question. Verily, if we are mistaken, we belong to a
goodly company! We have plenty of comrades to keep us in
countenance. We can bear a laugh at the number or quality
of our friends. Let the wits, then, exhaust their raillery at
our expense; let the prejudiced shake their heads and sneer;
let the timid and the cautious hold back for a season in doubt.
Truth, eternal truth, must be our motto. The more we dive
into the subject, the more shall we have to learn; the more
the science is practised and employed, the more will the
philanthropist have reason to rejoice at the virtues of the
discovery :— and the more will the humble and thankful
Christian be enabled to exclaim, " It is the gift of a merciful
and allwise God!"

CHAP V.

DANGERS OF MESMERISM, PHYSICAL AND MORAL.—DANGER OF MESMER-
ISING THE HEALTHY FOR AMUSEMENT.—CALMNESS, A QUALIFICATION
FOR A MESMERISER.—DANGER FROM IMPERFECT WAKING.—CROSS-
MESMERISM.—OBJECTIONS ON THE GROUND OF MORALITY ANSWERED.
—RULES FOR MESMERISING.—ATTACHMENT TO MESMERISER,—WHAT
IT IS.—"HORROR" OF MESMERISM.—DIFFICULTIES OF MESMERISM.
—HINT FOR YOUNGER MEMBERS OF THE FACULTY.

BUT we have another and a third class of opponents, widely
different indeed in the quality of their objections from either of
the two parties with whom we have been hitherto contending,
whose antipathy to Mesmerism professes to arise from a consideration of its *dangers*. It is not on the irreligious character
of Mesmerism that they dwell; at that view of the question
they shrug their shoulders and sneer, as if they themselves had
never advanced it. It is not that they are unbelievers in
Mesmerism : the facts brought home to their knowledge are so
staggering, that they are ashamed to remember that they ever
had their doubts. It is of the *dangers* of Mesmerism that they
now speak: "It is so fearful a power," they say,—"so liable
to be abused,—so pregnant with mischief,—no one is safe,—
no one can answer for what may happen,—its practice ought
to be prohibited :"—and all this is gravely stated by those with
whom, but a few weeks before, we had been fighting, *totis
viribus*, in assertion of its reality.

Deleuze, in his practical work, says, "The antagonists of
magnetism, after having decided that it did not exist, have
declaimed against the dangers that accompany it."[*] Every
Mesmeriser will confirm this statement from his own experience.

[*] " Les antagonistes du magnétisme, après avoir prononcé qu'il n'existe
pas, ont déclamé contre les dangers qui l'accompagnent."—DELEUZE, *Instruction P.*, p. 265.

It has happened to all of us, over and over again. I was on a visit with some friends last summer, whom I in vain endeavoured to convince of the truths of Mesmerism; an incredulous but polite smile settled on their faces: so perceiving that the subject was unwelcome, I passed on to another topic. I met them again in the course of two months. It was now their turn to begin: they were full of the subject: but it was altogether of its dangers that they now harangued. "Dangerous!" I calmly observed, — "you surprise me: how can a thing that does not exist be dangerous?" "Oh," was the reply, "*everybody knows that there is something in Mesmerism, and it is so very dangerous.*"

The transition of these views on Mesmerism is as abrupt as Napoleon described the passage to be of the sublime to the ridiculous: "it is but a step." Extremes, in fact, are always meeting. One day there is nothing in Mesmerism: the next, a great deal too much.[*]

The first French commissioners, whose Report is supposed to prove the non-existence of Mesmerism, also speak of its dangers, and decide positively that its effects may be most serious. A novice in the first elements of logic would see, that a thing that does not exist, can be neither useful nor dangerous; and hence we derive an additional corroboration, that it was not the purpose of the commissioners to do more than disprove the theory of the fluid.

That Mesmerism has its dangers must be admitted: what good is there in nature free from some attendant evil? what is there that folly or wickedness may not abuse? Still I am persuaded that the actual amount of these dangers is very greatly exaggerated. The invisibility of the agent, our ignorance of the true springs of man's organisation, the novelty of

* Dr. Gregory, Professor of Chemistry in the University of Edinburgh, whose strong conviction of the truth of Mesmerism is such a triumph to the cause, says, in his admirable pamphlet on the *Scientific Spirit in which the claims of Mesmerism ought to be examined,* "We cannot fear the perversion of that, the existence of which we deny. If, therefore, Mesmerism be altogether the result of fraud and imposture, these evil consequences must be imaginary." p. 11. — (Neil, Edinburgh.) Every student of Mesmerism should read this unanswerable paper.

the remedy, and our natural timidity at the employment of a new mysterious treatment, all these circumstances would cast a deeper shade of colouring over that danger which may really exist: — but having taken much pains to examine the subject, and discussed it often with some of the most experienced Mesmerisers, I feel assured that the apprehensions generally entertained are to a great degree without foundation. Still it must be owned that Mesmerism has its dangers: and as a work that professes to meet all the popular objections would be incomplete without some allusion to them, — we will state what they are, and how they may be met.

The dangers may be divided into the physical and the moral.

I would begin, however, with the remark, that Mesmerism is not a plaything for the idle and the curious. It is not meant as a pastime for a dull day in the country. Because a sharp frost has set in; and the hounds cannot meet at cover, or a deluge of rain has imprisoned the listless sportsmen, and the young squire, to kill the dreary morning, tries his hand in the new art, and mesmerises his sisters or their lady's-maid, and something unpleasant occurs, is that to be laid to the door of Mesmerism?[*] It would appear from certain anecdotes, that animal magnetism is to supply the place of some of these old Christmas amusements, of which our altered habits have destroyed the charm; and thus "philosophy in sport" is to become really a part of an evening's entertainment. How absurd and monstrous all this is! And then grave ladies very naturally look solemn and forbidding, and make a few not unreasonable remarks on the impropriety of Mesmeric experiments. But who would think of vaccinating a whole family for a little domestic diversion? who dreams of insinuating the lancet's point into the arm of some plethoric uncle, to see how the good gentleman would feel after a little festive depletion? And why is Mesmerism to be an exception to every rule of conduct on such a subject? As Mr. Colquhoun observes most judiciously, "In attempting to produce the magnetic phenomena, I would eminently caution individuals against all experiments of

* Many of my readers may have heard within their own circles somewhat similar stories to those referred to in the text.

mere curiosity. Whatever ludicrous ideas many persons may
have been hitherto in the habit of associating with this subject,
I can seriously assure them that experience has proved magnetism to be no trifling matter. . . . . We must not recklessly
attempt to handle the thunderbolt, or to play with the lightning
of heaven. Like every higher gift conferred upon us by the
Creator, the magnetic faculty ought to be exerted with judgment and discretion, and *only for benevolent purposes*."* "We
do not know," says Dr. Hufeland, "either the essence or the
limits of this astonishing power: whoever, then, undertakes to
direct this power, let him enter upon the duty with the most
profound respect for the principle which he endeavours to set
in operation. Above all, *let him beware of Magnetising in
sport.* In medicine, the most indifferent remedy is injurious to
persons in health; still more so an agent which is perhaps the
most active and energetic of all remedies." All these observations deserve serious attention: I would say even further, that
everything of a useless or jocose character connected with the
practice should be discountenanced in the strongest way: children should be especially warned against "playing at Mesmerism:" and if the above is what is meant by the opponents
of magnetism in their remarks upon its dangerous consequences, I agree with them most cordially,—and have always
done my utmost within my own circle to discourage such improper and discreditable trifling.

As it is, however, especially desirable to discourage in the
strongest way the practice of Mesmerism, for mere amusement,
a few more extracts from other writers are here added.

Dr. Elliotson says, "when persons inquire of me, whether
Mesmerism is not a dangerous thing, I always reply, that I
am happy to say it is. They look astonished, and I continue,
—because, if it were not dangerous, it would not be a real
power in nature. A nonentity, an unreal, though alleged,
power of nature can do no harm: but all real powers of nature
will work readily for evil if misapplied. The lights in our
houses, the fires which warm us, the heat, without which we

* Isis Revelata, vol. ii. p. 188.

could not exist and all living beings would be a dead frozen
mass, may burn up our bodies to a cinder, may destroy our
property, nay, whole cities, yet we take a candle to go to bed,
and we light fires in our rooms. The knives at our tables
could be plunged into our breast by the person who sits next
us, or by the servant behind our chair: yet our tables are
spread daily with knives. Mesmerism may be abused like anything else: like medicine, used through design or ignorance,
as a poison, or in too violent a manner, and like the surgeon's
wounding instruments plunged unskilfully into parts, and, perhaps, making fatal havoc."*

Dr. Elliotson then mentions three rather serious cases, which
had lately come to his knowledge, to "prove the danger of
playing with Mesmerism, and at the same time to show to those
who regard it as nothing, that it is something."

Dr. Esdaile also says, " *Experimenting on the healthy ought
to be discouraged,* as it is only undermining healthy constitutions for no possible advantage. The artificial disease is not
so light or transitory a matter as it seems to be reckoned by
many Mesmerisers, who go about upsetting the nerves of every
one they can lay their hands on. * * * It is proper that ladies
and gentlemen, who beg to be mesmerised for fun, should know
this; and then they will probably choose some other kind of
amusement."†

Upon the impropriety of mesmerising *persons in health,*
Dr. Esdaile says elsewhere, "People say to me, 'I should like
to ascertain if I can be mesmerised: do try.' I reply, 'you
very probably cannot; and I should as soon comply with your
desire to feel the effects of opium as mesmerise you without a
cause: when you need it, you will probably be benefited by
it.' If Mesmerism be forced upon a person in a state of
health, it is very likely to do mischief;—for any attempt to be
better than 'well,' is pretty sure to make one ill."‡

Dr. Bell, who in 1792 wrote a treatise on Magnetism, says
"I would never advise a trial to put people, who are in good

* Zoist, vol. iv. p. 388. Article " Mesmerism not to be trifled with."
† Esdaile's " Mesmerism in India," p. 246.
‡ Ibid., p. 12.

o 8

health, into a crisis to please others; for you may put them in a state of catalepsy or epilepsy." * * * "Power united with ignorance is like a loaded pistol in the hands of a child." *

Teste also states it as his opinion that it is "probably not *devoid of danger* to magnetise an individual in *perfect health.*"†

This part of the subject, then, I at once dismiss as foreign to the question. The abuse of a power is no argument against its use: and because Mesmerism is not a fit game for foolish girls to play with, this is no reason why it should be pre-eminently hazardous, when adopted seriously as a remedial art.

Still, even in this line, Mesmerism may have its dangers, especially when practised by the ignorant and the timid. A nervous Mesmeriser is worse than a nervous patient. The calm collected manner of the judicious Magnetist will soothe the most agitated sleeper; but even the tranquil repose of the deepest slumber may be disturbed by a sympathy with a frightened and unpractised manipulator. But what is there strange or unusual in this? why are not experience and competency equally necessary in Mesmerism, as in everything else? who employs a raw surgeon for a formidable operation? who sends for an untried dentist to extract a difficult and decayed eye-tooth? Skill, practice, knowledge, are qualifications that are requisite in every department; and in no treatment are coolness and presence of mind more essential than in the direction of the Mesmeric power; a fact which ought to be evident to all when they reflect that this agent "penetrates the depths of the organism and the internal life of the nervous system, and may even affect the mind itself, and unsettle its ordinary relations." This is the language of the great Dr. Hufeland himself, in the cautions that he gives to the unwary Magnetiser. But even with the drawback of inexperience and ignorance, I know not that Mesmerism is so dangerous as much of the common medical practice of the present day. When we remember that such tremendous poisons as prussic acid and arsenic are among the favourite remedies of the modern school; that our lives are at the mercy of an incautious physician in

* Bell on " Animal Electricity," p. 19. This is now a scarce book.
† Teste, translated by Spillan, p. 250.

the first act of prescribing; that an error in weight of the deadly ingredient may alter the whole character of the compound; that a careless chemist may convert the most judicious prescription into a draught of death; that a sleepy nurse may administer the wrong medicine;—who can think of these and similar contingencies, and not tremble when he sees the physician with the pen in his hand? * These things are mentioned, —not to prove that Mesmerism has not its dangers;—but to show the timid and unthinking opponent that the very system to which from custom he steadily adheres, has its evils and its hazards also, perhaps even greater than those of our ill-understood art.

Still Mesmerism has its dangers.† Among them I would more especially mention those that may arise out of the alarm of an inexperienced practitioner. If a change quite unexpected should take place in the sleeper, — if the trance should be prolonged to an unusual duration, — if convulsions, or fits, or violent pain (all ‡, in every probability, symptoms of the desired action) should come on,—the inexpert Mesmeriser might take fright; his fright would act sympathetically upon the sleeper; great excitement and agitation would be the result; this again would react on the Mesmeriser; till, from the mutual effect on each, very serious consequences might be produced. The health of the patient might be affected most alarmingly: but all this would be the fault, not of Mesmerism, —but of the

* Mr. Colquhoun, in his Preface to Wienholt, observes, " Opium, arsenic, foxglove, mercury, prussic acid, &c., are exceedingly dangerous things; yet these are publicly sold in all our apothecaries' shops, and are daily used in the ordinary medical practice. It is part of the object of animal magnetism to supersede the use of these dangerous drugs, by introducing a milder and no less efficacious mode of treatment. ' Thousands,' said Dr. Franklin, ' are slaughtered in the quiet sick room.'" (p. 17.)

† Teste, speaking of the dangers of Mesmerism, which he thinks are very serious, observes, that it seems "as if the best things should have their counterbalance in the dangers which their use brings with it." (p. 297.)

‡ Inexperienced Mesmerisers are apt to be alarmed, instead of encouraged, by the appearance of the symptoms alluded to in the text. Gauthier, in describing favourable signs of Mesmeric action, says, " it accelerates the progress of maladies, —brings out old pains, hastens on a crisis which is to produce the cure, and proves its remedial power by ceasing to produce results after that the patient is restored to health."— Traité Pratique, p. 6.

ignorant nervous operator, who had undertaken a duty for which he was not prepared.

In all these emergencies, the calm [*] judicious Mesmeriser sees nothing to fear: he knows that the most violent hysteric action is often the sign of a welcome crisis;—he knows that the most prolonged sleep—a sleep even of days—will wear itself out at last; he knows that the most threatening language and aspect of the sleep-waker (like that of a person in a deranged condition) can be best met by coolness and kindness: he is consequently firm, collected, gentle; his calmness and firmness act healthily on the patient; and, however great may have been the excitement of the Mesmeric state, the patient is sure to awake out of his slumbers refreshed and strengthened, with the mind beautifully composed, and the whole system renovated to an extraordinary degree.[†]

It is here not unadvisable to give a caution by the way. If the sleeper cannot be awakened by the usual methods, and the uneasiness of the Mesmeriser has acted with an unpleasant or exciting effect, to *send for a medical man*, who disbelieves in the science, and would treat it as a common normal state, *might be followed by the most serious consequences.* I cannot impress my readers too strongly with the necessity of bearing this caution in mind. Calmness and patience would bring all round.[‡]

---

[*] Gauthier says, " Calmness is one of the first qualities for magnetising. With a Mesmeriser, who retains his *sang-froid* and presence of mind, the invalid will always come out of a crisis, that nature or the disease brings on, successfully." (p. 22.)

[†] I was myself present on an occasion when the alarms of the Mesmeriser at the prolonged sleep of a patient produced most embarrassing and prejudicial effects. Fortunately, I was able to take the case in hand, and all terminated favourably. My composure composed the agitated sleeper. The only cause for fear arose from the fears of the Mesmeriser.—The Abbé J. B. L. mentions a case, where an incautious proceeding seriously disturbed the sleeper. " I changed my action,"—the Mesmeriser narrates, —" I made my passes more slowly, more calmly, and more *gently*, and an expression of happiness soon spread itself over the countenance of the sufferer." (p. 100.)

[‡] In *Zoist*, vol. iv. p. 404, is an instance of mischief arising from calling in a medical man, who was an unbeliever. Gauthier says, " *Whatever may be the crisis*, be not alarmed: if you will but wait *patiently and calmly*, nothing evil can or will happen to the sick person." (p. 214.)

Another point on which inexperience may be thrown off its guard, and through which very formidable results might arise, is the danger of an imperfect partial waking. With some patients it is not always easy to distinguish at first the half state from full and restored consciousness: the patient seems perfectly awakened, and says he is so; and the unpractised operator would be apt to leave him. This is a condition of real danger: the patient has no more self-control, or management of his actions, than a child or idiot, and yet for a time will converse most sensibly, and recognise every person present. I have seen this distinctly in two patients. It happened to me one time with Anne Vials, whom I could not manage thoroughly to awaken: she said she was awake; and she walked about the room, and ate and talked as usual. I was on the point of leaving her, being persuaded that she was awake, when the sound of something peculiar in her voice caught my ear; I recognised it to be the tone of the sleeping, and not the waking state (for the tones are often different); and I soon had reason to discover that she was not awakened. The French call this state " un somnambulisme imparfait." Townshend, in his " Facts," mentions a case of the kind. It is not uncommon, and should be watched; as the patient might commit some action, serious in its consequences not only to himself but to others. [*]

Cross-Mesmerism, which means the influence of two or more Mesmerisers or persons at one and the same time, is also a condition that the inexperienced Magnetist should be taught to avoid. To some patients, indeed, the effect is only disturbing and inconvenient; but with the very sensitive it is occasionally followed by serious results; with a large number, however, there is not apparently any adverse action,—and they seem indifferent under the operation.

Cross-Mesmerism is of two kinds. The first occurs when

---

[*] See Townshend's " Facts," p. 75.—Deleuze says, " At the close of every sitting, be careful to arouse the patient thoroughly, so that he do not remain in an *intermediate state* between sleeping and waking." (*Instruction Pratique*, p. 293.) Dr. Elliotson says, " She had not been fully awakened; and too much care cannot be taken to see that patients are perfectly awake before they are left."—*Zoist*, vol. i. p. 311.

the patient is actually asleep. Among his other excellent rules, Deleuze says, "Never suffer your patient while asleep to be touched by any one who is not *en rapport* with him; neither place him *en rapport* with another, unless it be to do him some good, or that he desires it." (p. 291.) Gauthier says, "Watch carefully that no stranger meddles in your treatment without your permission; and never allow him to touch your patients." (p. 347.)

The last writer gives a valuable caution to the Magnetist regarding the vulgar curiosity of the impertinent sceptic;—for, on the subject of Mesmerism, it must be ever borne in mind, that our opponents often consider themselves as set free from the usual courtesies of society, and at liberty to play what experimental tricks they please,—not reflecting that their tests for the detection of the untrue are being tried on the *sick*. "The brutal assault," narrated by Miss Martineau, (p. 85 of her Letters), has been already quoted, where a "gentleman violated the first rule of Mesmeric practice, by suddenly and violently seizing the sleeper's arm, and shouting out that the house was on fire." And I myself experienced something of the 'same kind, whilst mesmerising Anne Vials, though not of quite so outrageous a nature. In both these cases, however, it may be as well to add that the attacks "entirely failed"; the patients heard nothing, and saw nothing, and proved the truthfulness of their condition. But this was fortunately owing to their own insensibility or indifference to foreign influence, rather than to the delicacy of the gentle philosophers.

Gauthier, therefore, says, "If you absent yourself an instant,— if you turn your back even for a moment, you may be sure that these men (sceptics, medical or otherwise,) will not have sufficient command over themselves to restrain their curiosity, when they know that they are about to impress an influence on the patient. You ought never, therefore, to omit full caution with them. Human nature never changes; and scepticism and curiosity in all times produce the same fruits."[*]

Dr. Ashburner says, "I have repeatedly witnessed such bad effects from cross-mesmerism, that I cannot too strongly warn

* Gauthier: Traité Pratique, p. 358.

ignorant and rash persons from practising it. Some foolhardy Irish surgeons have, it is said, incurred an awful responsibility, by each, within a few hours, mesmerising a poor nervous girl." Dr. A. mentions a patient of his own, who, on one occasion when cross-mesmerised, slept eleven hours, and awoke with an intense headache."[*]

Dr. Elliotson says, "We ought carefully to ascertain, not only that the patient may be left by us, but that he can allow the presence or proximity of another. If he cannot, and we leave him asleep in the charge of some one, *great mischief may be occasioned*."[†]

In the People's Phrenological Journal, No. 42., a serious case of cross-mesmerism is narrated by Mr. Holmes, in which a state of delirium was induced, that did not perfectly pass away till after the expiration of four or five nights.

The second sort of cross-mesmerism occurs, when the patient is not actually asleep, but under magnetic treatment, and the original Mesmeriser, not being able to attend, sends a substitute in his place, with whom the physical peculiarities of the sick party do not sympathise. This is not uncommon. Experience shows, that it is not every Mesmeriser that primarily suits every patient; and still less so, after that the treatment has once set in. The sensitive temperament of the patient is then delicately alive to a change in the influence that is imparted; much distress is exhibited; and the progress of the cure may be even retarded, and perhaps a relapse occasioned,—at any rate, great disturbance caused to the whole system. Caution, therefore, is requisite, if the friendly aid of a second Mesmeriser be called in; though, at the same time, I am inclined to believe, that, with the majority of patients, no prejudicial effects would be visible.

Several other minor points might be mentioned, such as the danger of mesmerising upwards,—the danger of discontinuing a treatment in certain cases, &c., for information on which I

* Letter from Dr. Ashburner to Dr. Elliotson in Zoist, No. 14. The letters of this accomplished and experienced friend to Mesmerism are full of curious and suggestive matter.
† Zoist, No. 14. p. 473.

would refer the reader to Gauthier[*], and to the eighth chapter of the "Practical Instruction" of Deleuze, a most useful book for the young Mesmeriser.

Still I repeat that the physical dangers of Mesmerism are very greatly exaggerated; and I would conclude this part of the subject with a noticeable fact: that in spite of the number of ignorant Mesmerisers that are taking up the subject,—in spite of the number of most delicate patients that have been placed under its influence,—in spite of the number of opponents that are anxiously on the look-out for a disastrous result,—no well-authenticated fact of great and serious mischief has yet been named. I rather wonder that it is so; Mesmerism must, like everything else, have its drawbacks and its dangers. Still nothing very formidable has yet been publicly mentioned: now and then we read in the newspapers of a "fatal effect;" but in a few days we find a paragraph saying that the patient is better than ever. Now and then we hear in our own circle of something deplorable, which, on examination, proves to be a mistake. I was told the other day of a gentleman who had greatly injured the eyesight of one of his children by Mesmerism. I called and asked if it were true: he had never even mesmerised one of his children; and nothing had been the matter with their eyes. And thus it generally is; and several friends who have taken some pains to make the inquiry have never yet been able to establish one case of serious injury or evil: still my opinion is, that Mesmerism has its dangers, and some, too, of rather an anxious kind. I say, therefore, to the inexperienced Mesmeriser,—"Be cautious, be circumspect; you are playing with a powerful and ill-understood agent; and you are bound for the sake of the patient's safety to adopt every precaution that prudence can suggest."[†]

But there are certain dangers touching la morale to which Mesmerism is supposed to be peculiarly open, and respecting which allusion is often made in conversation. Much ignorance

[*] Gauthier, p. 351, &c.
[†] "I never heard," says Miss Martineau, "of any harm being done by it where as much prudence was employed as we apply in the use of fire, water, and food."—Letters, p. 82.

also exists on this point; and here, too, it is necessary to distinguish clearly as to what is intended by the charge.

If it is meant, that under the pretext of mesmerising, in a case where Mesmerism is not required, parties can avail themselves of the occasion to commit an offence contre les bonnes mœurs, I am not careful to enter upon the objection. Men sometimes go to church from the most improper motives; men sometimes read the Scriptures with no other view than that of finding food for ribaldry and unbelief; still, as has been often said, who would shut up our churches or burn our Bibles on that account? Again, we say the abuse of a thing proves nothing against its value. If parties, in sport or in thoughtlessness, throw themselves into the power of an unprincipled acquaintance, with them lies the fault, and they must take the consequences. Still I have my doubts whether Mesmerism does afford the easy opening for misconduct, with which it has been taxed. The deep sleep, or torpor, which would place the sleeper so completely at the mercy of the Mesmeriser, as to give an opportunity for evil, does not occur every day;—and more generally, if not always, the Mesmeric state produces, on the part of the patients, such a high tone of spirituality, and sense of right, as to make them less than ever disposed to an acquiescence in what is wrong.[*]

Still, into this view of the question I do not enter. Our question is, whether, in the treatment of the sick, and in regarding Mesmerism as a serious remedy, the influence be open to objections on the score of morality[†] and les bienséances? I

[*] Mr. Pyne says truly in his excellent little work: "If a magnetised person is in the earlier states of coma, the mind is as sufficiently active to repress evil as it is in ordinary circumstances:—if in the higher condition of sleep-waking, its impressions are withdrawn from the senses,—the judgment is refined,—and, in short, the soul is in a condition of the highest morality."—Vital Magnetism, by Rev. T. Pyne, p. 59.
[†] We must not forget that the practice of Inoculation was equally called "immoral" in its earlier days. "I have shown," says the Rev. T. Dalaber, "that inoculation is absolutely inconsistent with the virtue of our minds, and the rights of our fellow-creatures;—" "I have shown the manifold immorality, and undoubted iniquity of this device;—" "—that it exposes the soul to more important peril than what men dread from the disease,"—and so on for several pages. (p. 86.)—Inoculation, an Indefensible Practice, a pamphlet published in 1754.

answer, in the most unhesitating way, to no objections whatsoever. In Mesmerism, as in everything else, certain precautions and regulations are, of course, to be adopted; and in default of those precautions, why is the science to be blamed for the neglect of its own rules? Who sends for a low pettifogging attorney to make his will, or conduct an important lawsuit? who deposits his money with a banker that offers ten per cent. interest with no visible capital at command? who admits an unprincipled physician into his house? Only let similar safeguards be employed in Mesmerism; and nothing need be feared. Not only should the Mesmeriser be a person of character, of known and established principle; but even then it is the rule that the process should be conducted in the presence of a third party. All Mesmerisers require an attention to this rule where it can be observed. Patients have it in their power to have any of their relations present when they like.— Let this regulation be remembered and carried out; and where is the objection? Not only is every needful security obtained by this course, but "the appearance, even, of evil" is avoided; and the good work cannot be ill-spoken of, or misrepresented by the malicious neighbour or the *candid friend*.

Deleuze and Gauthier both urge the importance of the patient having a relative or friend present. Mr. Newnham says, "It is a standing rule with medical men that, on certain occasions, the presence of a female friend is requested, as a guarantee, &c.,—and therefore in the process of Magnetism, the same medical men would require the presence of some friend of the patient,—male or female, as might be more agreeable, &c. And thus," he adds, "ends the dreaded moral evil, which we have thought it necessary to combat in detail, because it is one of the most favourite weapons employed by the enemy."[*]

* Human Magnetism, p. 117. The opinion of Mr. Newnham, as an experienced surgeon, is especially deserving of attention on this head. He says elsewhere, "Magnetism confers no power of mischief, which was not previously attainable by other means, in the hands of wicked persons, especially through the instrumentality of opium, and who ever thought of opposing the exhibition of opium by medical men, for the cure of disease?" (p. 115.)

Another objection is, that even in the presence of a third party the process is one *qui blesse les convenances*; and that the treatment is what a father or brother would feel a pain in witnessing. Never was there a more unfounded mistake. I have seen a good deal of Mesmerism, and with different Mesmerisers; and never observed anything to which the most scrupulous delicacy could object. An evil-disposed chemist may administer a valuable drug in an improper way, and with an improper object;—but what argument is that against the drug? Choose a Mesmeriser of character, and choose a confidential friend or relative for a witness, and you have every guarantee that the management of the case will be such as the most fastidious would require.[*]

Another objection is, that the sleeper is placed in an undesirable state of feeling in regard to the Mesmeriser; that there is an attraction towards him, something amounting to affection, or even love; and that this state of mind or feeling reduces the patient to an improper dependence on the will of another. That, in the Mesmeric state, the sympathy between the Mesmeriser and the sleeper is powerful and extraordinary, we all know; it is one of the most curious phenomena.[†] The sensibility, that is then produced, is singular in the extreme. But the feeling is rather that which exists between two sisters than anything else; it is a feeling which has regard to the happiness, and the state of moral being of the Mesmeriser; which is alive to injuries or pain inflicted on him; which *desires his well-being here and hereafter*. Dr. Elliotson observes, in one of his most interesting papers, that "the Mesmeric state has,

* Mr. Colquhoun observes, "To those who knew and have witnessed the processes, the ludicrous falsehood of the objection must be perfectly apparent. Indeed, there is much less indecency and much more delicacy, than in the ordinary medical practice." (*Preface to Wienholt*, p. 15.) Mr. Newnham has also completely refuted this foolish prejudice and objection. (p. 113.)

† Professor Gregory, in the excellent pamphlet before quoted, says, "With regard to the influence of the Mesmeriser over his patient, in some cases it appears to be great, in others limited, in others again it is absent. The abuse of this power can only be dreaded by those who admit its existence, and there is no reason to suppose that it is more liable to abuse than other powers or agencies, none of which are exempt from the liability to abuse. The best security, in all such cases, is not *ignorance but knowledge*." (p. 11.)

even if characterised by affection, nothing sexual in it;—but is of the purest kind, simple friendship, and indeed exactly like the love of a young child to its mother,—for it seems characterised by a feeling of safety when with the Mesmeriser and of fear of others."* In some cases, I should say that the feeling rather resembled the not uncommon regard that is entertained towards a successful medical friend. There is, for instance, gratitude for pain removed, in accomplishing which the Mesmeriser has been the humble instrument;—there is the pleasure of seeing one, who has been kind and useful;—there is admiration for his benevolence and active virtues:—but that the attachment goes beyond this,—or what Dr. Elliotson describes, —is assuredly a mistake. Nay, as was before remarked, so far from the Mesmeric sleep producing a state of feeling inconsistent with what is right, it is considered by the most experienced operators, that a great increase of the moral perceptions is created and brought out; and that if the Mesmeriser were capable of commanding an improper or reprehensible act, the patient would revolt from an obedience to his will, with a language and manner even more decided and peremptory than when in a waking state. Puységur in his Mémoires (p. 168.), and Deleuze in his Letter to Dr. Billot (Billot's works, vol. ii. p. 34.), both give some remarkable and most interesting instances, in exemplification of this truth. Their facts are really beautiful illustrations of what Mr. Townshend says, viz., that "the state of Mesmeric sleep-waking is a rise in man's nature; —that the mind, separated then from the senses, appears to gain juster notions, and to be lifted nearer to the fountain of all good and of all truth." (p. 113.) Foissac states the same thing. And from what I have myself seen of the increase and development of the *intellectual* faculties during the sleep, I am quite prepared to believe in the existence of that *exaltation of the moral being*, which the best authorities have described as so invariable. Be this, however, as it may,—and be the relation between the Mesmeriser and the patient however peculiar,

* *Zoist*, vol. iii. p. 55. See also Mr. Newnham's *Magnetism*, p. 115, where this subject is examined.

the whole sympathy and attraction are at an end and forgotten the moment the sleeper is awakened into actual existence.*

Another objection is the facility with which unconscious parties can be put to sleep against their will. It is said, that "no one is safe,—no one can feel sure as to what may happen, and that a powerful Mesmeriser has his whole acquaintance under his command." This is a view entertained among the nervous and the timid;—but one more groundless can hardly be mentioned. Except in certain most rare cases of extreme sensibility, the Mesmeric sleep could not be induced against the will or consciousness of the party mesmerised. Certain conditions are requisite. Silence and stillness are among the most indispensable. It may often require half an hour of the most profound repose, before any somnolency can be obtained; and with many patients the Mesmeric action must be renewed for several days in succession before any effect be procured. The whole objection, therefore, is so absurd, that no notice of it would be necessary, were it not that the opinion on this point is so very universal, and one that has led the superstitious to their worst apprehensions against the science.†

Somewhat akin to the last objection is another class of feelings that should not be passed over; I mean a vague undefined "horror" of Mesmerism generally, a mysterious dislike to it,— an opposition which the party objecting would find difficult to put into a tangible shape, but which yet fills the mind with an unpleasant sensation respecting it. This is distinct from an opinion of its irreligious or Satanic character: without adopting that view of the subject, many persons regard Mesmerism with an indistinct and painful abhorrence. Here, again, we must distinguish and clearly understand what they *do* dislike. If

* "The remains of sleep soon went off, and the feeling then completely subsided." (*Zoist*, vol. iii. p. 55.) In respect to this feeling of affection or gratitude, whichever it be, Dr. Foissac says, that he had "never perceived any difference between the patients he had been fortunate enough to cure,— whether by medicine or Mesmerism." The feeling was equal under both treatments.—*Rapport*, p. 390.

† Even if the above charge were, in some degree, true, what comparison would there yet be with the tremendous powers at the command of chloroform? The facilities for evil, that may arise out of that otherwise inestimable discovery, are most formidable to contemplate.

they dislike the abuses to which the practice is liable, if they dislike to see it made the subject for trick and foolish experiment,—we can inform them that all right-minded Mesmerisers participate strongly in their feelings, and hold such conduct as most revolting and wicked. But if they dislike to see a racking pain removed by it,—to see the feverish sleepless invalid enjoying a balmy slumber by its aid,—to see the nervous excited patient restored to comfort and repose,—surely their feelings can only arise from prejudice, or rather from the novelty and freshness of the art. It is nothing else than what is even yet experienced among the uneducated classes respecting vaccination. Large numbers entertain a "horror" of this remedy. How often has the wife of a labouring-man told me that she would not have her child infected with the disease of a cow! It is objectionable to her, only because it is strange. And so is it with the present aversion to Mesmerism. Habit and observation will soon remove this feeling. The strangeness will pass away. People will soon perceive what a simple, easy, and natural process Mesmerism is; and when, day after day, they shall be privileged to witness some dear and beloved relative relieved or comforted by its means,—or when they themselves, after the agonies of pain, shall have found a respite or a cure,—their horror will soon be turned into gratitude to the Author of all good, and with myself they will exclaim that Mesmerism is the gift of God!

But though the dangers of Mesmerism have been magnified into an importance which they do not deserve, and which, for the most part, could be avoided by prudence, still our science has its difficulties. These difficulties somewhat arise from the infancy of the practice, and which the experience of a few years will tend to diminish; still they are considerable. It is easy to say to some unhappy sufferer, whom all the usual methods of the healing art have failed to benefit, "Go and be mesmerised,"—the difficulty is to find a Mesmeriser.* They

* The simplest and easiest remedy for meeting the above difficulty is for the healthy members of a family to mesmerise the sick ones. This plan would also silence many of the previous objections. Fathers and mothers, husbands and wives, brothers and sisters, should respectively employ mesmerism as the domestic "medicine of nature."—And to assist them in the process, instruction is given in the concluding Chapter.

are not so easily obtained. Added to which the treatment of a chronic case generally demands a sacrifice of time, which, even if men have the inclination, they have not always the leisure, to bestow. Experience and knowledge are also indispensable: I should be sorry to place a very delicate patient into the hands of an unpractised Mesmeriser. Temper, patience, and presence of mind, are also requisites; and as we before stated, character and right principle must not be forgotten. Here then are a number of qualities desirable for the formation of a competent Mesmeriser, and which are not to be procured at a moment's warning. And this, for the present, throws a difficulty in the work. It retards its course of more extended usefulness. Still time will correct this inconvenience. What the public demands, the public will always find provided ere long. As there is every certainty that Mesmerism will shortly take its rank among the established branches of the medical art, a supply of qualified practitioners will be soon forthcoming. Our difficulties are but temporary. Many junior members of the profession will devote themselves to the study, and obtain a standing in society by their experience and success. Others, whose time is less at their command, will only give a general superintendence; while the actual treatment will be conducted by pupils, specially instructed for the work. Nurses will be taught to mesmerise. Students in the hospitals will gradually bring themselves into notice by a useful exercise of their power; and when the drag-chain, which hinders the progress of the good cause, shall be removed by the retirement of the present Lecturers and Managers, these invaluable public institutions will become, at the very request of the subscribers, schools for the practice of the Mesmeric science. In short, everything looks fair and promising. Our obstacles are abating every day. Prejudice is becoming more and more silent. Fanaticism is retiring to a few select quarters. Ridicule is losing the sharpness of its edge. The timid begin to speak. The opponents display greater anger and abuse. A general interest is awakened. We have evidently reached a crisis. Our difficulties have been long and many: but

"Time and the hour run through the roughest day!"

L 2

CHAP. VI.

OPPOSITION TO MESMERISM FROM ITS PRESUMED MIRACULOUS ASPECT.—SECRET APPREHENSION OF THE CHRISTIAN.—GERMAN RATIONALISM.—NEW SCHOOL OF INFIDELITY ON THE DOCTRINE OF NATURE.—SALVERTE'S "OCCULT SCIENCES."—AMERICAN "REVELATIONS."—"CHARLOTTE ELIZABETH" AND MR. CLOSE ON MIRACLES AND MESMERISM.—DR. ARNOLD'S OPINION.—THE MESMERIC CURES AND THE MIRACLES OF THE NEW TESTAMENT COMPARED.—TOUCH OF THE MESMERIZERS.—WHY DID MIRACLES, IF MESMERIC, CEASE?—ARGUMENT FROM ARCHBISHOP OF DUBLIN.—MESMERIC PREDICTIONS.—CLAIRVOYANCE NOT MIRACULOUS.

BUT a more anxious consideration remains behind. The very truthfulness of Mesmerism carries along with it a perplexing apprehension. Its dangers may be proved in great measure chimerical;—its difficulties may be surmounted;—its curative powers may be admitted in all their magnitude;—the charge of an evil agency may be rejected as the product of that heated fancy which invades the mind at the appearance of novelty;—and yet well-regulated minds may approach the discussion with a distressing reluctance. Another argument presents itself. The subject appears to trench on the most sacred ground. It threatens to work a revolution in the most awful questions that can interest man. It unsettles the very groundwork of his faith. Such extraordinary statements are advanced,—such unexpected laws are developed in nature,—such mysterious facts are given,—that old accustomed principles of belief are shaken to their centre, and the piety of the Christian trembles for the result. A startling consequence is at hand. If the facts of Mesmerism be not miraculous,—if they be no otherwise marvellous than as their strangeness makes them so, and if custom will soon reduce this marvellous-

ness to an every-day occurrence,—how do all these positions bear upon the miracles related in Scripture? Are we not lowering their value? Is not the very keystone, on which our faith is built, loosened, if not removed? If the course of nature be not suspended by the action of Mesmerism, how can we show that the wonders of old time must not fall back to the same shrunken proportions, and that the truths of Revelation do not totter at their base?[*]

This is no unreal charge wantonly thrust forward for controversial display, and creating the very evil it professes to deprecate;—but the expression of an actual living opinion which is beginning to assume a serious shape and being. It is no longer whispered in the *salons* of science that the tendencies of Mesmerism go to uphold the Deist in his unhappy belief, the proposition is triumphantly advanced in the publications of the infidel; and the Christian himself often feels an anxious misgiving which deters him from a bold investigation of the fact. The position has been strongly stated to me by the two opposite sects. "If," said a friend, "you really have faith in the reality of the wondrous cures of which you make mention,—do you not see the dangerous ground you are treading?—You cannot stop where you will. If I believe in Mesmerism, I must disbelieve all that I have hitherto held as sacred and divine." "Follow out your convictions," said a gentleman of the other school, "and flinch not at their consequence. The reputed miracles of Scripture were but the result of strong Mesmeric power. Christ only raised the dead by Mesmerism." And thus has it ever been in the history of the world. And thus has every new discovery been dreaded or vaunted, according to the respective point from which it has been viewed by the friends or adversaries of religion. Thus was it with astronomy,—with chemistry,—with geology,—with phrenology.—The Bible speaks of the rising of the sun; but Copernicus and Galileo were charged with upsetting the Bible, for they proved that the sun was the centre of its system, and

* I here cannot help quoting an admirable remark by Jacob Bryant, which I lately met with: "I never suffer what I do not know to disturb my belief in what I do."—*Observations on different Passages in Scripture.*

consequently did not rise to gladden the earth. The theory of another hemisphere was heretical for a season, and Columbus was in his turn taxed with weakening the validity of Scripture. Cuvier, in like manner, was treated as the antagonist of Moses: and Gall was accused of leading his followers to a belief in the coarsest materialism. And thus it went on for a season. Men trembled at the truth; and the truth itself lay hid behind the mists of a partial knowledge and discovery. Soon, however, a brighter state of things came on. Profounder researches dispelled the anxiety of the timid. Faith and science were not found incompatible. Revelation and matter had but one and the same divine original. The first of philosophers were among the humblest of Christians; and the most aspiring student of the laws of nature has not blushed to bow in lowliest adoration before the Word of Life. And thus will it be with Mesmerism. The discovery of this mighty power will form no exception to the other departments of science. He, who spake as never man spake, wrought also as man has never been able to imitate: and while the Scriptural reader must feel in his heart an internal evidence [a] of the truth of that book on which he places all his hopes, under the conviction that doctrines so pure, so lovely, could proceed from nothing short of a heavenly source, even so will he perceive in the miracles of his blessed Lord an inseparable pledge of the divinity of His mission, for that no one could do such things as Christ did, except God were with him!

The question of Scripture evidence, it has been before observed [b], has within these few years shifted ground. The charge of dishonesty, of exaggeration, or of falsehood, is now but seldom advanced against the Gospel Historians. The

[a] " In truth, however," observes the lamented Arnold, " the internal evidence in favour of the authenticity and genuineness of the Scriptures, is that on which the mind can rest with far greater satisfaction than on any external evidence, however valuable." * * * " It has been wonderfully ordered that the books, generally speaking, are their own witness." — Rugby Sermons, p. 252.

[b] See Preface to second edition, p. 7. " Christian Truth," says Dr. Hawkins, the present learned Provost of Oriel College, when speaking of the examination of the Christian Evidences, " is a subject ever new, and of the deepest interest to each individual man in each successive generation." — Bampton Lectures, p. 235.

Apostles are no longer described as either enthusiasts or impostors. The argument of Hume on the insufficiency of human testimony is thrown back into the shade. A new position is adopted by the adversary. The facts recorded in the New Testament are at once admitted, — the narrators are allowed to be truthful intelligent men, — but the wonders they relate are referred to the operation of an *adequate and natural cause*, — a cause of which the spectators at the time had not the remotest suspicion, — but which is amply sufficient to explain away the existence and effect of the seemingly miraculous. All that is needed, it is said, is to "separate the kernel of truth from the shell of opinion," and to trace in each individual case, the possible or probable foundation of fact.

The modern school of German Rationalism [*], no small or inconsiderable sect, invented and adopted this exposition. Everything that savours of the supernatural can, according to their views, be explained by some "rational" elucidation. Nothing needs be coarsely denied, or presumptuously disbelieved. Semler, a learned divine of the University of Halle, who died in 1791, and who, among other works, published an "Apparatus for a *liberal* interpretation of the New Testament," was the founder of this theory. Eichhorn, Professor of Theology in the University of Göttingen, who died in 1827, and was a voluminous writer, improved upon the notion. [†] But Paulus has, in our own days, been the favourite authority on the subject. He carried out the original idea with the most unexpected solutions. According to his ingenious system of unravelling a difficulty, some scientific, or philosophical, or natural cause was at the bottom of all those wondrous facts, which had hitherto confounded the cavillings of the sceptic, or compelled the obedience of the faithful. And his explanations were caught at with eagerness, and generally adopted. That carnal heart, which is so at enmity with everything of a divine character, applied the views of Paulus to the whole

[*] Occasionally this school of theology, i.e. those who account for all the miracles on natural principles, are called Neologians.

[†] One of Eichhorn's works on the subject was an Introduction to the New Testament, published at Leipsic, in 1814.

range of Scripture evidence, and built up a species of semi-Christianity. In the north of Germany, and in the Roman Catholic no less than in the Protestant churches, this rationalistic interpretation openly obtained. Disciples were soon found in France, in England, and in the United States of America, — as is seen by several publications on the subject.[*] And whilst for different classes of miracles different explanations were suggested, — for the miracles of healing and for some others of an analogous and corresponding character, Mesmerism was almost universally esteemed the natural and adequate solution.

As the language of other writers will bring these statements more clearly home to the apprehension of the reader, a few extracts from some recent works shall be now given in illustration.

In an article in the Edinburgh Review on Christian Evidence, — as late as October, 1847, — it is said, "in the case of the Scripture miracles, some have been led to adopt the principle of endeavouring, in each particular instance, to seek for an explanation derived from the operation of *known natural causes.* * * * According to his (Paulus) view of them (the miracles) they were events which were regarded as miraculous in *that* age and country; — but which ought to be regarded in a very different light by the more advanced intelligence of our times. We ought, therefore, to construe them into extraordinary natural events; — or into results whose causes have been simply omitted in the narrative; — or into the mere effects of *superior skill and knowledge*, which the Evangelist has described, in the popular language of the day, as supernatural interpositions."[†]

Salverte, a popular but superficial French writer, in a work called the "Occult Sciences," which has reached a second edition, and been also translated into English under the title of the "Philosophy of apparent Miracles," asserts that "if we

---

[*] Milman's History of the Jews contains some slight indications of the prevalence of this theory, in his explanation of certain of the Mosaic miracles. The remarks of the lamented Hugh James Rose, on German Rationalism, must be fresh in the memory of many.

[†] Edinburgh Review, No. 174. for October, 1847, p. 413.

put on one side that which belonged to jugglery, to imposture, or to the delirium of the imagination, there is not one of the ancient miracles which a man skilled in the modern sciences could not *reproduce.*"[*] "It is reasonable," he adds again, "to suppose that *some individuals* had the physical knowledge and power suitable for working a miraculous act, in the time and in the country where historical tradition had placed the miracle;" — and then he observes again, that "it is absurd to refuse to believe, or to admire as supernatural, that which can be explained on natural causes."

In some lectures, recently delivered at the chapel in South Place, Finsbury Square, and since published under the title of "German Anti-supernaturalism," Mr. Harwood, the lecturer, though preaching, apparently, in favour of Strauss's views, takes occasion to unfold the interpretations of rationalism. "The spirit of legend," says he, "would have many and many a nucleus of fact to work upon. Some miracles, *miraculous-looking incidents*, there must have been in an age like that and among a people like that. Nothing but one prolonged mental miracle could have hindered miracles from taking place almost daily, in the presence of one who was believed or imagined to be the Christ of God. No doubt, many demons were cast out: probably paralytics not a few were wholly or partially restored, as by miraculous voice or *touch*: possibly some few all but dead may have lived again upon the divine, 'I say unto thee, arise.' Perhaps Jesus himself was more *than once startled by the discovery of powers which he had scarcely been aware that he possessed.*"[†]

These quotations sufficiently illustrate the tendencies of the rationalistic school, — though it will be seen, that Mesmerism is rather alluded to than named. Other writers have, however,

---

[*] "Il n'est point de miracles anciens qu'un homme versé dans les sciences modernes ne pût *reproduire.*" (*Sciences Occultes*, seconde édition, p. 461. &c.) In his 90th cap. Salverte makes some further observations on the miracles of healing, on the raising of Jairus's daughter, and on the powers of Elisha and of St. Paul.

[†] Harwood's German Anti-Supernaturalism, p. 68. Some extracts from the same work are given in the Preface, p. 7. Other expressions might be quoted, as, for instance, where in the language of modern Deism, the Saviour is spoken of as "that wonderfully gifted Being Jesus of Nazareth." (p. 96.);

spoken more expressly; and the influence of this agency is at once claimed as the secret source of the Divine manifestations.

Richter, Rector of the Ducal School at Dessau, an influential German critic, and the author of "Considerations on Animal Magnetism," and who died about three years back, taught that "the miracles of the New Testament were performed by this extraordinary power." M. Théodore Bouys, who published in Paris a work on the same subject, endeavoured to prove the same thing. Professor Rostan, who drew up the article on Magnetism in the Medical French Dictionary, asserted therein that a "mass of the miraculous facts of old find a satisfactory, a physiological and natural explanation" in Mesmerism. M. Mialle, a copious and popular French writer on the subject, strongly declares the same opinion, and enters into reasonings to prove the assertion. Other writers could be mentioned:—but we will come at once to a recent and remarkable publication, in which the above views are expressed in explicit language.

The work referred to is one that originally appeared in America, and has been just reprinted in England, called "The Principles of Nature and her Divine Revelations." It is in two large octavo volumes, closely printed, is written with much power, and has attracted large notice in some literary circles, both across the Atlantic and in this country. Professor Bush of New York, and other scientific men, have shown themselves greatly interested in its contents, and in the manner of its production. The work professes to set forth the "Revelations" of an illiterate young man, named Andrew Davis, which he dictated in the Mesmeric sleep with a fluency and clearness most extraordinary. As a "voice to mankind," it pronounces, authoritatively, upon the most abstruse subjects, embracing theology, cosmogony, natural history, and science. Into the derivation and authenticity of the work it is not necessary to enter. Whether it be the combined result, in part of a trans-

* "The Principles of Nature, her divine Revelations, and a Voice to Mankind," by and through Andrew Jackson Davis, the Poughkeepsie Seer and Clairvoyant. (Chapman, Strand.)

ference of thought from the Mesmeriser and others,—in part of a suggestive and assistant imagination,—and in part of previous knowledge surreptitiously obtained, all mingled together in wondrous harmony and poured forth under the condition of an excessive exaltation; whether this be a correct view of the origination of the book, is not important to the argument:—the point for present consideration is this, that great attention has been paid to the statements of the work,—that Professor Bush declares that for "grandeur of conception and soundness of principle" it is almost unrivalled,—that other critics speak nearly the same language,—that its readers and admirers are numerous,—and that it reflects the opinions of an influential section. Mr. Chapman, the English editor, says that it is "a work of no ordinary theological pretension." To that portion, therefore, of its theology let us briefly turn, where the Clairvoyant speaks of the miracles of the New Testament. It is painful in the extreme to be thus driven to record so many objectionable and offensive passages: but nothing would be gained by concealment. The book is extensively read and quoted: and the more plainly that such obnoxious notions are set forth, the more easily are they met,—and the more quickly disposed of.

The Clairvoyant says, that "Jesus seemed to possess an intuitive knowledge of the medicinal properties of plants,—of mineral and animal substances,—of their use, and of the proper time and manner of their application in the curing of various diseases. He possessed also a great physical soothing power over the disordered or disconcerted forces of the human system. This was because of his superior physical endowments. Hence it is related in various places in the New Testament that he laid his hands upon persons and they were cured." (Vol. ii. p. 562.)

And again he says, "Such deeds of charity, sympathy and benevolence, (i. e. the miracles of healing,) are to be admired in the character of any person who ever has lived, or who ever will live on earth; but further than this they are of no importance, and demand no veneration nor approbation. For they are simply the good and just deeds of any person who is natu-

rally (which means *mesmerically*) qualified for their accomplishment." (p. 512.)*

Now these rationalistic views have, perhaps, not unnaturally, raised up a distinct class of objections to the practice of Mesmerism,—in opponents, whose inaccurate perceptions have confounded misrepresentations against a study with the study itself. "Is it no evil," says a hostile writer, calling himself Senex, "that from the deductions of this science, *the arm of infidelity is so strengthened*, as to induce men to assert, that the miracles of our Saviour, however stupendous, were performed by the same art, though, we are told, then not generally known?" † In another pamphlet, which I have already noticed, called a "Dialogue between a Mesmerist and a Christian," it is said, "the doctrines founded on these imitations of the miracles of our Lord, go to explain away the divine character and end of his miracles; and thus to undermine the truths on which our faith and hope rest. * * * Some of the advocates of Mesmerism have not hesitated to say that by means of a "virtue," common to all human bodies, "the miracle of healing was effected," &c. (p. 21.) Mr. Spencer Hall, in his "Mesmeric Experiences," has referred to the same opinions: "so striking," says he, "have been some of the effects of Mesmerism in this way as to cause many to regard it as a *sort of scientific divinity*, and to consider it the parent of all attested miracles; a view," he adds, "from which I unequivocally express my dissent." (p. 25.) And the late Mrs. Tonna (Charlotte

---

Elizabeth), and Mr. Close, of Cheltenham, and Mr. Bickersteth, of Watton, have all three deemed the argument worthy of a notice, and referred to it in their writings.

The latter observes: "Infidels have ventured to say that the miracles of Mesmerism are superior to those of our blessed Saviour; and yet," adds Mr. Bickersteth, "we must not, on that account, deny that Mesmerism is an *immense blessing* from God."*

"Charlotte Elizabeth," asserts that the marvels of Mesmerism are, through satanic agency, such close *imitations* of the miracles of Christ, as to undermine the first principles of the Christian faith: and she refers to some "book on Mesmerism, written by a Frenchman, who, after stating that Mesmerism prevailed among the ancient Egyptians, reminds his readers that Jesus was in Egypt, and there learned the Mesmeric art by which he effected the miraculous cures recorded in the Gospels."†

The Rev. F. Close, in his excellent lecture on the "Nature of Miracles," says,—"he might be asked what he thought of the astonishing phenomena of Mesmerism. Were they miraculous, or were they not? This seemed, at first sight, a *very hard question to answer*: still he thought that a solution might be given." And, after discussing the point at some little length, he concludes with observing, that "he felt persuaded that there was nothing miraculous in Mesmerism, and no interference of the evil spirit" in its wonders. Mr. Close here seems to me to pass over the more general and more formidable argument. It is not so much taught that Mesmerism is miraculous,—as that the miracles are little else than Mesmeric phenomena.‡

Dr. Arnold, too, in his Sermons, has more than once considered the subject deserving of a remark. "I mention this," he says,—"because I am inclined to think that there exists *a lurking fear of these phenomena* (of Mesmerism), *as if they*

---

* Nothing is more marked than the change in the language of Deism, since the time of Voltaire and the Philosophical Dictionary, as those different quotations above prove. The divine mission of the Saviour is, indeed, equally denied: but the coarse and irreverent sneers, with which he was then reviled, have passed away; and the excellency of his moral code, and the beauty and soundness of his views, are the constant theme of admiration. Christ is now spoken of, in this new and spreading school of infidelity, as the wisest and best of men,—as a benevolent, and "highly-gifted" individual. This altered phraseology is the more fatal and ensnaring from its subtility and respectfulness, reversing that mischievous aphorism of Bucket, of "vice losing half its evil by losing all its grossness." Many who would be shocked by the ribaldries of Paine and the French Philosophers, are caught by the smooth plausibilities of German Rationalism.

· † Extract from "Scripture on Phreno-Magnetism," by Senex, (Simpkin and Marshall.)

---

* See explanatory Letter from Rev. Edward Bickersteth, in No. 17, of Zoist, p. 71.

† Letter to Miss Martineau, by "Charlotte Elizabeth," pp. 7, and 13.

‡ See Mr. Close's Lecture on Miracles, delivered at the Cheltenham Literary Institution, p. 23.

might shake our faith in true miracles;—and, therefore, men are inclined to disbelieve them, in spite of testimony; a habit far more unreasonable, and far more dangerous, to our Christian faith than any belief in the facts of Magnetism." [a]

These extracts, from such various and very adverse writers, all show the prevalency of the opinion, that I now propose to enter upon. They, at least, prove that the notion is not the exaggerated invention of my own fancy,—nor the feeble suggestion of a few inconsiderable enthusiasts. Churchmen of the most diverse schools, rationalistic professors, unbelievers in revelation, and friends and opponents of Mesmerism, have alike regarded the subject as deserving of attention, and have alike pressed the consequences deduced from it into the service of their respective views. Nay, Dr. Arnold, as it has been seen, collected from his experience, that this "lurking fear" of the magnetic phenomena went so far as actually to indispose men for the investigation and admission of their truth. He thought that he could perceive that they were afraid of diving into the depths of nature, lest they should encounter an inconvenient disclosure in their course;—that they hung back from believing in one fact, lest, as a sequence, they must disbelieve in another. All this, it is repeated, shows the prevalency of the opinion,—and an opinion, it may be remarked in the next place, that does not at the first blush appear very unnatural. For some of the cures and marvels of Mesmerism have been so startling, and so contrary, indeed, to the ordinary operations of physics, that the bulk of mankind, who seldom are at the pains of distinguishing between conflicting, though seemingly homogeneous effects, are caught by the primary presentation of an object, and hasten to some unphilosophic conclusion about its nature. A medley of ungeneralized ideas passes through the brain; the true and the false, the same and the similar, are jumbled together without precision or distinctness;—and so one man pronounces that the new phenomena are but identical

* Arnold's Sermons, vol. iii. p. 246. "These facts," he observes again, "are mere wonders in our present state of knowledge: at a future period, perhaps, they may become the principles of a new science; but they neither are, nor will be miracles."—Ibid.

with the olden miracles;—another, that they are diabolical imitations;—while the third, and major part, shrink from the very name and study of the science, lest they should stumble on some untoward and distressing discovery. All this, it may be again observed, does not, in the first instance, appear either unnatural or inexplicable: but it is, therefore, the more necessary to meet the question at once in all its bearings and deductions,—and by a careful and complete analysis of the real nature of our facts, settle the doubts and scruples of the perplexed Christian once and for ever. *

What, then, it may now be asked, is the resemblance that exists between the miracles of the Saviour and the wonders of Mesmerism? We answer confidently, none whatever. An impassable gulf divides them. Both, indeed, proceed from the same Eternal Being; but the Mesmeric phenomena are nothing else than the product of a simple power in nature; while the marvels of Scripture arose from an interruption of those laws by which the government of the universe has been administered from creation: and this position, with God's grace, I proceed to prove.

I commence with a consideration of those miracles, to which only the wildest dreams of some enthusiastic Mesmerisers pretend to have made approach. And here, it will be observed, we assume that the reader is a Christian,—that he believes that the facts recorded in the Gospels did take place and are true, and that his only question is, how far the Divine origin of those facts is shaken by what has occurred in these latter days. Into the previous matter of evidence, therefore, we do not enter. Paley's incomparable work has exhausted the sub-

* Many other writers who have referred to these deistical views could be mentioned. The Rev. T. Pyne, in his work on Vital Magnetism, says, we must "carefully guard against the supposition of the miracles of Scripture having been performed by this art; for among them are many circumstances recorded to which Magnetism could never aspire, &c." p. 18.— Mr. Colquhoun, in the last chapter of the Isis Revelata, observes, that "the doctrine of Animal Magnetism does in no degree interfere with our belief in real miracles, &c. &c." (Vol. ii. p. 104.)—And the Christian Remembrancer, in a long article in favour of the science, in the April number for 1847, discusses briefly the fear entertained by some, of "Magnetism rivalling the miracles." (p. 366.)

ject, and refuted every doubt. To Paley, therefore, we refer the wavering heart. But our present inquiry is, whether there be any *counter-claims* on our attention, from facts evincing equal power, and supported by evidence equally conclusive.*

The "beginning of miracles, with which Jesus manifested forth his glory," was the *change of water* into *wine.* He did not command the six stone water-pots to be first emptied of the water, and then replenished them with wine;—but he ordered the empty vessels to be previously filled with water; and from these vessels, which were "filled up to the brim," the servants were instructed to draw forth, and bear to the governor of the feast; and a quantity of water, being supposed, upon the smallest computation, to be above a hogshead, was discovered by the guests to be converted into wine.—Mesmerism could have no agency here. The fact admits of no other explanation than that of being a miraculous and supernatural work.†

---

* Those who are indisposed for the study of Paley's longer work, will find an admirable compendium of the whole subject in a small volume, called "Lectures on the Evidence from Miracles," by the Rev. R. C. Coxe, the present learned and excellent Vicar of Newcastle. (Rivingtons.)

† And yet this is the miracle, that the well-meaning and lamented "Charlotte Elizabeth," by a confession of the facts, singled out as the one which she considered that Satan was *imitating* through certain powers of "*willing*" in a Mesmeriser. "Whether you," she says to Miss Martineau, "are conscious of it or not, this last incident, (that of the sleeper imagining some mesmerised water to be wine,) was devised by Satan to pour contempt, or to throw a soul-destroying doubt, on the miracle of Cana in Galilee. You or your companion in these perilous doings acted upon a suggestion of the evil one, to *will* a glass of water into wine; and though no change took place, perceptible to any mortal sense, the spirit had power over the possessed girl to *imitate* in her the effects of a draught, &c." (*Letter,* p. 18.) Now a slight examination of the circumstances in the two facts will explain the complete difference between them. In Miss Martineau's story, the Mesmeriser willed one single individual, who was *fast asleep,* and under strong mesmeric influence, to fancy that a glass of water, that she was sipping, was a glass of sherry. But there was no sleep at Cana of Galilee. The governor of the feast, and the guests, to say nothing of the attendants that drew the water, were all wide awake, and saw the colour of what they were drinking, a fact irrespective of, and in addition to, the change that they perceived in the quality. If the mesmeric fact be a *satanic imitation,* it is a most feeble and disturbed one. To have a parallel case, a Mesmeriser must *will* a room-full of friends and servants, whose senses shall be in an active state of wakefulness and discrimination, not only to imagine that a tumbler of what they see to be water is actually wine, but wine of a very superior vintage.

We next come to the miraculous draught of fishes. This occurred twice: once at the commencement of Christ's ministry and once after his resurrection. Twice had the fishermen been toiling all the night, and *caught nothing.* At the command of Jesus, they let down their nets, and inclose the first time so extraordinary a draught, that their nets brake, and their boats were beginning to sink. On the second occasion, they were hardly able to draw the net to land for the multitude and size of the fishes; and yet it is mentioned by the Evangelist, as an additional wonder, that the net was not broken. Now we cannot, perhaps, strictly describe a fact like this as *beyond nature,* for such a thing *might* happen; but it is not *according to nature.* Nothing like it has ever been seen, before or since. It is, therefore, contrary to the order of nature,—contrary to the general laws of nature. And when an event like this, which no natural causes have produced at any other time, occurred twice in the history of one man, we are justified in saying that it could be no peculiar or fortunate coincidence,—but a preternatural fact, which can be classed under no other head than that of the miraculous.

The next miracle to be noticed is the instant stilling of a tempest on the Lake of Gennesareth,—a tempest so violent that the waves were breaking over the ship. Dr. E. Clarke, in his travels, mentions that when adverse winds, sweeping from the mountains with the force of a hurricane, meet the strong current of the waters, which is formed by the river Jordan passing through the lake, a dangerous sea is at once raised. Now some such a hurricane Christ and his disciples encountered; and he stilled it in a moment; for there was a "*great calm.*" The "raging of the water," and the violence of the winds, subsided at once. Now this was clearly miraculous. By a singular accident the wind might have been suddenly hushed at the very same moment that Jesus spoke, but this fortuitous calm would not also have extended to the waters. Whoever has been to sea, or whoever has witnessed a storm at sea, knows full well that it requires a certain interval of time for the waves to cease to swell after the winds have ceased to blow. It is never a great hurricane in one moment, and a

glassy surface in the next. The fishermen, unaccustomed to such a transition, "marvelled," as well they might, and demanded, among themselves, "what manner of man" Christ was. And the only answer is, a Man from God! Where is Mesmerism here? [*]

The feeding of great multitudes, on *two occasions*, with a few loaves and fishes, surpasses all bounds of exaggeration also. There could be no false perception here. The statement does not admit of the supposition of a fortunate experiment. As Leslie says, that "one small loaf of bread should be so multiplied in the breaking, as not only in appearance and to the eye, but truly and really to satisfy the appetites of a thousand hungry persons, and that the fragments should be much more than the bread was at first," is a fact which can admit of no explanation. And while we do not know the precise point at which the powers of nature terminate, as in the case of Mesmerism, we can declare, unhesitatingly, that such a multiplication of food is beyond the reach of a natural cause, and that here we have again a manifest interposition of the power of God.[†]

The walking upon the sea is a plain fact which admits of no explanation. It is a statement in which there could be neither

---

[*] "So, too, in the storm, not only did the awakened Saviour make at once a great calm, hushing, in an instant, winds and angry waves,—but immediately the ship was at the place whither they went."— *Rev. T. Pyne's Vital Magnetism,* p. 22.

[†] Some pretend to see a satanic "imitation" of this miracle in the well-known mesmeric sympathies of taste, as when a mesmeriser puts bread, or ginger, or sugar, &c. into his mouth, and the sleeping sympathising patient tastes it. To apply the phraseology of "Charlotte Elizabeth," it is considered an "infernal travestie on the work of the Lord Jesus Christ, in which horror gives way to a burning indignation of soul." Now in this "satanic imitation," to pass over the number of souls that partook of the food, "five thousand men, besides women and children," there are one or two other points wanting; the satisfying of hunger, and the filling the baskets with the remainder.

Let it be observed, once for all, that it is not I who am first suggesting an odious comparison between these opposite facts. The very naming them together is as revolting to myself as it is ridiculous in reality. I am simply replying to the different objections and arguments of religious and well-meaning opponents of Mesmerism, who originally started them, and gave great publicity to their views.

---

mistake nor exaggeration. The ship was "in the midst of the sea," and he walked to them. He "walked upon the sea." The ship was twenty or thirty furlongs distant from the shore, i. e. more than three miles, and he walked to them. St. Peter also walked upon the sea to meet him, and, "beginning to sink," was saved by Jesus catching him by the arm. The miracle is mentioned by three Evangelists, and most fully by St. Matthew. The same word in the original, which is used by St. Mark, in his sixth chapter (verse 47.), for describing Jesus as being "on the land," is used by him and St. John, when they speak of him as walking "on the sea." [*] No statement in the New Testament will admit of a closer or more critical examination than will this. And what confirms the miraculous character of the action is the fact, that the disciples seem to have been more impressed by this than by any preceding miracle, for they "worshipped" him, St. Matthew says, in consequence, and declared that "of a truth he was the Son of God."

"The Transfiguration of the Saviour is a fact, also, which admits of no softening explanation. It happened not at night, but in broad day;—not in a corner,—but on the very top of a mountain. The brightness and glory were more than the faculties of the spectators were able to endure. A celestial voice was heard, speaking to Jesus. The disciples were so overpowered with all that took place, that they flung themselves with their faces on the ground, and so remained till the Saviour touched them and bade them rise. And St. Peter expressly refers to the wonders of this day, as a special proof that the Gospel was "no cunningly devised fable." [†]

---

[*] This is mentioned, because some rationalistic interpreters have said that Christ was walking upon the shore, by the sea, and not upon it. Their explanation will not bear a moment's criticism. It is the suggestion of men unacquainted with Greek, and who have not studied the context.

[†] In the "Dialogue between a Mesmerist and a Christian," containing "a suitable and earnest address to all true Christians" against Mesmerism, a profane and fancied "imitation" of this miracle is dwelt upon and reprobated, but which I shall not offend my readers by reciting. Let it be sufficient to say, that there is no proper resemblance between the points compared; neither is it one which, conversant as I am with Mesmerism, I ever before found referred to, till I met with it in this tract, by "Philadelphus." These exclusively Christian writers in their opposition to "unchristian Mesmerism,"

The drying up of the fig-tree is a fact to which no Mesmeric power makes the most distant approach. Jesus spoke, and the fig-tree withered away instantly from the roots. "How *soon*," said the disciples, "is the tree withered!"

The raising of the dead, on three distinct occasions, is explained by the modern unbeliever as the revival of a sleeping person out of a trance. The different facts of each case put together contradict the opinion. Jesus meets the dead son of the widow of Nain, humanly speaking by *accident*, as he is carried out on his bier. He at once approaches and bids the young man arise; "and he that was dead sat up, and began to speak." Now, on the supposition that the mother and the numerous friends of this young man (for "much people" were in attendance, and the body was not inclosed in a coffin, but carried openly on a litter, as is the way in the East), on the supposition that all were deceived, and that the young man was only entranced, can we suppose, with any degree of reason, that in the two remaining instances the relations and domestics were also under a delusion? Let us take, then, the case of the ruler's daughter. Jesus is *suddenly* invited by Jairus to his house to heal his child. In the meantime death seizes his victim; and so undeniable are the signs of dissolution, that the family are anxious that Jesus should retire and be no further inconvenienced. "Trouble not the Master, for she is dead." It would be a singular coincidence if this also were a trance. But Jesus, *before he has even entered the house*, or seen the body, pronounces that the maiden shall live and be "made whole." But we have a third instance: the raising of Lazarus.* Lazarus had been in his grave four days. When the stone was removed

call into being some odious phantom, put ideas into our heads, and language into our mouths, such as never existed, and then charitably conclude their pamphlets in teaching, as proved by themselves, that "Mesmerism is, in fearful reality, the assertion of the will and of the power of Satan." (p. 34.)

* "Paulus of Hiedelberg says that the Bible narratives must be acknowledged as records of real occurrences, but that these occurrences, which were miracles merely in appearance, always admitted of a natural explanation. For instance, Lazarus was awakened, not from death, but only from a state of asphyxia, for Christ was no worker of miracles, though he may have been an excellent physician, &c." — *Wolfgang Menzel's German Literature*, translated by Gordon, vol. i. 196, "On Religion."

from the cave, and as soon as Jesus spoke, that instant Lazarus came forth, bound hand and foot, in grave clothes, and his face fastened over with a napkin. The restoration was instantaneous and complete. He did not merely move, and speak, and die again. He did not gradually, and with further assistance, come to himself; but he, whose corpse was supposed to be already in an offensive state of decay, walked forth at once from the tomb, returned home to his family, and lived, and was seen alive a long time after. Now, upon an examination of the above, this train of questions suggests itself. What probability is there, that *all* the attendants and relatives in these three cases were equally under a deception? Is it meant that all who die are only in a trance; and if not, what reason is there to show that these three persons were exclusively in a trance more than any others? How should Jesus, if only a man, know *before he had even seen them*, that Lazarus and the ruler's daughter were only entranced? Supposing, after all, that they had been dead, and did not rise forth, would not the power of Jesus have been proved null and void? The same remark applies to the son of the widow of Nain. Jesus, as a mere man, dared not have risked the chances of a failure, unless it be said that a trance is a more common occurrence than a death. The unbeliever, however, says that these three persons were not really dead, but only in appearance. From their own statement, here then were three of the most curious coincidences,—and all in the course of two years. The mere recurrence of the fact refutes the theory. This is the dilemma: if they were really dead, *none but a divine power could raise them, and that by a miracle;* —if they were only entranced, how could Jesus, if but a mere man, know it? and not knowing it of a certainty, how would he venture on the hazardous experiment of placing his reputation on the issue of such a chance? Never was an hypothesis built on a more untenable position.

We will not enter upon an examination of the question that naturally presents itself in the next place, as to whether the Saviour was himself also in a trance. No one fact is better established in the whole Gospel history, than the re-appearance of Christ after the crucifixion. If that fact be not true, there

is an end of human evidence for ever. Was He also, we ask then, in a trance when hanging on the cross, and when laid in the tomb by Joseph of Arimathea? The question answers itself: it is too monstrous to need refutation.

Here, then, we have examined in detail a class of miracles in the New Testament, to which the proudest results of the Mesmeric power offer not the most distant resemblance. And let no one say, that this examination was idle, — that it is foreign to the subject, — that we "fight, as one that beateth the air." Nothing is useless, by which the faith of the believer may be strengthened, and the misgivings of the anxious heart be quenched as they arise. The extracts that have been given from anti-mesmeric writers, prove the opinions that are afloat, respecting "the manifest tendency of Mesmerism to undermine the first principles of the Christian faith." Many, it is added, who "go to laugh at a mesmeric exhibition, may remain to doubt, to disbelieve the Gospel, and to perish."* The facts, it is said by others, are old, but the principle is newly discovered. And knowing myself that Mesmerism is a living reality, — knowing that its powers reach to an unsuspected extent, — knowing that the faith of many has been disturbed by this discovery, I have thought it essential to analyse the question closely, and place the subject in its true colours. If I could not say how far Mesmerism *does go*, I have at least shown how far it *does not go*. The inquiry has commenced by an examination of facts, to which no approximation, even in the faintest degree, has ever been made by the Mesmeric power. If the matter stopped here, sufficient would have been said to prove the Divine Mission of the Lord Jesus, and to show that He was a teacher sent from God. But we now proceed to an investigation into those miracles of a curative character, to which a greater resemblance with this new power is supposed to exist.

And here it is at once asserted, that the Mesmeric cures are something very extraordinary. For the convenience of the present argument, we do not fall back from that position. They have often been most wonderful. The treatment has

* "Charlotte Elizabeth's" Letter, p. 14, 15.

often and often been efficacious, where no other remedy could succeed. This is admitted in the fullest and most unequivocal manner. Independent, moreover, of the general power, which is common in a degree to most men, certain persons have been physically gifted with a peculiar virtue of a very unusual character. A denial of the fact cannot alter it. The evidence on this point is too authentic to be questioned. Valentine Greatrakes, an Irish gentleman who lived in the seventeenth century, — De Loutherbourgh the well-known painter, Gassner a Roman Catholic priest in Suabia, an English gardener named Levret, and several other parties could all be mentioned, whose powers of cure by manipulation and magnetic action were something very peculiar.* Their patients were most numerous. All sorts of diseases were relieved by them. The then Bishop of Derry, speaking of Greatrakes, says, "There is something in *the power more than ordinary.*" Still with the very largest allowance for the extent and variety of the effects, they all fall very far short of being miraculous;—they all fall very far short of the Gospel wonders. "The cure often did not succeed, but by reiterated touches; the patients often relapsed; he failed frequently; he can do nothing where there is any decay in nature, and many distempers are not at all obedient to his touch."† This was said of Greatrakes; and

* In the Monthly Magazine, vol. xxv. and xxvi., is a reference to a Mrs. Bostock, of Nantwich, Chester, who possessed "an extraordinary sanative gift." She had generally hundreds of patients, and her power was regarded as miraculous. A baronet applied to her to raise his wife from the dead.

† In the Rawdon Papers, Lord Conway says in a letter to Sir George Rawdon, speaking of Greatrakes, that "some diseases he doth dispatch with a great deal of ease, and others not without a *great deal of pains*" (p. 213.). There are two letters from Greatrakes himself in the Rawdon Papers.

"Greatrakes' reputation arose to a prodigious height for some time," says Granger, "but it declined almost as fast, when the expectations of the multitude that resorted to him were not answered."— *Note in Rawdon's Papers,* p. 211.

There is an account of Greatrakes, by Glanvill, in his strange book on witchcraft, p. 53. The Dean of C. writes to Glanvill, saying, "some take him to be a conjurer, some an impostor, but others again enter him as an apostle."

In the Zoist, vol. iii. p. 96, there is a further account of Greatrakes, in a letter from Dr. Elliotson, with a lithographed "Portraiture of him,

the same applies to every other Mesmerist of whom I have ever heard. The most successful practitioner has never laid claim to the possession of an infallible and universal power. He has never pledged himself beforehand, in every possible case, to produce a cure. If he have succeeded in ninety-nine cases, he has failed in the hundredth. If he have procured a lasting benefit in many patients, the relief is often but temporary in others. Here, then, in the *first place*, is the wide and immeasurable interval that separates the wonders of the Mesmeriser from the marvels of the Redeemer of Israel. No one ever sought His face in vain. No one ever went unto Him and was cast out unrelieved. The word of promise that went forth from His lips never returned unto Him void. His language was decisive and with authority; His touch was in its effect certain, foreknown, invariable; His sanative power extended to every pain, — to every complication of disease. Nothing can be more decisive than the testimony of Scripture on this point. To use Paley's happy expression, there was nothing *tentative* or experimental in the manner. "There is nothing in the Gospel narrative," says he, "which can allow us to believe, that Christ attempted cures in many instances, and succeeded in a few; or that he ever made the attempt in vain." And the Gospel history confirms this position. "He healed *all* that were sick." (Matt. c. viii. v. 16.) St. Luke says that "All they that had *any* sick, with divers diseases, brought them unto him: and he laid his hands *on every one* of them and *healed* them." (c. iv. v. 40.) St. Matthew, again, says that "He went about *all* Galilee, — healing *all manner* of sickness, and *all manner* of disease, among the people." "And they brought unto him *all sick* people, that were taken with divers diseases and torments, and those which were lunatic, and those

curing diseases and distempers by the stroke of his hand only," after an old print lately found in Cambridge.

Mr. Thoresby, in the *Philosophical Transactions*, 226. p. 332. A.D. 1699, mentions how Greatrakes "drove the pain from place to place, bringing it to the leg, and at last out by the toes." This is by no means uncommon in Mesmerism: I have done it myself with one of my parishioners who had a diseased knee.

Dr. Beal mentions, in the *Philosophical Transactions*, No. 12. p. 202., a blacksmith who cured by stroking with the hand like Greatrakes.

that had the palsy, and he *healed them*." (c. iv. ver. 23, 24.) Again, we read, that "*great multitudes* came unto him, having with them those that were lame, blind, dumb, maimed, and *many others*, and cast them down at Jesus' feet, and he *healed them*." (Matt. c. xv. v. 30.) There was no exception that we read of in any instance. Here then, in the first place, is one distinguishing characteristic of the Christian cures — the *universality* of the success wherever the attempt was made.

We now come, in the next place, to a *second* and most material distinction, the *class of cures* effected by either party. In Mesmerism, the diseases subdued have been of a very remarkable character; tic-douloureux, fearful epileptic fits, brain fever, derangement, deafness, weakness in the eyes, neuralgic pains of all kinds, loss of voice, paralysis, fevers, and a variety of other disorders; cures have been effected where all other means have failed; still all these fall immeasurably short of the miraculous effects recorded in Scripture.— Cures of a far higher order are there related; cures, where the limbs or members had been organically injured,—cures where the injury had dated from the birth of the party. And here to mark the difference more strongly, it is necessary to introduce a *third* and even greater distinction, viz. the period of time in which the benefit was produced. In Mesmerism the relief has been often most rapid; in a quarter of an hour pain has begun to give way, and has been even expelled; in a first sitting a disorder has been removed; yet, even rapid as has been the therapeutic power of the Mesmeriser, it is idle to compare it to the instantaneous — to the magical change that followed on the touch and the voice of the Saviour. Christ "spake the word," and quicker than thought a complete revolution took place in the brain, in the blood, or in the structure of the sufferer. What was wanting, was supplied; what was weakened, was renewed; what was broken, was made whole; and that, too, in an instant of time. In the twinkling of an eye, a mass of diseased and putrefying sores became "as the flesh of a little child," in the bloom of health. The combination is very noticeable, and marks the miraculous character. In Mesmerism I have heard of more than one instance, where a rheumatism

of many years standing has been cured at the first *séance*, as soon as the magnetic medium had passed into the patient's system; perhaps even greater and more expeditious effects may be named; still, let them be compared to the miracles of the New Testament in regard to the class of diseases and the instantaneous character of the cure, and what resemblance is there? *

Peter's wife's mother is confined to her bed with a *fever*; Christ takes her by the hand; the fever *immediately* leaves her; no lassitude, the usual consequence of feverish action, remains; for she arises and ministers to them at their meat.

Eleven specific cases of a cure of leprosy are recorded. The leprosy is a disease beyond all description fearful; by some it is thought incurable. The skin and flesh are one mass of corruption. To effect a cure, therefore, a change must take place in the whole current of the blood. In the first cure related, the leprosy "*immediately* departed." In the cases of the other ten lepers, they were all cured at once on their quitting Jesus, and in their way to the priests.

* The instantaneousness of the Gospel-cures is a most important distinction. Even Gauthier, the great French Mesmerist, points out this mark of difference. "That which was accomplished by Christ in a second, will take you a day, or a month, *or a year*." (*Traité Pratique*, 700.) So marvellous, indeed, is the distinction, that this new school of Rationalism is much perplexed in finding a way to explain it. The American youth, Davis, in his "Revelations," therefore, cuts the knot in the easiest manner possible. He asserts that when Scripture speaks of a thing being *instantaneous*, that it meant that it was "*gradual*." These are his own words. "There has arisen a vast amount of misapprehension concerning these miracles, from the *style* of the written word. Matthew and the other evangelists record the cause and effect as occurring in rapid succession—almost simultaneously. In the physical infirmities cured by Jesus, the effect is related as though it followed the cause *immediately*. All who are acquainted with physiological principles, and with the calm, gentle, and energetic movements of the human organisation, are persuaded, even positively convinced, that no cause can be brought to act so as to produce health as an *immediate* result, in case of any established disease. Therefore, notwithstanding the things recorded *were* performed, they were effected by causes agreeing with *the nature of the human system*; and the re-establishment of health, which actually occurred, was effected *gradually*, and by means adapted to the temperament of the individual, and the nature of the disease." Vol. ii. 512.

This is as if a philosopher in Cochin China, on hearing of the rapid transmission of news by an electric telegraph, should say that it was impossible, and that what was meant was, that it was by degrees.

Many important cures of paralysis are mentioned. One in particular is specified, where the sufferer was so completely deprived of the use of his limbs as to be carried by four men. He is cured *instantly* that Jesus speaks, and *walks* off, carrying his bed.

A cripple, who had been suffering from his infirmity and loss of limbs for thirty-eight years,—and a poor woman, who had been bent double for eighteen years, are both cured at once. The latter "was *immediately* made straight." The former was "*immediately* made whole, and took up his bed and walked."

What can be a more hopeless state than a dry withered limb? Nature seems dead in the part. All power is gone. A man with a withered hand comes to Christ: he is ordered to stretch it out, and "it is restored whole *as the other*."

Mesmerism has been of signal service in deafness, in blindness, and where the voice has been injured; but the benefit has been obtained by degrees; and in no instance has a cure been produced where the privation has arisen from a structural defect, commencing with the birth. Several cases are mentioned in Scripture of cures of blindness,—of blindness "from birth,"—of deafness and dumbness united from birth,—of deafness with impediment in the speech,—and so on, where the cure was *instantaneous*, and following the touch. In one case of blindness, the cure was effected more gradually; still it was cured; and half an hour, or an hour at the most, was the time occupied from the sufferer's first interview with Jesus, before his eyes were "restored, and that he saw every man clearly." To compare any of the benefits procured by Mesmerism with those marvellous cures of blindness and deafness, would be an absurdity, which none but those who have not studied them closely would dream of committing.*

Among other instantaneous cures, we may mention that of a

* "We have distinguished between the miracles of Scripture and Magnetism: for the latter makes no pretensions to such power as that of rendering perfectly sound a withered arm, or of instantaneously giving sight, with all the effects of experience (the greater wonder of the two) to one born blind."—*Rev. T. Pyne*, p. 90.

woman with an issue of blood of twelve years' duration, who came behind, and without the (humanly speaking) knowledge of Jesus, touched his garment, and was cured *directly*; that of a boy with violent epileptic fits; and that of the servant whose ear was cut off, the wound of which was at once healed by the touch of Jesus.

It may be as well to add, that in the xvth of Matthew, verse 30., where the Evangelist speaks of the "lame and maimed" being brought to Jesus, and of the "lame walking," and the "maimed being made whole," some of the best commentators are of opinion, that the word, which in our translation is rendered "maimed," signifies those who had not merely lost the use of their limbs, as the lame, — but *even the limbs themselves*; and that those deficient limbs were replaced, and the sufferers "made whole." Be this as it may, here is a succession of cures, standing out in pre-eminent majesty, both in the nature of the disease and the suddenness of the relief, — far — far above any that the annals of Magnetism can adduce, with a line of demarcation between them so broad and insuperable, that the most trembling Christian need not dread the faintest approximation.

A *fourth* distinguishing mark, attendant upon the cures related in the Gospel, is the permanency of their effect. There is no reason to suspect, from the slightest phrase that drops from any of the New Testament writers, nor from any charge that was advanced by the unbeliever, that the benefit was not as lasting as it was complete. No one can assert the same of all our Mesmeric cures. Many are indeed permanent; but with a large number the action requires to be renewed at intervals, especially in some diseases that are of a chronic kind.

Still the unbeliever replies, that Christ performed all his cures by the "*touch*." "They brought unto him those that were sick with divers diseases, and he *laid his hands* on every one of them and healed them." It was the Mesmeric "touch" they assert. Though there was no manipulating process adopted, still the Mesmeric power was possessed by him to such an unusual and excessive degree, that the mere touch was sufficient. That a virtue accompanied the touch of the Saviour is admitted.

It is, in fact, the very thing we assert. The question is, whether that touch was divine or human, — whether the touch of any other human being, not recorded in Scripture, ever wrought out the same effects? Supposing, even as some think, that the touch was Mesmeric, only exerted to a supernatural degree, the result would not be less of a miracle.[*] If God brings out a latent power in nature, and exercises it to an extent of which man is incapable, though the virtue itself be part of nature's forces, still its employment to this extreme degree would be an interference with our physical laws, and therefore strictly præternatural. This is the distinction between an energy that is ordinary or extraordinary. The former may be very wonderful, — but the latter is miraculous. And certainly, in confirmation of this view, it must be said that God works by means. To judge from analogy, He does not *create* a fresh power, where *sufficient* in nature already exists. When the Red Sea was divided by miracle, though dry land could have been produced at once by the simple word of his power, He rather caused the waters to go back by the effect of a strong east wind, which He called into unusual action for the occasion. And thus it may be with Mesmerism: Christ may have exercised a latent Mesmeric power to an extra and miraculous extent. For instance, when the poor woman with an issue of blood touched him secretly, and Jesus said that he "perceived that *virtue* was gone out of him," He *may* have meant that a supernatural portion of that magnetic virtue, which is imparted in a greater or less degree to every human being, had escaped from Him, and caused the benefit.[†] I mention this in defer-

[*] Mr. Spencer Hall, who always writes in a spirit of Christian faith and humanity, says, "true, since Jesus did not disdain to use even dirt and spittle as agents, and since he felt a 'virtue gone out of him,' on an occasion when another was benefited by touching him, I would not deny that, as Lord of all, he might use magnetism, or any other agent in creation, for the working out of his compassionate designs." (*Mesmeric Experiences*, 94.) The Christian Remembrancer, in the article before referred to, adopts the same view, and thinks that the Saviour might have exercised the "faculty," after a miraculous way. (April, 1847, 369.)

[†] Gauthier says: "La vertu magnétique, qui résidait à un degré incomparable en Jésus-Christ, existe à un degré inférieur chez tous les hommes, et chaque fois que le magnétiseur impose les mains, il sort une vertu de lui." — T. Pratiques, 16.

ence to the views of others, rather than as expressing my own opinion. *However*, in changing water into wine, or in multiplying five loaves to feed five thousand, there would appear a species of divine power exerted, having no connection whatever with this quality of "touch." His touch, therefore, may not have been meant for a medium of communication. It may simply have been an external action, identifying himself with the cure, and attracting the attention of the party more especially towards him.* Moreover, Jesus did *not* always touch the sick. In the cure of the sick of the palsy, of the cripple, of the withered hand, of the boy with epileptic fits, no mention is made of the "laying on of hands." And this brings us to a *fifth* and very remarkable distinction, the cure of three sick persons immediately and *at a distance*, whither this assumed Mesmeric virtue could not possibly, except by miracle, extend. Nothing in the annals of Mesmerism has a parallel to this. I certainly know of some instances, where a strong sanative and soothing power has been communicated at a distance by the transmission of a highly Mesmerised material, such as leather or cotton, and from which the benefit has also been at present permanent. But this curative effect was the work of weeks, of months, — of long incessant application. Let us, on the other hand, turn to the three cases recorded in Scripture. The first was the cure of a nobleman's son, who was dying of a *fever*, at the distance of more than twenty miles. The disease left him at the very hour in which Jesus said, "Thy son liveth." The second is the cure of the Centurion's servant, who was sick of

* On the external action of the hand, the Rev. C. Townshend makes the following pleasing and appropriate remarks : — "Gifts of healing, not less than of power, belong to the hand by prescriptive right. If the potency of the royal touch, in curing the king's evil, be but a superstition, let us remember that it took its origin from a holy source : Christ and his disciples laid their hands upon the sick, and they were healed. The miracles of our Lord were remarkably accompanied by actions of the hand, as if they were in some measure connected with that external means. In restoring sight and hearing, he touched the ears and eyes of the afflicted persons. Even the imparting of the gift of the Holy Spirit followed the imposition of hands ; and this external ensign of a spiritual agency is still retained in our church. Who that has undergone or witnessed the beautiful rite of confirmation but has felt its power" (p. 199.).

a palsy and "ready to die," who "was healed in the self-same hour that Jesus spoke," — without his passing under the roof. The third was the recovery of the daughter of the woman of Canaan, at once and at a distance, by the mere word and command of Jesus. Whatever the sickness was, whether derangement or epileptic fits, it matters not ; the fact was, she was cured, and cured without touch or even approximation of the Saviour.

Here, then, are five characteristics, which especially distinguish the curative miracles of Christ, and separate them from any resemblance to even the highest order of Mesmeric power.

1. The cure was universal.
2. The diseases were more desperate, and in some cases organic.
3. The cure was instantaneous.
4. The cure was permanent.
5. The cure was occasionally performed at a distance.

One other quality may be mentioned : the power was transmissive. The Apostles were invested with the same virtue to an equal degree. This can in no wise be said of those who possessed that peculiar healing power that we before alluded to. This cannot be said of Gassner, of Greatrakes, of De Loutherbourgh, or of others. The power died with them. It was not imparted to followers or friends. Not so in the Christian dispensation : the Disciples were empowered equally "to lay hands on the sick," and the promise was, "and they shall recover." We read of "many wonders and signs being done by the Apostles." We read of a *multitude* out of the cities round about Jerusalem bringing sick folks to the Apostles, and *they were healed every one!*" More especially, we are told, of the cure by Peter and John of the impotent man in the temple, that was lame from his birth, whose ankle-bones and feet received strength immediately ; of the cripple at Lystra, "who had never walked" from his birth, and also stood up at once and leaped, at the mere word of St. Paul ; and of the father of Publius, who lay sick of a fever and was healed by

the same Apostle. Other wonders might be named; but this is sufficient to enable us to ask this question, If Christ only wrought his cures by the exercise of the same natural power that Gassner and others employed, why was he able to transmit the same virtue to his followers, while with Gassner and Great-rakes no successor appeared?

But here comes a fresh argument, that decides the question at once. It is said, that this virtue was *transmitted*, — or, in other words, that the curative process, whatever it was, was *taught* by Jesus to his disciples, — and by them to many others: if so, how came these supposed miracles of healing to cease? and would they not rather have *increased* in each successive generation? As this argument, however, is given in the most clear and forcible language by the Archbishop of Dublin in his tract on Christian Evidences*, I avail myself of his permission to render it in his own words.

"I have said that the works performed by Jesus and his disciples were beyond the unassisted powers of man. And this, I think, is the best description of what is meant by a miracle. *Superhuman* would perhaps be a better word to apply to a miracle, than *supernatural*; for if we believe that nature is merely another word to signify that state of things and course of events which God has appointed, nothing that occurs can be strictly called '*supernatural*.' Jesus himself accordingly describes his works, not as violations of the law of nature, but as works '*which none other man did.*' But what is in general meant by 'supernatural' is something out of the ordinary course of nature, — something at variance with those laws of nature which we are accustomed to.

"But then it may be objected that we cannot decide what *does* violate the ordinary laws of nature, unless we can be sure that we are acquainted with all these laws. For instance, an inhabitant of the tropical climates might think it contrary to the laws of nature, that water should ever become hard; since he had never seen ice. And when electricity was first discovered, many of its effects were contrary to the laws of nature, which

* Christian Evidences, printed for the Society for promoting Christian Knowledge.

had been hitherto known. But any one who visits colder regions may see with his own eyes, that water does become solid. And any one who will procure an electrical machine, or who attends lectures on the subject, may see for himself the effects of electricity.

"Now suppose Jesus had been a person who had discovered some new natural agent through which any man might be enabled to cure diseases by a touch, and perform the other wonderful works which He did, and through which any one else might have done the like, this would soon have become known and practised by all; just like the use of electricity or any newly-discovered medicine, and from his time down to this day every one would have commonly performed just the same works that He did. He might, indeed, have kept it to himself as a secret, and thus have induced some to believe that he wrought miracles. But so far from acting thus, He imparted his power, first to the twelve Apostles, and afterwards to seventy others; and after his departure, his Apostles received the power of not only performing mighty works themselves, but also of bestowing those gifts on all the disciples on whom they laid their hands, as you may see from Acts, viii. 14. 23.; Acts, xix. 6.; Rom. i. 2. &c.

"There must have been therefore, in the early church, many hundreds, and probably many thousands, performing the same sort of works as Jesus and his Apostles. And if, therefore, these had been performed by means of any natural agency, such as any one else might use as well as they, the art would soon have been universally known: and the works performed by the disciples of Jesus would have been commonly performed by all men ever after down to this day.

"But the Jews were convinced, with good reason, that the works of Jesus were beyond the powers of unassisted man. And it may seem strange to us that they did not all come at once to the same conclusion with Nicodemus, when he said, 'No man can do these miracles which thou doest except God be with him.'"

"But," says the anxious inquirer, "you have at present made

no allusion to the most wondrous parts of Mesmerism. *Clairvoyance*, internal vision, the predictive faculty, are all passed over; and these are the phenomena that more than any partake of the miraculous character."

Of the predictive faculty there is some difficulty in speaking. Many remarkable facts have certainly been stated, on the most respectable authority; and he would be a bold and hasty man, who should presume to reject them, without having fully certified himself as to the defect in their evidence. But strange as some of these predictions appear, to place them in the same category with the prophetic writings of the Old Testament, — to compare them with the fulfilment of facts which had been predicted hundreds of years before, is preposterous. They somewhat approach the character of the stories of *second-sight* among the Scotch. It would be difficult to discredit *all* the anecdotes that are related under that head; and many other singular predictions have occurred in the history of the human mind, to which different medical and metaphysical works have referred. How far, in certain states of disease, the mind becomes more spiritual and acquires a peculiar character of exaltation and of subtle judgment, so as to decide more clearly as to the *probability* of an event, I leave to physiologists to determine. Such, at any rate, is my own opinion. Still all this, even at the best, is widely different from the prophetic character. The anticipation of an event, a few weeks previously, is very remote from a prediction of several centuries; and in fact, this sort of foresight bears no more relation to ancient prophecy, than do the wonderful cures of the Mesmeriser to the miraculous effects recorded in the Gospel.

These predictions, then, as far as I have been able to judge, go no further than the foretelling a result that is about to arise from circumstances *then in action*, at the time of the somnambulist's vision. The increased subtlety of the clairvoyant's perceptions foresees the conclusion from facts fermenting towards their issue. In other words, the future is known through its then existing cause: for a *clear* acquaintance with the present infers what *must* arise in the sequel. This would also appear to be Mesmer's opinion, and the opinion of many other experienced Magnetists. The power is remarkable enough: but infinitely distant from the nature of prophecy.[*]

Of Clairvoyance, or the faculty of seeing through opaque bodies, of reading without the use of the eyes, and so forth, wonderful as these facts appear at first, and utterly discredited as they are by many who believe in the other marvels of Mesmerism, it is not needful to say so much as might be expected, for two reasons.

First, they bear no resemblance whatsoever to anything recorded in Scripture. Nothing of the kind is mentioned in the Gospel history as one of its miracles. Christ never appealed to any such fact, as a proof of his divine legation.[†]

But, secondly, however wonderful or incredible they may appear, there is not one single fact of this nature, occurring in the Mesmeric state, but the same or a similar fact has been found to exist, spontaneously, in the condition of natural somnambulism. Those who will study the subject, will see this assertion unequivocally proved. I have given this statement before. In certain stages of extreme or peculiar disease, nature has found a vent, by throwing the patient into an abnormal condition. In this condition very singular phenomena have appeared. Very many cases[‡] could be cited of clairvoyance in that particular state. In these cases, Mesmerism was unknown to the parties, or was not applied artificially. These phenomena were the result of hysteria or natural Mesmerism. At any rate, they appeared spontaneously and in a state of disease; and as such they relieve the Mesmeric wonders of the character of the supernatural, and bring them down to the level of ordinary occurrences; and any comparison, therefore, between

---

[*] Mesmer says, "prévoir l'avenir, c'est sentir l'effet par la cause." See Gauthier, T. P. p. 601. See also l'Abbé J. B. L., where he speaks of the means of distinguishing between a divine revelation, and an exalted penetration into the future.—p. 611.

[†] If Mesmerism had been the agent by which Jesus and his disciples wrought, how happened it that coma, clairvoyance, prevision, rigidity, insensibility to pain, and other phenomena, never presented themselves in the process? We read of nothing of the sort. This is an additional proof that there was no Mesmeric influence in the action.

[‡] See Appendix, L

the latter and the miracles of Scripture, would be misplaced and superfluous.

I trust that the anxious and the scrupulous may now feel more assured on this important subject; and perceive the wide distinction that exists in the matter. The question is capable of a much more detailed analysis, and of receiving a fuller and more conclusive proof. But enough, and perhaps more than enough, has been stated;—much, too, that is wearisome, much that is old, much that is self-evident. But I seek not to please a sect, or give knowledge to the well-instructed. This little work is for the use of the ignorant or the timid; and while I am anxious by its publication to "do good unto all men;" I more especially write for the "household of faith." Many amiable and virtuous minds have been deterred from giving Mesmerism that candid trial which its importance deserves, from no other feeling than a silent unuttered fear as to its bearing on Revelation. To say that such a feeling is not right, —that a love of truth ought to be predominant at all hazards, is easy of utterance, and perhaps correct in reality. Still it is a feeling that deserves respect. And it is to meet this feeling, and remove these scruples, that the materials of this Chapter have been put together. How far they may be successful time will show. That there was a necessity for the attempt, there cannot be a question. And my hope is, that many a perplexed and doubting heart, whose faith had been staggered for a little season at the presumed mysteriousness of our new science, may be led to a more accurate understanding of its relative merits;—and comparing natural things with things that are really superhuman, may see more clearly the transcendent superiority of all that has been related of Christ, beyond any antagonistic claims affecting equal power;—and, with a belief more and more strengthened by a diligent and prayerful investigation of the truth, may be enabled in all sincerity with Nathaniel to exclaim, "Rabbi, Thou art the son of God! Thou art the King of Israel!" [*]

---

[*] In a recent address at Exeter, before the Devon Pathological Society, Dr. Shapter of that city actually spoke of the "blasphemies of Mesmerism being quoted as part of the medical art," meaning, as it was understood, by that

CHAP. VII.

EXPLANATION OF MARVELS AND FANCIED MIRACLES.—ECSTATIC DREAMERS AND REVELATIONS.—THE MAID OF KENT, THE PROPHETESS OF THE CATHOLICS. — MARGARET MICHELSON, THE PROPHETESS OF THE COVENANTERS.—THE SHEPHERDESS OF CRET.—THE BOHEMIAN PROPHETESS.—SISTER GERMAINE OF BRAZIL.—MARTHA BROSSIER, THE WITCH OF PARIS.— THE ENTRANCED FEMALE, OR WESLEYAN PROPHETESS.—JOHN EVANS AND THE DEMON OF PLYMOUTH DOCK.—LORD SHREWSBURY'S TYROLESE ECSTATICA. — REVELATIONS OF THE "SEERESS OF PREVOST." — "REMARKABLE SERMONS" OF RACHEL BAKER. — "DIVINE REVELATIONS OF NATURE," BY AN AMERICAN CLAIRVOYANT. — THE MESMERIC PROPHETESS. — THE SLEEPING HAYMAKER. — THE SLEEPING SOLDIER. — MESMERIC ACTION CONTAGIOUS. — MAXWELL AND BACON ON MAGNETIC SYMPATHY AND VIRTUE.

BUT though Mesmerism do not shake, in the most distant degree, the belief of the intelligent Christian in the reality of

---

phrase, the pretensions of the science to some miraculous character, or rather its "imitations" of the divine power.

"Even the blasphemies of Mesmerism!" What can the Baconian lecturer mean? By what process of "induction" has he landed on this notion? Mesmerism may be false, or exaggerated as to its value, but wherein is it more blasphemous than any other of those adjuncts in the healing art, which the doctor himself employs? Mesmerism is simply an application of a power in nature towards the mitigation of disease, and nothing else: is this blasphemous? An assumption of religious zeal and of religious language when we wish to raise a prejudice against an adverse party, is an old game, and a plausible, but not remarkable for its charity. "The wrath of man worketh not the righteousness of God:" in other words, Christian feelings are not advanced by a lecturer stepping unnecessarily out of his path to brand an adversary with the nickname of "blasphemer," under the sanctimonious guise of a horror of his opinions.

Dr. S. is a self-dubbed follower of Bacon: here is a quotation from his favourite author, which he seems to have overlooked.

"It was a notable observation of a wise father, that those which held and persuaded pressure of consciences," (a phrase, which Bacon previously explains as meaning, the 'making the cause of religion descend' to some opprobrious purpose,) "were commonly interested therein themselves for their own ends."—Essays, III.

Scripture miracles,—it furnishes the Philosopher with a useful clue towards the understanding of much that has hitherto been mysterious.* In the history of man, many facts have been recorded, of which a clear explanation has yet been wanting. In all ages of the world, we have had a succession of marvels, at which the ignorant have been alarmed, the wise have been staggered, and the superstitious excited.† False prophets, pretended miracles, wonder-working saints, have, from time to time, arisen, disturbing and deceiving the very elect. Though heathenism and idolatry have had their prodigies in abundance, to the authority of which their votaries have appealed in confirmation of their creed, the Church of Christ has been more especially rife with pretensions of the same order. The charge of trick and delusion on these occasions has been advanced in every generation;—sometimes correctly,—not unfrequently, however, with inconsiderate haste.‡ The unbeliever has detected much that was false;—the scientific have traced much to the effect of imagination; and so the inconsequential conclusion has been adopted through convenience, that imposture was at the foundation of all the rest. And yet to those who had impartially examined the various recorded statements, this summary decision was not always satisfactory. A miracle, or miraculous train of incidents, is, for example, announced. After a time an

---

* As, in a variety of curious facts to be adduced in this chapter, I am constantly saying that Mesmerism will explain them, let it be understood once for all, that I do not *always* mean that the parties had been mesmerised, but that their condition was identical with the Mesmeric state.

† "If we look through the records of past times, we shall find many extraordinary facts not to be accounted for, nor yet, therefore, to be disbelieved, but still which are simply extraordinary; WONDERS NOT MIRACLES; things which excite surprise, but which lead to nothing."—*Arnold's Sermons*, vol. iii. p. 345.

‡ In Professor Gregory's "abstract" from Reichenbach, there is a curious and satisfactory explanation of certain ghost-stories, or "corpse-lights in churchyards." "Many nervous or hysterical females must often have been alarmed by white, faintly-luminous objects in dark churchyards, to which objects fear has given a defined form." Reichenbach gives a most interesting explanation, and adds, that "it was not altogether erroneous when old women declared that *all had not the gift to see* the departed wandering about their graves, for it must have always been the *sensitive alone*, &c."—The number is reduced to the whole account for the elucidation.—p. 67.

---

inquiry is pursued. The sceptic and the unprejudiced take the question up. A mass of falsehood and folly is discovered; and yet, after a large deduction on that head, there often "remained a residuum of something strange and perplexing" to the most philosophic. Of course, all this was, in the end, placed to the account of "imagination," and so the question was disposed of for a season;—but the real analysis of the difficulty was incomplete and partial.*

Most divisions of the Church have, in their turn, appealed to their own especial marvel. A miracle has not been wanting to prove the most opposite doctrines. Wherever there has been the coarsest ignorance, there has generally been the greatest prodigy: and the number of these "lying wonders" has been in proportion, not so much to the quality of the faith, as to the enthusiasm of the party, and the multitude and character of the respective followers. As Bacon says, in his Advancement of Learning, "This facility of credit, and accepting or admitting things weakly authorised or warranted, hath too easily registered reports and narrations of miracles wrought by martyrs, hermits, and other holy men, which, though they had a passage for a time by the ignorance of the people, the superstitious simplicity of some, and the politic toleration of others, —yet, after a period, when the mist began to clear up, they grew to be esteemed but as old wives' fables, impostures of the clergy, and illusions of spirits, to the great scandal and detriment of religion."†

---

* Dr. Arnold observes, "A man may appear ridiculous, if he expresses his belief in any particular story, to those who know nothing 'of it but its strangeness. And there is no doubt that human folly and human fraud are mixed up largely with most accounts of wonders. Yet, to say that ill recorded wonders are false, from those recorded by Herodotus down to the latest *reports of animal magnetism*, would be a boldness of assertion wholly unjustifiable and extravagant. * * * We should consider whether the accounts are of force enough to lead us to search for some law hitherto undiscovered, *to which they may all be referred*, and become hereafter the *foundation of a new science.*"—*Lectures*, 189.

† "If some *fables* have been received as *truths*, there are probably many *truths*, disguised by circumstances, which have been generally *rejected* as *fabulous.*"—*Colquhoun's preface to Wienholt*, p. 15, where some instructive instances and experiments are referred to.

One point, however, is deserving of notice. Whatever accumulation of falsehood has been super-added in the progress, the original fact, from which the pretended miracle has taken its rise, has in general been a genuine and undoubted occurrence, for which a natural or secondary cause may be discovered. Most corrupt as is human nature, this statement may be adopted with but occasional exceptions. Nor is it difficult to follow out a transaction of the kind, till it altogether assumes the colour of complete imposture. A singular fact, for instance, occurs in a secluded spot, and amongst an ignorant population. It is soon spoken of as supernatural. The first to visit and inquire into the details is the spiritual pastor of the flock. He hears much that is incomprehensible to him. But little removed in intelligence above his own superstitious congregation, he adopts their theory, and sees with their eyes. The fact becomes a miracle with him.[*] God has visited his people; and as the especial minister of God he takes the management of the case under his peculiar care. Nothing has thus far occurred but what is fair and natural. Soon, however, a temptation assails him; for the admiration of the populace begins to flag; the wonder is ceasing to be wonderful. The good man fears that the salutary check upon sin and immorality, which the suddenness of the marvel had effected in his neighbourhood, is losing its charm. A little excitement is necessary: a small additional wonder, therefore, is ingeniously brought out. The success is complete: the credit of the miracle resumes its hold; the power of religion takes deeper root: and thus the supposed goodness of the object, and the real benefits of the deception, warp his judgment and lead him on. The same round, however, must again be shortly run. And thus, step by step, the pious fraud grows beneath his hand; unintentional deceptions are added in virtue's spite; the man himself has become rather "what he cannot change, than what he chooses;"—and at last the original wonder has swelled into a monstrous amount of

[*] "It is not every wonderful thing, contrary to the laws of nature, so far as we know them, that becomes immediately a sign of divine power."— *Arnold's Sermons*, vol. iii. p. 245.

wickedness and imposture; and religion and the cause of truth are perilled by the detection.[*]

Now, for many of these marvellous occurrences, Mesmerism can afford a natural explanation.[†] From my own experience, I can state that very many facts, which have been accepted as miraculous, and secured the wonder of a superstitious multitude, have been but the transcript of the same class of incidents as have occurred within the walls of my own house. Natural Somnambulism, or Mesmerism, (for they are both but different phases of the same condition,) will explain many points of the "supernatural" which were previously inexplicable to the inquirer. Nor is it necessary, on all occasions, to assume that any additional prodigies have been appended to the first wonder. Oftentimes the whole transaction has seemed, on Mesmeric principles, nothing but a probable and natural chain of facts: good faith, and honesty of purpose, have prevailed throughout;— the original marvel remained as it began; and a charge of imposition would be wanton and unphilosophical.[‡]

More often, however, the temptation to deceive has been too successful with sinful man. His unconquerable love of spiritual power has acted fatally on the evil propensity within. And where this power could be maintained by the encouragement, or connivance, or practice of deceit, the Old Adam has too generally surrendered to the seduction. This is the fact with all creeds and all religionists. It is monstrous to make it an

[*] Southey says that "the *physiologist* may peruse the legends of the saints with advantage." — *Vindiciæ Eccl. Angl.* 144.

[†] In some interesting papers in the Zoist, by Mr. Lloyd, called "Allusions to Mesmerism in the Classics," full of various research, and showing extensive reading, there are several passages in point. The writer well remarks, "the examination leads to the result, that the new discovery of the science, is, to a considerable extent, a *re-discovery*." The opening observations will repay a perusal. — *Zoist*, vol. iii. p. 157.

[‡] Miss Martineau, in describing some of her sensations, when under the influence of Mesmerism, observes; "then, and often before and since, did it occur to me that if I had been a *pious and very ignorant Catholic*, I could not have escaped the persuasion that *I had seen heavenly visions*. Every glorified object before my eyes would have been a revelation; and my Mesmerist, with the white halo round her head, and the illuminated profile, would have been a saint or an angel." (*Letter*, p. 15.) Let this striking fact be remembered and applied to some subsequent histories.

exclusive charge against one particular Church. That a greater variety of pious frauds has been detected among the priesthood of the Romish church is referable to the fact, that their sway has been most predominant during the darkest ages of Christianity. As Archbishop Whateley says in one of the most useful of his works, "The Origin of Romish Errors," — "This tendency to fraudulent means is not peculiar to any sect, age, or country — it is the spontaneous growth of the corrupt soil of man's heart." *

In illustration of the above, a fact can be stated on the best authority. I received it from a lady, whose name I am not at liberty to mention, — but whose position in society is a guarantee for the correctness of the story. She received it from a sister of the patient, and was herself acquainted with the names and residence of the parties. An invalid had for seven years lost the use of his legs, it is believed, by rheumatism. A Wesleyan minister in the neighbourhood, who had discovered in himself the power of relieving pain by the Mesmeric process, long, however, before Mesmerism had become generally known, called upon the sufferer, — offered to do all he could to heal him, and said that "he hoped to be as useful to him as the Prophet Elisha." The man, of course, was but too willing to place himself in his hands.† And, after a succession of manipulations, a genial warmth came on, followed by a complete restoration of the limbs. In short, the sufferer was wonderfully cured.‡ The immediate cause, we know now, was

---

* Chapter on "Pious Frauds," p. 143.

† That truly English writer, Defoe, says, "as no cheats are so fatal to those which come profaned with introductions of religion, so no cheats are so easy to prevail, or so soon make impressions on the people." — System of Magic, p. 64.

‡ Southey, in his Life of Wesley, vol. ii. p. 215, refers to a cure performed by a life-guardsman, which Wesley published as "plainly miraculous." Southey says, "it must either have been miracle or fraud;" and then shows his own opinion, that it was the latter. To this Coleridge appended a MS. note. "As to the fact itself, Southey's 'must — either — or —' is grounded on imperfect knowledge of the complaint here described. It was a case of that class which have been found most often and most influenced by stimulants of imagination, sudden acts of active volition, and by repeated friction, touching, kneading, and the like." Coleridge, it is well known, had deeply studied the question of Mesmerism, especially amongst the Germans.

Mesmerism; for such results are not uncommon; but the thing was inscrutable to all around, and was deemed miraculous by the patient and many of his friends. The Wesleyan minister was regarded by the ignorant populace as a prophet, or, as Bacon expresses it, a "holy man," in consequence; and as his spiritual influence was mightily increased by the transaction, our good preacher winked at the delusion, — but in reality was more of a deceiver than many a calumniated monk in the church of Rome. *

De Foe, in his "System of Magic," speaks of "an artificial or rational magic, in which men cured disease by charms, by herbs, — by such and such gestures, striking the flesh in such and such a manner, and innumerable such-like pieces of mimicry; working not upon the disease itself, but upon the imagination of the distempered people, and so effecting the cures by the power of nature." † De Foe evidently refers to some facts, with which he was acquainted by tradition or observation: the quotation is a curious one: but our writer, in his remark on "imagination," undervalued that "power of nature," on which he was dwelling.

But it is on that class of strange appearances, which has received the name of the Devotional Ecstasis, that Mesmerism throws an especial light. In all ages, heathen and Christian, a peculiar species of physiological effect has been observed, from time to time, to present itself in young and sickly females, — which has assumed the character of the miraculous or the divine. Sibyls, prophetesses, inspired priestesses, ecstatic dreamers, magical maids, devout nuns, entranced females, have all followed in succession, and received their particular appellation from the accident of the country or religion that claimed them, and of which they became the temporary boast.‡ All

---

* In the Abbé J. B. L. (Chapter 19.) some similar facts are given, especially in extracts from a "Traité des Superstitions," by J. B. Thiers. The accounts are curious and instructive. Gauthier, in speaking of these facts, and in describing how Mesmerism passed from the hands of the Pagans into those of the Christians, calls it a "Catholic magnetism." The Catholics, it will be seen, have no exclusive claim to the title.

† Works, vol. xii. p. 42.

‡ "Nevertheless certain facts, furnished by the history of sibyls, pytho-

these female prodigies have invariably been regarded as divinely commissioned; and while their symptoms, language, attitude, and dreams, have all partaken of one uniform character, the doctrines they have upheld have been as opposite as the poles. *Disease was the secret of the whole matter.* I do not believe that one single instance of this class of ancient or modern miracles can be adduced, in which the party had not been originally, and often for a long time, in a most unhealthy condition.* Let this fact be followed out, and it will be found correct. In this diseased state, nature often relieves itself by throwing the patient into an hysteric and sleeping state. This somnambulistic condition is nothing else than Mesmerism spontaneously produced, — as the symptoms and phenomena clearly indicate. They are but one and the same; with this difference, that in artificial Mesmerism, a sympathy with the Mesmeriser is superadded, and a curative action obtained. I do not mean that these peculiar phenomena occur in every case of Mesmerism; on the contrary, they are very rare: but when they do take place, they are so precisely similar in their character and affection to what occurs in common somnambulism, that no material difference exists between them. Of course, as in the natural ecstasis, they are not all equally marked: some are stronger in one point than in another; some are of a very short duration; — some are very beautiful — some are very painful to witness; — still they all belong to one family; and whether resulting from a natural or artificial action, may universally be traced to the working of disease. The very same phenomena, which I have myself witnessed in the case of Anne Vials, and which have occurred with her over and over again, have been brought forward as proofs of the miraculous nature of several appearances in different entranced females.† Dr. Elliotson, in the fourth number of the "Zoist," mentions a

masses, convulsionaries, and ecstatics, will perhaps be more easy to be understood, at least in their second causes, when we shall know more of the phenomena of artificial somnambulism." — *Abbé J. B. L.,* p. 106.

* Michelet, speaking of a case of this class, says, " there was nothing in this relating to theology. It was merely a subject of physiology and medicine." — *Priests and Women,* p. 91.

† See Chapter III. page 193.

---

similar case in one of his patients, where a beautiful ecstatic fit of holy rapture was brought on in the Mesmeric trance, and which, amongst an ignorant people, might have been used for any superstitious purpose.* In other cases, which will be mentioned, the patient is invested with an apparently prophetic character, and a species of divine knowledge seems to be conferred upon her.† In all these cases, naturally or artificially induced, there is almost always, during the period of the paroxysm, a very great exaltation of the intellectual faculties, an unusual clearness of mind, — a high tone of moral feeling, — a spirituality not only in appearance but in language, and occasionally that peculiar power of foreseeing the *probable* result of certain circumstances *then in action,* which, when the effect corresponds with the expectation, assumes the semblance of the prophetic. In fact, as has been truly observed, the crisis is so strange, and the characteristic phenomena so remarkable, that "the same individual, when awake, and when somnambulist, appears like two entirely different persons." ‡ It is not, therefore, at all to be wondered at, that a young and ignorant girl,

* Zoist, vol. i. p. 449. Mr. D. Hands, Surgeon, of 22. Thayer Street, had also a patient, whom I have more than once seen in an ecstatic and devotional attitude from Mesmerism. In Mr. S. Hall's "Mesmeric Experiences" is a description, by Mr. William Howitt, the popular writer, of "Little Henry," whom Mr. Hall cured of a curious affection of the brain. Mr. Howitt says, "the effects produced on him by music are in particular striking. They throw him into attitudes which would form the finest models for the sculptor and painter." (p. 30.) Having myself seen Mr. S. Hall place Henry in the Mesmeric sleep, I can bear witness to the accuracy of Mr. Howitt's description. "His countenance at times acquires a pathos, a sublimity, or an expression of fun, that are singularly beautiful."

† Of a similar character are the "Divine Revelations of Nature," by the American youth, Andrew Davis, the "Clairvoyant," to which I referred in the last chapter; and the Revelations of the "Seeress of Prevost," communicated by Dr. Kerner, of Weinsburg.

‡ I shall shortly refer to the "Remarkable Sermons" of Rachel Baker, delivered during her sleep, in the State of New York, in 1814. She was an ignorant girl, only fifteen years of age, by no means "endowed with a sensible mind," but who, in her "night-talkings," showed herself most learned and eloquent in the doctrinal parts of Calvinistic Christianity.

I have already (p. 30.) quoted from Dr. Moore, the case of Dr. Haycock, who preached so powerfully in his sleep, but was unequal to it when awake. Dr. Moore mentions two or three other cases of similar exaltation; and refers to an opinion of Dr. Copland, that the Italian Improvisatori are in a peculiar state of ecstasy at the time of their pouring forth their ideas.

when thrown by disease into this devotional ecstasis,—at one moment looking up with heavenly smiles, and clasping her hands together as if praying,—at another, uttering the most strange and mysterious opinions, with a degree of knowledge, and freedom, and decision, of which she is perfectly incapable when awake, should be regarded by the uneducated as a supernatural being. And when certain phenomena, such as an absence of pain, lengthened sleep, vision of persons or things with the eyes closed, should be superadded to these other appearances, it is, perhaps, to be expected that some such an opinion should possess the minds even of the better informed. Deceived themselves by the incomprehensible character of the sleeper's condition, they end in deceiving others. And thus a diseased habit of body, which a larger acquaintance with physiology can now readily explain, became accredited as a miracle, or denounced as Satanic, according to the accidental creed of the parties interested in the interpretation."

The object, therefore, of this present Chapter is twofold.

First, to show that the Mesmeric condition is not an eccentric, anomalous state, abhorrent from all previous experience and tradition, and oversetting, if true, the acknowledged laws and operations of nature;—but rather analogous to,—or, to speak more correctly, actually identical, in its phenomena and in its essence, with much that had been recorded by physiologists and divines long before Mesmer and his treatment had been born or thought of.†

Secondly, to divest a variety of wonders in past, and present

---

* The sceptic takes a different line. Hume, in his famous Essays, rejects all such statements as "impossible." Speaking of the cures performed at the tomb of the Abbé Paris, he says: "What have we to oppose to such a cloud of witnesses but the absolute impossibility or miraculous nature of the events which they relate? and this, surely, in the eyes of all reasonable people will alone be regarded as a sufficient refutation." The modern physiologist knows, however, the possibility of far more wondrous facts.

† I am not pretending to any originality in offering this argument: the opinion has been long established among Mesmerists. See Elliotson's Physiology; Colquhoun's Isis Revelata, chapters xvi. xvii. and xxii.; and especially Townshend's Facts, book iii. on "Conformity of Mesmerism with general Experience." The French writers all take the same view. It is hoped that the sceptic, on observing this identity of Mesmerism with antecedent marvels, will be disposed to give a readier credence to our simpler tales.

---

and even future times, of their seemingly superhuman character;—to relieve many innocent parties of that charge of imposture with which ignorance taxes them; and to reduce the mysterious and the uncommon to the Mesmeric level of every-day nature. In attempting this, I must here and there rob a religious visionary of some pleasing illusion, by showing how his favourite prodigy has been, at times, manifested in behalf of an heretical antagonist: but I have no intention of infusing into the inquiry the bitterness of theological controversy. I see enough of the melancholy result of polemics within the pale of my own Church, to lose any temptation, that the occasion might offer, of assailing the erroneous conclusions of those that are "without." With Meric Casaubon, "I meddle not with policy, but *nature*; nor with evil men so much, as *the evil consequence of the ignorance of natural causes.* * * * My business shall be, as by examples of *all professions in all ages*, to show how men have been very prone upon some *grounds of nature*, producing some *extraordinary*, though *not supernatural*, effects, *really*, *not hypocritically*, yet falsely and erroneously" to deem themselves or their co-religionists inspired; and my wish is "to dive into the dark mysteries of nature, *for probable confirmations* of natural operations, falsely deemed supernatural." *

With this object, I proceed by divers extracts and instances, to show how Mesmerism, Hysteria, and natural Somnambulism, reciprocally throw light the one on the other.

Without going back, however, to the olden days of Greece or Rome, we may procure many an example out of the annals of the Church. Take Hume's "History of the Holy Maid of Kent," in the reign of Henry the Eighth. "Elizabeth Barton had been subject to hysterical fits, which threw her body into unusual convulsions †; and having procured an equal disorder in her mind, made her utter strange sayings, which, as *she was scarcely conscious of them during the time*, had soon after en-

---

* Treatise on Enthusiasm, 1655, chap. i. p. 4. Casaubon, in his preface, speaks of religious zealots "embracing a cloud or a fog for a Deity,"—"pro Junone nubem."

† Strype, in his Memorials, says, "the maid was visited with sickness; and in the violence thereof would fall into fits."

tirely escaped her memory. The silly people in the neighbourhood were struck with these appearances, which they imagined to be *supernatural*." The vicar of the parish began to "watch her in her trances, and note down her sayings." Knavery soon followed the first delusion. The maid was taught to assume a more extraordinary language, and to counterfeit stranger trances under the dictation of her spiritual director. "Miracles were daily *added* to increase the wonder; and the pulpit everywhere resounded with accounts of the sanctity and inspiration of the new prophetess." She was afterwards apprehended, the forgery of her miracles was detected, and the public was undeceived.

Now it is clear, from the attendant circumstances, that this was a case of natural Mesmerism. The poor girl had been subject to hysterical fits, the effect of disease. In these fits she fell into a deep trance or sleep: in this sleep the usual exaltation of mind came on;—she "uttered strange sayings," of which strange sayings, when she awoke, she was quite unconscious. This common occurrence in the Mesmeric state the world deemed "supernatural;" and a designing priesthood "persuaded the people and the maid herself that her ravings were inspirations of the Holy Ghost." *

As the mistaken views of the multitude in this instance caused the death of Elizabeth Barton,—and the imprisonment, and, perhaps, ultimately the execution of Fisher, Bishop of Rochester, this case has acquired an historical importance.

The above ill-used girl was a Roman Catholic prophetess: our next example shall be taken from the Calvinistic fanatics of Scotland,—in a case which is equally stamped with the Mesmeric characters.

When Charles I. was endeavouring to force Episcopacy upon the reluctant citizens of the northern province of his kingdom,

* Burnet says, "she forgot all she had said in her fits; yet the crafty priest would not let it go so, but persuaded her that what she had said was by the inspiration of the Holy Ghost."—Vol. i. p. 275.

Lingard says, "she herself insensibly partook of the illusion, and the rector of the parish advised her to enter a convent. In her new situation her ecstacies and revelations were multiplied."—Henry VIII., p. 206.

it is well known what passionate feelings were excited in the fervid breasts of that determined people. The whole nation was in an uproar. Hume says, "We must not omit another auxiliary of the Covenanters, and no inconsiderable one; *a prophetess*, who was followed and admired by all ranks of people. Her name was Michelson, a woman full of whimsies, partly hysterical, partly religious, and inflamed with a zealous concern for the ecclesiastical discipline of the Presbyterians. Thousands crowded about her house. Every word she uttered was received with veneration, as the most sacred oracles. The covenant was her perpetual theme. Rollo, a popular preacher, and zealous Covenanter, was her great favourite; and paid her, on his part, no less veneration. Being desired by the spectators to pray with her, and speak to her, he answered, that ' he durst not, and that it would be ill manners in him to speak while his Master, Christ, was speaking in her.'" *

But the fullest description of this curious case will be found in the Royal or "Large Declaration," which was put forth for the purpose of traducing the Covenanters and their adherents. "There was a maid, whose name is Michelson, her father was a minister, and when he died, left her young: she hath for many years been *distracted by fits*. Upon this young maid's weakness, some were pleased to work, and to report her for one inspired with a spirit of divination: and finding, that out of her blind zeal she was wonderfully affected with their covenant, and that in her raving fits her words tended all, or, for the most part, to the admiration of it,—and perceiving that she was *well-skilled in the phrases of Scripture*, and had a good memory, they thought her a fit instrument to abuse the people, and cried her up so, that the multitude was made believe her words proceeded not from herself—but from God. All sorts of people watched and stayed by her, day and night, during her *pretended fits*, and *did admire her raptures* and inspirations, as coming from heaven. She *spake but at certain times*, and *many times had intermissions of days and weeks*." Opponents to her said, "there was nothing *supernatural*, she had a good

* Hume, vol. vi. p. 337.

U

memory, and a *very good expression of herself;* she knew what she was speaking, and while speaking, if she were interrupted by any questions, she *made very pertinent answers to them.* — Most of all she spake tended to the Covenanters' ends : when she spoke of Christ, she called him the Covenanting Jesus."

"Many thought that the crying up of this maid did look like a Romish imposture." *

Her "good expression of herself" while speaking, and the "pertinency of her answers," in her fits and trances, all clearly point to the condition that this poor girl was in, and to its identity with Mesmeric sleep-waking. The circumstances of the case are similar to those of Elizabeth Barton, except that the one was a Catholic and the other a Calvinist.

Our next instance shall be also drawn from the pages of Protestant History, in which the Mesmeric type can be still more evidently traced. When Louis the Fourteenth revoked the Edict of Nantes, and withdrew the protection of the state from the reformed Church, the most extraordinary excitement was stirred up in the south of France, in the mountainous district called the Cevennes. The whole population went mad with religious zeal. They preached, — they prophesied, — they quaked ; — in short, the most marvellous state of things came on, — so that to the eye of the ardent Protestant a divine revelation and assistance appeared vouchsafed to the cause. All the parties, however, fell asleep first, before they began to preach.

In the midst of the general excitement, one especial case of miraculous illumination was singled out. Isabeau Vincent, a young girl, aged seventeen, was constantly falling into a state of deep sleep, from which it was at times impossible to arouse her. They called to her with a loud voice, — they pushed her, — they pinched her, — they pricked her till they drew blood, — they burned her, — but nothing awoke her. She was soon regarded by her Protestant neighbours as a prophetess. For in her sleep she sang Psalms, and chanted long hymns, and made

---

* *Large Declaration, by Charles I., London,* 1639, one of those Tracts, for which, like the *Eikon,* the royal martyr obtained the credit of authorship. The "Declaration" is supposed to be written by a Divine who was afterwards rewarded with the Deanery of Durham.]

---

admirable prayers, and recited texts of Scripture, — which she expounded, and from which she formed her prophetic declarations. When she awoke, *she remembered nothing of what she had said or prophesied during the ecstasis.* And one other remarkable point in her condition was, — that she rarely awoke of herself, — but required assistance, and told those about her to awaken her. *

[Isabeau was called "the Shepherdess of Cret." In a "Relation of several that Prophesie in their Sleep," a writer, who calls himself "a physician and philosopher, naturally incredulous," states, that "he examined the eyes, pulse, the beating of the heart of the shepherdess, five different nights, and asks, that notwithstanding the agitation she is in all the night, she has her pulse as quiet as one that is in a deep sleep, and *her body insensible.* She has preached from the 3rd of February to the 28th of May, but does not find herself the least weary, *rising as fresh in the morning* as if she had neither said nor done any thing (during the night). She never opens her eyes in speaking : — and *speaks in a shriller tone than when she ordinarily talks."* †

Turner in his "Providences," also speaks of this case, — beginning with "reflexions upon the miracle that happened in the person of a shepherdess of Dauphiné," ‡ and then gives the famous "Pastoral Letter" of Jurieu upon the subject. Peter Jurieu, it is well known, was a celebrated French Protestant divine, who died at the beginning of the eighteenth century. His theological and polemical writings, more particularly his "Preservative against Popery," were so highly valued, that he was sometimes called the "Goliah of the Protestants," — and we are, therefore, naturally curious to learn what this giant in controversy thought of the "reformed" wonder. Jurieu, then, was evidently caught by it. He considered Isabeau "in-

---

* "Ces extases ne paraissaient que comme un profond sommeil, duquel il était impossible de la tirer. On l'appelait à haute voix, on la poussait, on la pinçait, on la piquait jusqu'au sang, on la brûlait, rien ne la réveillait." — Bertrand. *T. du Somnambulisme,* p. 362.

† Tract in the British Museum, called a " *Relation of several, &c., that Prophesie and Preach in their Sleep, containing a Relation of the Prophets of Dauphiné,*" 1689. p. 13.

‡ Turner's Providences. Folio, p. 161.

v 3

spired," to use his own words: he says, that "there is a great character of Divinity in what she utters," when asleep. When he saw her, he described her as being "in an entire and absolute privation of all sense." "She puts her arms out of bed, and with them forms *certain graceful and well-ordered gestures.*" "She was observed, after her waking, to return to her natural simplicity, and to the *ignorance* of a poor shepherdess," —and to forget all her inspired preachings, and the improvement in the character of her language and ideas.

While the Protestants thus regarded her as miraculously inspired, the neighbouring priesthood endeavoured to exorcise her with Holy Water. The Curate of Bordeaux came to see the case, and also to examine others that were thus diabolically possessed. "He pressed the finger, and sorely pricked a young maid of fourteen years old, who notwithstanding felt nothing of it."* We have, however, seen, that in the case of Elizabeth Barton, the very same trances and prophecies were deemed fraudulent by the Protestants, but the inspirations of the Holy Spirit by her own people.

Now an experienced Mesmeriser sees the clue to the whole story of Imbeau Vincent. There is nothing in her case, but what he has occasionally met with. The deep sleep, and the insensibility to pain and to noise, come first of all;—and then we have the change in her condition, when she begins to preach and sing psalms, with an exaltation of the faculties, and an improvement in the language, and an alteration in the voice, and the utter absence of fatigue after most violent exertion,—and the gracefulness of her attitudes, and the forgetfulness of every thing that she has said or done, when she is awakened from her ecstasy. All these incidents in her history were purely Mesmeric, except in their origin. Nature brought them out spontaneously in a simple ignorant shepherdess, but the practised Mesmeriser has more than once induced them by his manipulations and influence.

We have another remarkable prophetess in the reformed church, Christian Poniatova, of Bohemia. Her convulsions, trances, and visions took place in 1627, at the time that a sharp

* "Relation of several," &c. p. 14.

persecution was set on foot against the Protestant part of the Bohemian community. Her visions had reference to the prosperity and fortunes of the reformed church. Her sleep was most profound; during which she fell into an ecstasis. She then predicted several events; and she seems to have had in that state a certain species of *prevision*, such as Mesmerised patients occasionally possess. Her Protestant partisans regarded the whole as a miracle, and the girl as divinely inspired. But here is the noticeable point: when she recovered her health, the *supernatural* disappeared. The malady and the miracle went away together. She afterwards married, and was no longer regarded as a prophetess.*

Mr. Colquhoun, in the "Isis Revelata," gives us another case that occurred in Brazil, where a girl, named Sister Germaine, in 1808, was attacked by an hysterical affection, accompanied by serious ill health:—"She was in such a state, that she was no longer able to rise from her bed, and subsisted upon a regimen which could scarcely have supported the life of a new-born infant." And now comes the miraculous part. The poor invalid fell into a deep trance: her arms grew stiff, and were extended in the form of a cross, and in this position remained for hours. Other circumstances, usual in this sort of ecstasis, took place; the whole was declared to be a miracle. Sister Germaine was regarded as a saint; and the concourse of pilgrims to visit her was immense. And now let us notice the close connection between natural and Mesmeric somnambulism. The priest stated, that "in the midst of the most fearful convulsions, it was always sufficient for him to *touch the patient* to restore her to perfect tranquillity. During her periodical ecstasies, when her limbs were so stiff that it would have been

* Bertrand, Traité du Somnambulisme. In regard to this simultaneous departure of the malady and the miracle, we have another proof of its connexion with Mesmerism. Gauthier says, "*The best proof of a perfect state of health is the cessation of somnambulism, and of the action of magnetism.*" —Traité Pratique, p. 590. And M. Casaubon says, "To all these natural diseases and distempers enthusiastic divinatory fits are incidental. I do not say that it doth happen very often: but when it doth happen, as the disease is cured by natural means, so the enthusiasms go away, I will not say by the same means, *but at the same time.*"—Treatise on Enthusiasm, cap. ii. p. 59.— Casaubon was evidently a cautious and close observer of nature.

easier to break than bend them, her confessor, according to his own account, had only to touch her arm, in order to give it whatever position he thought proper." Every Mesmeriser who has had a patient in a rigid or cataleptic state can understand and believe the above narrative.*

In the reign of Henry IV. of France, a case containing some startling phenomena had its origin in the town of Romorantin, and subsequently occasioned much disturbance at Paris, from its connection with religious animosities and the edict of Nantes. The narrative is given by the great historian De Thou.†

Martha Brossier, the name of the girl, was seized with fits, and violently convulsive movements, and fell into a state of delirium and ecstasy. Marvellous prodigies were performed by her in this condition. The ultra-Catholic party, anxious to trouble the king and unsettle the country, in consequence of the toleration recently conceded to the Protestants, fastened upon this case as a proof of divine displeasure, and a signal instance of diabolical possession.‡ The girl is carried before the Bishop

---

* A learned writer in the "Church of England Quarterly Review," for April, 1843, in an article on this subject, has collected the names of several ecstatic nuns and females of the church of Rome. The reviewer mentions some cases in which the imposture was clear, and admitted afterwards by the parties: and hence he infers that all the other instances were "sheer imposture," in like manner. Imposition, however, will not explain all the facts. It explains much that was added on in the progress of the work, after the priests had found the trances profitable; but that the original state of many a "prophetess," which led to the delusion, was a natural and diseased action none can doubt, who have given to the subject of Mesmerism a philosophical study. See Appendix II.

† Thuanus, tom. v. liber. 123. The case is also alluded to by several other writers. Bayle, in his Dictionary, has a long article upon her: his sceptical mind regarded the whole as a cheat.

‡ De Foe, in that strange but orthodox book, "*The Political History of the Devil*,"—written indeed with good intentions, though too often in an irreverent style,—has a chapter about "the cloven foot walking about without the devil," or, in other words, a dissertation to show that "Satan is not guilty of all the simple things we charge him with." Much of it is very germane to the uses of Mesmerism. "How," says our author, "does the devil's doing things so foreign to himself, and so out of his way, viz., showing a kind of a friendly disposition to mankind, or doing beneficent things, agree with the rest of his character?" Part ii. chap. 7. De Foe professes in the Introduction to "give the true history" of Satan,—"to show what he is, and what he is not; where he is, and where he is not;—when he is in us, and when he is not."

---

of Angers. The good Bishop laughs at the idea of Satanic influence;—but not understanding the character of the disease, and believing the case to be an imposition, secretly advises the father to take Martha home, and let the matter die a natural death. But the father was in the hands of those who wish any thing but quiet, and at their suggestion he removes his daughter to Paris. There the Capuchin Monks take the matter up, and asserting that the unhappy girl is tormented by an evil spirit, try to exorcise her. The Archbishop of Paris now comes forward, — and calls in five of the most celebrated physicians of the metropolis to advise: these differ in opinion: the majority asserting the case to be one of fraud, — Duretus, an instance of Satanic agency. The parliament next steps into the arena, and guided by the judgment of the first four doctors, decides that the girl is an impudent impostor. This adds fuel to the flame. The greatest tumult is occasioned. The clergy and Archbishop, indignant at the matter being thus taken out of their hands, appeal to Rome; and had it not been for the prudence and tact of Henry, the affair might have had the most serious results. The King, however, manages to close the matter peacefully; and the "famous imposture," as Bishop Lavington calls it, of Martha Brossier ends like others of its order.*

Some of the phenomena recorded in this case require a notice. The first is, the girl's insensibility to pain. Meric Casaubon mentions that "pins and needles were *thrust* in at the fleshy parts of her neck and arms, and that the girl never seemed to feel it." De Thou records the same fact. Duretus, the physician, drove a needle into Martha's hand between the thumb and forefinger, and not the slightest movement was made, nor any blood followed. Duretus, therefore, judged it to be a case of Satanic possession, in compliance with the old opinion, which has always regarded the absence of sensation as an evidence of witchcraft, an opinion, it may be added, that only ether and chloroform have succeeded in removing.†

---

* Bishop Lavington, p. 257. M. Casaubon, cap. iii.

† It is a question, supposing that the excellent Professor Simpson had been living but a century or two back, whether the elders of the Scotch Kirk, so famous for their inquisitorial intermeddlings, would not have dragged him before their synod to answer for his discoveries.

Secondly, the girl, according to De Thou's narrative, remained, for a moment or two, suspended in the air without support, from some lightness of body peculiar to her condition. Fullo, Abbot of St. Geneviève, stated that Martha, though held down by six strong men, lifted herself up four feet above their heads, and remained so some short time. The priests, not so unreasonably, pronounced this diabolical. Marcescotus, however, one of the physicians, examining into the fact, thought it partly fraud, and partly according to nature, or *rather not beyond nature*[*], and he gives his reasons for the opinion. Incredible, or rather impossible as the above fact appears, we shall find more than one instance of something of the kind occurring in cases of this description.

Thirdly, the last peculiar point, is that the girl, in her sleep-waking state, spoke languages, of which, when awake, she knew nothing. She spoke Greek and English. Duretus, the physician, thought this a proof of diabolical possession (quod linguam præter naturam exercuisset).[†]

Martha Brossier and her father, on their return home, died in great misery and want, through the popular feeling against them. That there was fraud mixed up with the latter stages of the proceedings, is too probable; but that, in the first instance, it was a genuine case of Mesmeric-hysteria, there can be no question.

We will now come to later days—to certain modern miracles among the Wesleyans and Roman Catholics, which have excited considerable interest and sensation in their respective churches.

Among the Wesleyans[‡] there have been recently two or three wonders,—some of which are too ridiculous to be noticed;

[*] " Eam, supra eorum, qui captam tenebant, se capita efferentem, in nervo aliquamdiu constitisse, præter naturam non esse." See Appendix III. for remarks on this incident, and for several other alleged facts of the same kind.

[†] See Appendix IV. upon this fact.

[‡] See Appendix II. for earlier cases among the Wesleyans, from Wesley's Journal, &c.—Coleridge in his Table-Talk observes, "The coincidence throughout of all these *Methodist* cases with those of the *Magnetists* makes me wish for a solution that would apply to all," &c. Vol. i. p. 107. The coincidences is so complete, we reply, that it shows that the physical condition is the same.

but there is one which, from the notoriety and credit it has obtained,—the manner with which public attention has been invited towards it, and the effect it has produced upon the religious feelings of their own body, is more especially deserving of examination.[*]

"The History of an Entranced Female" is a narrative drawn up and attested by the Rev. R. Young, Wesleyan Minister. This little work was sold by the accredited organ of the Wesleyan Book Committee and of the Conference, with their connivance, if not their permission; and so far the story received their indirect sanction. The circulation was immense. It reached a twenty-seventh edition; and the revelations of the prophetess were considered so important that the faith of whole Wesleyan congregations was in a state of warm excitement respecting them.

It was simply a case of hysteria, or natural Mesmerism, as a few words extracted from the narrative will show. The somnambulist "had *been very ill*, and was supposed to be *dying*." Here is the first point to be remembered. At last she fell into a trance. "In this state," Mr. Young says, "she appeared to die. But after lying, with no signs of life, save a little froth from the mouth and a slight warmth about the region of the heart, for nearly a week, she opened her eyes. *And now began her remarkable disclosures.*" It is unnecessary to examine these disclosures. There is no reason to suppose either trick or imagination in the transaction. It is a case of pure ignorance on the part of the writer and of his Wesleyan supporters. Like the Holy Maid of Kent, and several Mesmerised patients, the "Entranced Female" was simply in a state of exaltation, moral and intellectual, and had clearer and more active perceptions than in her ordinary condition.[†]

In 1820, a case occurred among the Wesleyans at Plymouth Dock (now Devonport), which created immense sensation in

[*] Sold by Mason, Paternoster Row.

[†] See a clever useful little book in refutation of several of these absurdities, called "Modern Miracles condemned by Reason and Scripture," by Philo-Veritas. (Painter, 342. Strand.) Still the writer has not gone to the bottom of the subject, or understood the real cause of the phenomena.

that neighbourhood. The phenomena were of a Mesmeric type, and were ascribed, as usual, to Satanic power. A small book, called "The Demon, or a case of Extraordinary Affliction, and Gracious Relief, the effects of Spiritual Agency,"[*] was published by Mr. Heaton, the minister of the congregation, — in which the facts were described. This book had a large sale, — and was followed by a tract by the same author called, "Further Observations on Demoniacal Possession,"—in which the "praeternatural" character of the symptoms were again urged. This tract reached a second edition. Some of the circumstances, indeed, were most singular: and as a medical gentleman, who attended the case, called the malady a "very extraordinary, *unnatural, unaccountable*" thing, and as Mr. Heaton, the minister, who tells the story, lived next door to the patient, and had every opportunity of examining into its truth, the facts may be considered well authenticated and deserving of notice.

John Evans, a boy between nine or ten years old, had been some time in the Plymouth Dispensary, for the treatment of fits and loss of speech. Here he was blistered and bled repeatedly. One Sunday, after service at Windmill-Hill Chapel, Mr. Lose, the father-in-law, came to Mr. Heaton with a message, that the boy was very ill, and wished him to come and pray with him. Mr. Heaton went accordingly, and was shocked at the "extraordinary affliction" of the poor child. We will give his own words. "The boy could not speak, but was perfectly sensible, — was violently convulsed, — fixed his eyes, staring upwards, — then stood motionless, his muscles appearing on a painful stretch, his arms close to his side, and stiff as the branches of a tree, and then became relaxed." Mr. H. began to pray, but the boy was agitated by prayer, and "at the name of Christ convulsions came on, — he showed antipathy to every thing sacred, — and was enraged at the sight of the Bible,"—but could not approach nearer to Mr. H. to scratch and bruise him, than within four inches, with all his efforts! Every day there came on "convulsions, — and dancing, and horrible fits, and shrieking and noise, — ending with limbs

[*] Sold by Mason, Paternoster Row.

stiffening like a tree or a corpse." "Of epilepsy, there were some very strong symptoms, nevertheless there were others which distinguished his case from being merely epileptic, — he would in his fits go through *difficult and dangerous* manoeuvres with apparent ease, self-command, and *perfect safety*, as he could not possibly perform when he was properly in his senses." "Whatever he did, — whatever he suffered during his paroxysms, he had *no recollection of*, when he came to himself." "At one time, the spirit of hartshorn was applied to his tongue, — at another, a needle was thrust deep into his flesh, neither of which he appeared to regard. This was done by a medical gentleman, solicitous to find out the real nature of the case. Several persons tried the lad's sensibility, by suddenly shaking him, beating him with a cane, &c. When he has been making his aim at the door (walking towards it), a handkerchief has been held before his face: *still his eyes were fixed*, and his course was undisturbed. When he came to himself, he was as one *awaking from a profound sleep*. The boy said, 'I was like as though I was fast asleep, and didn't dream neither; I don't remember anything.'" In his fits, he performed the most difficult exploits, — things which other people could not, — and which he himself could not, when not in the fit. "He would dance strangely and with ease on the surface of the room." "Some of his attitudes were of the most *graceful and elegant* kind; — then again he would become stiff and motionless as a corpse, and continue in this state for an hour and twenty minutes, — with his eyes fixed. His uncommon stiffness (rigidity) was the most surprising thing: some one put his hand under his head to raise it, but it could only be raised as the body was raised with it. We placed him upon his feet; he rested his whole weight on the *point of his toes*; — but even this did not make him bend his joints."[*] "Men of science," says Mr. H., "were puzzled, and medical men hesitated to give an opinion; — for to say that he was epileptic, was to give but a mere scrap of the truth of the case: — good sense must determine whether or not the supposed superhuman actions, performed by the suspected demoniac, be *physically* possible to the

[*] See Appendix III.

patient in disease or health:" and our author arrives at the conclusion that it was a clear case of Satanic possession.

After a time, a solemn assembly of Wesleyan ministers was held at the house to offer prayers for the recovery of the boy, and for the final subjugation of the power of the demon; when, suddenly, and as if in answer to their supplications, the attacks ceased,—a normal state came on, and a complete cure followed: the child subsequently suffered a relapse, but recovered through the same means and after the same way.

Such is, briefly, Mr. Heaton's strange story. Of the reality of its facts, there is no reason why any doubt should be entertained. The points, which the author considered as proofs of demoniacal possession, and which "puzzled the men of science and the medical attendants,"—may be clearly traced to a condition identical with that of Mesmerism. It is unnecessary to repeat the characteristics; the reader by this time must be familiar with them. The boy's brain, too, was evidently in a state, in which the imaginative faculty was capable of being powerfully acted on,—as was seen by his agitation and horror, at one time, of prayer;—and at another, by his recovery after its use. Epilepsy, catalepsy, Mesmerism, and imagination, will explain Mr. Heaton's "Demon."*

We will now examine some recent and no less memorable occurrences in the Roman Catholic community: which have produced an equal excitement, and have equally been referred to as proofs of the supernatural. It has long ago been observed, that in enthusiastic belief of the marvellous, the Wesleyans and Romanists are sister churches.†

We must first return to Mr. M'Neile, and give his views on the question; for strange to say, he has in some manner alighted on a certain portion of the truth, and seen the real connection between the artificial and the natural ecstasy. "This pretended

* Mr. Heaton, among his arguments to prove the demoniacal character of this case, gives us a reason which is so amusing for its logic and naïveté, that it deserves a transcript. "A preternatural affliction will betray itself by some preternatural symptoms; and without much danger of error, we may conclude that preternatural effects must have a preternatural cause." (p. 8.) This reminds one of the ratiocination exposed in the first chapter.

† See Bishop Lavington's well-known and most useful work.

science," says the sermon, "is precisely the thing that my Lord Shrewsbury has put forth, to prove that popery is the true version of Christianity. What is his Ecstatica which he has written such a book about? You have heard of the Ecstatica and Addolorata,—the two young women whom he saw on the Continent: they were Mesmerised. His description of them *exactly corresponds* with the description we have of these Mesmerised persons. He tells us of a young woman, who was in a state of ecstasy, wrapt in prayer, devoted to the Virgin;—her eyes were open, but she had no natural sensibility of what was going on without. He says that "*a fly was seen to walk across her eyeball*, and she never winked; she was totally insensible of everything that was going on, except one thing: he says, that she manifested consciousness at the approach of the consecrated host." "Now here is a state, pleaded by a popish writer as a proof of divine influence, as a proof of divine origin of his creed." "Now this belongs to the mystery of iniquity."—And so far the sermon. Now what Mr. M'Neile considered as Satanic, and my Lord Shrewsbury as divine in the above transactions, I must beg leave to reduce to a humbler character; and stripping the facts altogether of the marvellous, show to be merely an action of nature in a state of disease.

In that most delightful province of southern Germany, where the simple character of the inhabitants, and the ever-varying charms of mountain, valley, and torrent, would tempt the idle traveller to linger for weeks, two young girls have lately been the subject of much observation from the peculiar character and condition of their health. Those who have traversed that picturesque route in the Tyrol, which leads from Brixen to Trent, want not to be reminded, how every nook and turn of the road swarms with the emblems of Roman Catholic worship. Superstition puts on its most persuasive form. Images of the Virgin, of the Saviour, of the crucifixion with all its attendant accidents, stations for devotion, and hermitages, meet the eye of the passenger in uninterrupted succession. In no part of the Continent have I ever remarked so many of the externals of devotion as in the smiling vales of the Tyrol; and the primitive habits of its mountain peasantry have been strongly

moulded under their influence. As Southey says in his Colloquies, "Religion may be *neglected*, but cannot be *forgotten* in Roman Catholic countries;" and the reader is requested to bear this observation in mind, as throwing light on certain phenomena, of which strong religious feelings were the source."

These two young girls, the Ecstatica of Caldaro, and the Addolorata of Capriana (as they are now termed) had both been subject to much ill health. The former "had had *various attacks of illness* during her early years." The Addolorata "had been attacked *with violent and complicated illness* about the age of seventeen." Both at last fell into a trance. Both became "Ecstatic." And in that state such singular phenomena exhibited themselves, the effect of an excited mind upon a diseased habit of body, that the appearances were pronounced by the surrounding country to be miraculous. The priesthood at once took the case under their protection; but there is no reason to believe that any imposture or trickery were superadded by them. They were as honest as they were ignorant. All they did was to magnify the importance of the facts, and to give the largest currency to the intelligence. Multitudes flocked from all quarters as on a pilgrimage. Amongst them came my Lord Shrewsbury and suite; and several Protestant gentlemen, who were all staggered by what they saw.

Lord Shrewsbury, believing the facts to be supernatural, published that account to which Mr. M'Neile referred; and from his little pamphlet, we will select the more prominent points. "We found her," says the Noble Lord, speaking of the Ecstatica, "in her usual state of ecstasy, — kneeling upon her

* Sir Joshua Reynolds observes in one of his Discourses, " He might have seen it in an instance or two; and he mistook *accident for generality* ;" — a blunder, which Mesmerists are too prone to commit. Still, with this caution before me, I cannot help recording an observation, which has struck me, respecting the tendencies of the Reformed and of the Roman Catholic religions to develop themselves, in the Somnambulistic condition, according to their peculiar systems. The characteristic of Protestant churches is *preaching* ; that of the Roman Catholic, *contemplation of images, &c.*, as helps to prayer. Roman Catholic Somnambulists have generally fallen into the ecstatic and devotional attitude; while sermons and revelations have usually proceeded from the lips of the Reformed Sleeper. Sometimes, however, the very reverse has been the case : — it may, therefore, be all " accident."

bed, with her eyes uplifted, and her hands joined in the attitude of prayer as *motionless as a statue.* . . . . There was much of grace in her attitude." "Our first feeling was that of awe at finding ourselves in her presence." She appeared "motionless." "When in this state, she neither *sees nor hears* : all her senses are absorbed in the object of her contemplation; she is entranced; but it is neither the trance of death, nor the suspension of life, but a sort of supernatural existence, — dead indeed to this world, — but most feelingly alive to the other." " *She had not the least perception of our presence.*" "Her confessor by a slight *touch* or *word* caused her to fall back upon her pillow." "Her confessor proposed that he should awaken her entirely from her trance." "In an instant the most perfect animation was restored to her." "The circumstance which struck us, was the extreme facility with which her confessor transformed her from a state of perfect unconsciousness, as to sensible objects, to one of ordinary life." — "She has been known to remain for hours in this state," — "yet a *gentle touch* from her confessor, or any ecclesiastic with whom she is acquainted, is sufficient to dissolve the charm at once."

"A. M. de la Bouillarie visited her on his way to Rome, and found her kneeling in a state of ecstasy, when he saw a fly walk quietly across the pupil of her eye, when wide open, without producing the slightest emotion."

The Addolorata was much the same. "She frequently lay entranced for a considerable time." "It was *under these circumstances* that during one night her whole head was encircled by small wounds." "Fourteen days after the crown of thorns she received the stigmata in the hands and feet." "As a piece of deception," — says Lord Shrewsbury, "it is both morally and physically impossible." These are the main points in these two Roman Catholic miracles, with the addition of what has already been mentioned, "the consciousness of the approach of the consecrated host," — the fact of Maria Morl being raised off her knees, when physically all but incapable of motion, and *resting* only on *the tips of her feet*, — and the fact of the sheets never being stained by the blood, while, notwithstanding, there is a strong smell of coagulated blood in the room.

"Now," says Lord Shrewsbury in conclusion, "the infidel may scoff at all this, but the designs of God are accomplished." There is, however, no inclination to scoff at the sincere opinions of any man, when it is said in reply, that these supposed miraculous appearances are the same in character, as what the Wesleyan and the Protestant maidens of the Cevennes and of Bohemia exhibited in their persons, due allowance being made for the differences of religion, and the various habits of mind and body; nay, they are much the same as what numerous spectators have witnessed in the house of Mr. Atkinson, and what I have seen occurring under my own roof.

I have not a shadow of doubt, that if Mr. Atkinson had wished to found a religious sect, and, secluding Anne Vials from the world, had habituated her for years to conversation, and objects, and persons, and books of an exclusively religious character, and never permitted mundane transactions to be brought to her notice, either in her waking or sleeping state, that the most extraordinary effects might have been produced, and the most monstrous doctrines have been built up at his suggestion. He might have retreated with his ecstatic dreamer to some romantic vale, — startled the superstitious neighbourhood by her attitudes, her devotions, and her miraculous sufferings; and crowds would have flocked to witness the spectacle, and imbibe his creed; and gaping tourists might have perplexed their readers with lucubrations on the phenomena. But Mr. Atkinson is a philosopher and lover of truth: his habit is to illustrate, — to compare, — to explain; — with Bacon he delights in the "Interpretation of Nature," believing that "God hath fitted much for the comprehension of man's mind, if men will open and dilate the powers of his understanding as be may." He knew, for instance, that Lord Shrewsbury's description of his Tyrolese maidens might answer word for word, to much that has occurred with poor Anne. The fact of a fly walking over the pupil of the eye, when wide open, which seemed such a proof of the miraculous to M. de la Bouillerie, has happened with her two or three times. The fly even once stopped and cleaned its wings on the eyeball. I once saw the end of a pocket-handkerchief placed gently on the pupil, and

the lid neither winked nor moved at the touch. She was perfectly unconscious of the act.

In regard to the appearance of the stigmata and the small wounds on the head of the Addolorata, Dr. Elliotson and Mr. Atkinson both are of opinion, that they might be the effect of strong imagination and habitual contemplation upon a highly diseased frame [*] : if that view be *trop fort* for some readers, I can say, on the other hand, in spite of Lord Shrewsbury's assertion, that, as "a piece of deception, it is physically impossible;" that I would have engaged repeatedly to have made the very same marks upon the head and hand of Anne Vials without any consciousness on her part.[†] All Mesmerisers will confirm this declaration: at the same time, I see no reason to charge the Tyrolese priests with any artifice of the kind; the involuntary effect of imagination, after a preconceived idea, is so strong with some sickly sleep-waking females, that through the bare impression of the mind, nature might throw out the external phenomenon.

In the Foreign Quarterly Review, No. LXIII, is an example taken from Lavergne's "De l'Agonie et de la Mort, sous le Rapport Physiologique," &c. which strongly illustrates the probability of this opinion, and shows the effect of *habitual thought* upon *the state of the body:* "At this moment there exists in a village of the department of the Var, of which Brignoles is the chief town, a woman possessed by divine love. Since her earliest infancy this woman professes the most ardent love for

[*] See Appendix II. for extract from Ward's *History of the Hindoos*, for instances of the effect of imagination upon the fasting ecstatics of the East. I have to thank a writer in the Medical Times for reference to this work: "Practice of Hindoo Mesmerism." — July 1844.

[†] In Percival's *Cause Célèbres*, vol. vi. p. 171, is an account of a priest, Gaufridy, who seems to have possessed a magnetic power in his breath. He marked Madeleine, one of his victims, in her head, and breast, and many other parts of her body, without her consciousness. These stigmata sometimes disappeared and came back again.

An admirable article in *The Examiner* also directs our attention to a "parallel miracle, in the case of the novice Yetser, at Berne, 300 years ago, whose side, and hands, and feet were pierced, after he was made drunk with wine and opium, by the monks of his convent." See *Examiner*, Feb. 26, 1842. — This case may be found at length in Voltaire's *Essai sur les Mœurs*, &c., chap. cxxix.

Chloroform, however, may make us believe every thing.

the Saviour; the Passion *has always been her fixed idea*, the object of her aspirations and thoughts. She meditates and prays; and in her moments of ecstasy may have confided some of her visions to her friends. *When her prayer is at its height*" (in other words, when the ecstatic state is most fully developed) "a crown is seen to surround her forehead and the rest of her head, which looks as if it were opened by a regular tattooing, from each point in which a pure blood issues: the palms of her hands and the soles of her feet open spontaneously at the places where the nails of the punishment were inserted, her side offers the bleeding mark of a lance-thrust, and, finally, a true cross of blood appears on her chest. Cotton cloths applied to these places absorb the red mark.—This fact can be vouched for *by hundreds* in the country."

It may be desirable to add,—that Lord Shrewsbury, speaking of the Ecstatica, says that Görres, in his narrative of the case, relates that "so early as the autumn of the year 1833, her confessor observed, accidentally, that the part of the hands, where the wounds afterwards appeared, *began to sink in*, as if under the pressure of some external body, and also that they became *painful* and frequently attacked by cramps. He conjectured, from these appearances, that the stigmata" (i. e. the five wounds, like those of the Saviour, in the crucifixion)—"would eventually appear, and the result fulfilled his expectations. On the Purification, on the 2nd of February, 1834, he found her holding a cloth, with which, from time to time, she wiped her hands, frightened like a child at what she saw there. Perceiving blood upon the cloth, he asked her what it meant? These were the stigmata, which thenceforward continued upon her hands, and *shortly afterwards* made their appearance upon her feet, and to these, at the same time, was added the wound upon the heart." *

Now, when the Earl of Shrewsbury, with a piety which commands our respect, says that he considers these stigmata, &c.,

* A clever paper in the Dublin University Magazine for July, 1847, quotes Görres's *Seductious Triumphans*, and mentions a girl, named Elizabeth Hill, whose hands and stomach swelled, and thorns were found stuck in; and adds, that the Tyrolese were "swelled enormously" about the head, previously to stigmatisation. The writer evidently is of opinion, that there was deception in the case: it is not my opinion. See "Evening with Witchfinders."

"the most extraordinary objects in the world,"—It is necessary to remind him, that Görres mentions that "it is asserted by the directors of her conscience, and by her curate, that *in her ecstasies*, during the *last four years*, she had been employed in contemplating the life and *passion of Christ*. The most frequent object of her contemplations is the Passion of the Redeemer;—this produces the profoundest impression upon her, and is most vividly expressed upon her exterior. Particularly during the holy week, her whole being seems penetrated, and the images in her *soul act forcibly upon her frame*."

Now, when we find that this poor girl had from her childhood evinced an ardent love of God and a pleasure in prayer,—that her visits to the Franciscan church had been unremitting, that her *bodily sufferings began even in her fifth year*, that she was often on the brink of the grave, that no remedies ameliorated her health, that the root of the disorder remained undiscovered, and that therefore she became in consequence still *more pious*, meditative, and constant in prayer,—the physiologist obtains a clue to the wonder. "In her eighteenth year she again fell seriously ill, and when, after a whole year's suffering, she inquired of the doctor if it were quite impossible for her to recover her health, and he answered—that he could only alleviate her pains, she replied that she would do for the future without medical advice,"—and would receive with submission what God would lay upon her. Here, then, we see a physical preparation for what the ecstasis, or somnambulistic condition, brought out. She lived for four years during her ecstatic state in the contemplation of the Passion of the Saviour;—for more than four months before the appearance of the wounds, that part of the hands began *to sink in*, and became painful,—and the stigmata on the feet and heart did not occur till afterwards. In reading all this,—the result does not appear so very extraordinary: to use Görres's own expression,—"the images in her soul were acting forcibly upon her whole frame."

The history of the Addolorata shows the same preparation of mind and body for the same effect. "Domenica gave early indications of extraordinary piety. She was frequently found praying in the most secluded parts of the house. She received

her first communion with singular devotion, — and had expressed an ardent desire to do so at an earlier period." "At the age of seventeen she was attacked with violent and complicated illness;" — "her sufferings were so great, that her screams were often heard at a great distance;" "the holy communion alone relieved her, — after which she frequently lay entranced for a considerable time."

When the pamphlet mentions too, — that "under the very shadow of the large crucifix, which is *suspended over the head* of Maria Morl (the Ecstatica), the spirit of ecstasy is infused into her," and that "Domenica Lazari (the Addolorata) lies stretched upon her pallet *in face* of the representation of the death of the Saviour," though Lord Shrewsbury describes them as "two great and astounding miracles" — we see an additional assistance to the action of the mind upon the body, — and uniting with Mesmerism to explain the matter.

Lord Shrewsbury mentions in a note the case of another Ecstatica, in whom the wounds appeared, — who had been "*very ill*," and "*contemplating the sufferings* of the Saviour, — and, moved by sympathy, had demanded to suffer with him." * From all which occurrences, it would appear that this peculiar state is, after all, not so very extraordinary; for fifty other persons, similarly affected, are supposed to have existed in the Roman Catholic Church.

As to the consciousness of the Ecstatica, during her trance, of the approach of the consecrated host, though Mr. M'Neile thinks it an additional proof of the "mystery of iniquity," it is simply an instance of *clairvoyance*, which, though rejected at present as impossible by many unbelievers, is so exceedingly common an occurrence, that shortly it will occasion no wonder whatsoever. While the miracle of Maria Morl being raised off her knees, and resting only on the *tips of her feet*, when, physically, her strength seemed unequal to any effort, finds a parallel in Mr. Heaton's "Dæmon;" when John Evans, by the aid of Satan, "rested his whole weight on *the point of his toes*;" and in Martha Brossier, who was lifted up still higher, to the amazement of Duretus, and the Parisian fanatics.†

* See Appendix II. for this case.

† See Appendix III. for still greater wonders of this class.

After allowance, then, for the accidentals of religion, and the diversities of constitutional temperament, there is nothing in the Tyrolese phenomena of which the experienced Mesmerist has not seen or read indubitable indications. Some of the minor points, indeed, may be new and peculiar to these cases, but there can be no mistake as to the essential character of their main features; if animal magnetism has done nothing else, it has "cast," says Wolfgang Mansel, "a surprising light on the whole subject of Physio-psychology." *

Of a different class to the Ecstatics of the Tyrol is the case of Madame Hauffe, better known by the name of the "Seeress of Prevorst," a small town in Wirtemberg, and her native place. This lady was said to "*see*" and converse with the spirits of the dead, and to free them by her prayers from a purgatorial state. Upon her "Revelations," a new belief in the communications of the unseen world spread extensively in some parts of Germany. Eschenmayer, a well-known writer on Philosophy and Psychology, first attracted attention to her case by his communications.† Dr. Kerner, physician of Weinsburg, published, in 1829, a detailed account of her illness and visions, in a book that has recently been translated into English.‡ And we are told that many of the "*most pious*, cultivated, and enlightened men of Germany," have given much consideration to the case, from admiration of its phenomena.§

Mrs. Hauffe had long been a fearful sufferer, and was at last reduced to almost a skeleton. At an early period she had been remarkable for excessive sensibility, and at length became a natural somnambulist, and easily influenced by Mesmerism. In

* Chapter on Natural Sciences. The only point in the Tyrolese Ecstatics, of which I have not found something similar or analogous, is the reported fact of the "blood not staining the sheets," &c. &c. Supposing this to be true, it would not, by itself alone, prove the supernatural character of the condition, when every thing else had a physical explanation, but would rather point to the idiosyncrasy of the disease and its peculiar effects; but I have been told that this is the least well-authenticated fact in the story. Has a chemist or medical man inspected the fluid?

† Among other works, he wrote the "Conflict between Heaven and Hell, as observed in the Spirit of a Possessed Girl."

‡ The "Seeress of Prevorst," from the German of Justinus Kerner, by Mrs. Crowe, Authoress of "Susan Hopley," "The Night-Side of Nature," &c.

§ See a Letter to Editor of Critic. — June, 1845.

these conditions she saw sights, and poured forth revelations, which, in no other respects, are deserving of notice, but from the credit and importance attached to them. Her "disclosures," however, enter into some of the highest questions in religion. She distinguishes, with accuracy, the precise difference between the soul and the spirit, and points out their separate functions: she describes how infants grow in the other world: she speaks of the shape of the soul, and of the forms of spirits; instructs us as to the condition of the heathen, and of virtuous Pagans after death; and gives us, in short, "a great deal of other information about a great number of other things." According as this poor lady's revelations coincide with the views and belief of her readers and followers, they are deemed semi-inspired and authoritative. Dr. Bush, Professor of Hebrew, in New York, finds a confirmation of Swedenborgianism; certain German enthusiasts, the triumph of Christianity over an empirical philosophy; and Mrs. Crowe, a proof of her favourite doctrine, the existence of ghosts, and of spiritual appearances. "She was more than half a spirit," says Kerner, "and belonged to a world of spirits; she belonged to a world after death. She was a delicate flower, and lived upon sunbeams."

The awkward part in the "revelations" of these various vision-seers is the contradiction between the different doctrines they respectively countenance. It is with the purpose of pointing out this discrepancy, that their history is alluded to. They cannot be all true, nor all of a quasi-miraculous authority; the conclusion rather is, that they are none so. The case of the "Seeress of Prevorst" was, doubtless, a real one, and deserving of study; but there was nothing more in her disclosures than what may be often met with in communications of the somnambulist family. They give a lesson in physiology, and the matter is ended.

Rachel Baker, who preached in New York during her sleep, in the year 1815, is another instance of popular delusion from the same principle.* Learned Professors, Divines of divers persuasions, Doctors of Medicine, Quakers and Methodists,

* "Remarkable Sermons of Rachel Baker, delivered during her Sleep, taken down in Short-hand." 1814.

crowded round to catch the words that fell from her mouth, as something heavenly and miraculous. Her discourses were deemed so striking, that it was said generally that they could only be "dictated by an extraordinary agency of the Divine Spirit." Short-hand writers attended to take them down. A letter from America to this country stated, "several hundreds flock every evening to hear this most wonderful preacher, who is instrumental in converting more persons to Christianity, when asleep, than all the other ministers together, whilst awake." The tendency of her preaching was to uphold Calvinism and the Millennium.

Rachel Baker was born in the state of Massachussetts of Presbyterian parents, in 1794. She was so rigidly instructed in religion, that "she might be said to have known the Holy Scriptures from a child." "When she was about nine years old, the thoughts of God and eternity would make her tremble." In her 17th year, some religious ordinances impressed her with such ideas of her sinfulness and wretched state, that she became silent and reserved, taking little food, sleeping scarcely at all, bursting out into tears and occasional ejaculations, and appearing altogether on the brink of despair. Suddenly she commenced "night-talking." She was sitting in her chair, and had been observed to be nodding; when she began to sigh and groan, as if in excessive pain, and her parents thought that she was dying. Their alarm, however, abated, when she commenced talking. There was not much regularity in her observations at first,—and there was a mingling of "shrieks" and "anguish," with the concomitant language and demeanour of ultra-fanaticism. After some nights, however, her manner sobered down, and she became regular, and pathetic, and solemn. Her father, at length, carried her to New York. Here the greatest sensation was experienced. Multitudes crowded to hear her preach and pray. An intense excitement continued. A few, indeed, taxed her with being "an impostor of the first rank." But that an ignorant and young girl of slight mental capacity should "dream in" a course of enlightened theology, and show herself "not merely orthodox, but able and copious" in expounding, and "fervid and eloquent in her language," did seem to the

majority a fact so "*completely to defy human explanation*," that her revelations were regarded as miraculous, and the "immediate effusions" of the Holy Spirit of God.

The accidentals of Rachel's birth and education being strongly Calvinistic, the tendency of her preaching of course took that direction. She pronounced authoritatively that "those who had the true religion could never fall away,"—that "the chosen of the Lord could not do evil," but "*must* keep God's commandments," and that grace was indefectible. She spoke confidently of the millennium and of its establishment. And being asked, how it was that she, a woman, presumed to preach in opposition to the apostolic injunction, she unhesitatingly replied, "Shall a woman hold her peace, because she is a woman? Methinks, the Apostle meant not so—but meant that she should let her light shine before men. This is a mystery to you, my friends; but God forbid that I should be silent, for I only speak the truth."* Those "Revelations" were considered supernatural in the city of New York in the year 1815: we shall, in the next case, come to Revelations of an opposite character, which have been equally regarded as supernatural in the same place.

There was, however, the truthfulness peculiar to the somnambulistic condition exhibited in this case. Upon Rachel being asked repeatedly in her sleep, by different ministers, whether she had not "received a supernatural revelation," she invariably denied it, and resisted the temptation and the honour; but her denials were only attributed to humility and meekness.

A physician of New York, Dr. Mitchill, examined the case, and described its leading phenomena. They clearly indicate the mesmeric condition. "This somnium is of a devotional

* This is by no means a single instance of Scripture being made to bend to a Somnambulist's interpretation. The last Chapter showed how the immediate cause of Christ could not be immediate but were produced, according to another sleeper. These explanations remind me of something similar that occurred in my own neighbourhood. An ignorant expounder was requested to explain the Parable of the "Unjust Steward," and say why he was praised so by his Master. Our interpreter was perplexed for a moment. At last he hit upon it. "The fact is," said he, "that he was a *just* steward, and only called unjust to attract attention." This was not in sleep, it should be added.

kind, and of a very extraordinary character, and occurs once a day. The paroxysms begin at early bed-time. It commences with a sort of uneasiness of the spasmodic kind, anxiety in respiration, and hysteric choking. There is no chill nor coldness,—nor any febrile excitement. The transition from the waking state to that of somnium is very quick. During the paroxysm her pulse varies but little from the common beat. She takes the recumbent posture: and her face being turned toward heaven, she performs her devotions, with a fervour wholly novel and unexampled. Her body and limbs are quiet and motionless: they stir no more than the trunk or extremities of a statue;—the only motion the spectator perceives is that of her organs of speech. Her eyelids are closed: but the muscles of the eyes, on disclosing the lids, have been observed to be in tremulous agitation, and the balls to be inclined upwards. Her fingers are observed to be firmly closed for a few seconds: and the muscles of the back and arms to be rigid. She passes into a sound and natural sleep, which continues during the remainder of the night. In the morning she wakes as if nothing had happened, and is entirely ignorant of the memorable scenes in which she has acted. She declares that she knows nothing of them. And she complains of no pain, lassitude, nor of any disorder."

It remains to be added that her *language* no less than her *ideas* were greatly improved and heightened during the fit of somnium. They were, in fact, "far beyond her waking state." Another point was, that when awake, she maintained that she was not asleep during her paroxysms, though her condition was evident to the bystander. What became of Rachel Baker afterwards, I know not: she probably recovered, and the supernatural disappeared also.

The disclosures of Andrew Davis, "the Poughkeepsie Seer and Clairvoyant," in his "Principles of Nature and Her Divine Revelations," are regarded by the learned Professor Bush, of New York, as an instance of "supernatural knowledge, only to be explained by the influx of the minds of spirits into his mind." The Professor views this case "in a higher light than that pertaining to any other sample of the clairvoyant power."

Moreover, "he has no scruple to avow it as his firm conviction that the phenomena of Mesmerism have been developed in this age with the *express design* of confirming the message of Swedenborg, and of testifying to the truth of the doctrines he promulgated." And in publishing his own observations on the subject, the Professor "regards himself as entering into *direct co-operation* with the designs of Providence."* Now when a talented and religious writer can thus express himself on a particular case, and when numbers of other learned and clever men are also regarding it with deep attention, our curiosity is naturally stimulated to know something of the history. The "Revelations" of Davis, given in his sleep, have been published in two thick volumes, and recently reprinted in England.† Some extracts from the book were given in the last Chapter. A few more observations may not be without their use.

Andrew Jackson Davis, the young American in question, was accidentally present at some Mesmeric lectures, that were being delivered at Poughkeepsie. By chance he was selected for one of the parties, whom the operator was to try to send to sleep. All the manipulations, however, were unavailing. Some time afterwards, when his brain or nerves were in a more impressible state, a companion commenced the passes for amusement. Davis soon dropped off into the slumber:—and subsequently became somnambulist, clairvoyant, and an introvisionist. His power of seeing into the condition of the human frame so greatly increased, that he was continually consulted in disease, and his fame spread widely; and he also put forth many clever opinions in philosophy. This happened in 1843.

His faculties, in his somnambulist condition, continued so to advance, that in a year or two afterwards he was taken to New York. Here an immense sensation was created. The learned of the city flocked around him. Short-hand writers attended, as in the case of Rachel Baker; and he delivered, in his sleep, lectures on Religion, Astronomy, Cosmology, Geology, and, in

* "Mesmer and Swedenborg" by Professor Bush. New York, 1847. See Preface for these passages.
† "The Principles of Nature, Her Divine Revelations, and a Voice to Mankind" by Andrew Davis. (Chapman, Strand.)

short, upon almost every subject that the universe embraces. Like Goldsmith, in fact, *nihil erat quod non tetigit*, and perhaps almost like Goldsmith, *nihil tetigit quod non ornavit*, for his language, ideas, power and philosophy were of the most extraordinary kind. Viewed under whatever light they may, these discourses are a most remarkable effort of the human mind, and deserving of perusal;—and the question is, how did this very young man obtain all his learning?—for in his waking state, he is very ignorant and illiterate, and possessing, as it is said, no knowledge of science whatsoever. His advantages had also been of a limited kind;—he had enjoyed little schooling; and his occupation was that of a shoemaker's apprentice: *how, then, did this lad of twenty obtain a knowledge as profound, as it is extensive and minute?*

The Hebrew Professor of New York, it has been seen, considers the Revelations of so "astounding" a character, as to prove that Davis is "in a preternatural state," and specially commissioned by God to affirm the doctrines of Swedenborg. This opinion he shares with many. While the ultra-mesmeric party, in their extravagant estimation of the capabilities of Mesmerism, consider that the clairvoyant powers of the youth have arrived at so etherialised and sublimated a condition, as to give him the knowledge he possesses through an actual and quasi-personal inspection; in other words, that he knows all this to be true, because he sees it to be so. Under this light, therefore, they regard his lectures as of authority, —the authority of "nature" teaching through her own "voice." These, then, are the views of the extreme sections: a little examination may, perhaps, reduce the wonder to its real level.

Without denying the lectures to be very extraordinary, and not to be explained upon common principles, I am not prepared to say, that they are much more extraordinary, certain attendant circumstances being taken into consideration, than many of the Revelations that have previously been examined. Davis was constantly surrounded by very learned and philosophical visiters, and their presence would of course have its influence. Neither can I quite believe, with Professor Bush, that there has been no "cramming" in the matter: though I must admit

that all the cramming in the world *could not* so have filled the lad's mind, as to enable him to pour forth, from day to day, for several months, long lectures and digressions *de omni scibili*, and to answer with readiness and aptness the perplexing questions that were put to him. But I am persuaded that there has been a little surreptitious reading, nothing very deep nor extensive, but sufficient to lay a sort of basis to build upon. An unusual knowledge of detail exhibited by him in some branches of study leads me to this opinion. His friends, indeed, all assert that there has been no accessibility to books, and on this they speak very positively: but they themselves may be mistaken. It would be difficult for them to prove a negative. Many a young lady in our suburban seminaries has the "Mysteries of Udolpho," and "the Italian" at her fingers' ends, of whose ignorance in such polite branches of learning the presiding genius of the establishment would speak with every confidence. No quarantine can effectually shut out such intellectual smuggling. And so it may have been with young Davis.[*] Still even a far greater amount of reading than what I am prepared to tax him with, would come very short of explaining, in the case of a young man under twenty, occupied as he was all day, the prodigious, and indeed profound, stores of erudition which he occasionally developed. The Mesmeric principle, in its very highest condition, is of all solutions the only one which is able to clear up the difficulty. That very peculiar exaltation of the faculties [†] (to which I have so often referred), in an unusually

[*] Since the above was written, I have met with an account of Davis, given by the Rev. A. Bartlett, of Poughkeepsie, who says, that "he loved books, especially controversial religious works, whenever he could borrow them, and obtain leisure for their reading; and that he was fond of asking questions, and possessed an inquiring mind." Mr. Armstrong, however, with whom he was apprenticed, says that his reading was most limited, and confined to books of juvenile or narrative description. It is clear that his reading laid a substratum of information.

[†] Dr. Radclyffe Hall, in a letter before referred to, speaking of a case of Education, where the patient developed an increase of mental power, adds assuringly, "nor does it approach in wonderfulness the superhuman manifestations of increased intellectuality, described by Mr. Sandby and others." Dr. Hall implies that there has been exaggeration on our part. Here, then, is a case of exaltation for him to study. — *Lancet*, April, 1847.

The reader is also referred to some judicious articles in the "Critic" on the case of Andrew Davis.

intense and elevated state, accompanied by a transference of thought of no common force from those *en rapport*, may solve the problem, especially if we throw in the aid of "imagination" and "invention," for much that is evidently new and unborrowed. The history of Davis is either an infamous forgery from first to last, — or a miracle, — or a mesmeric marvel. The number and respectability of the witnesses completely forbid the first conclusion: there are sufficient reasons for our rejection of the second. Mesmerism in its noblest and most exalted phase can alone come in to throw light on the mystery.

So far from Andrew Davis being a divine instrument for the diffusion of Swedenborgianism, some of his statements are strongly opposed to its very doctrines. When, therefore, is he inspired? — and when not? So much for the miracle. Nay, some of his teachings are fearfully subversive of Christianity itself, especially in those passages which relate to the miracles of the New Testament, as was shown in the last chapter. He is orthodox on some points, and the veriest heretic on others. That an able man, like Professor Bush, should be caught by a temporary harmony of opinions, is one of those illusions which it is the object of this chapter to dissipate. Andrew Davis, in fact, in his eloquent volubility, utters much that is contradictory and inconsistent, and much also that is nonsensical; unfortunately those points are alone remembered, which coincide with the special prepossessions of his admirers. What, however, is true, is not new; — and what is new, I fear, is not exactly true. When the brain of Davis has been impressed by a Swedenborgian, the disclosures relate to the world of spirits and the glories of the New Church: when the impression comes from a Germanised scholar, the philosophy of the "inner life," and of Kant, and of Schelling, and of Oken, takes its turn. The "Vestiges of the Natural History of Creation," — the studies of Le Verrier and of Adams, — disquisitions on prophets and prophecy all follow in succession, like figures in a magic lantern, according as a cosmologist, an astronomer, or a theologian have influenced his organism. At one time, the young man is the regenerator of society, and sent into the world to forward some coming

reformation; at another, he discusses the origin and affinities of languages "with the most signal ability,"—in obedience to some action on his brain from a disciple of Fourier, or a philologist. Almost every thing, in short, passes under review, as the accidental *rapport* determines the order* : the lectures show, like an intellectual kaleidoscope, *very clever, very curious*, but *not at all convincing*; and the "Poughkeepsie Seer," having done his work, and worn out the impulses that excite this cerebral activity, will pass away as a meteor, like his predecessors before him, to give way to fresh "Voices from Nature," equally præternatural, and equally to be explained on some homogeneous principle.

Something similar to the "Revelations" of Davis, though greatly inferior in power, occurred a few years ago in one of our midland counties. A short description of the case appeared in Zadkiel's Almanack for the year 1845. The "Prophetess," as the party was considered, caused at the time much excitement and discussion. A clergyman, who took an interest in her, actually declared that she was "The *most illustrious female visitant of this earth since the time of the Virgin Mary!*" An examination, however, of the case will confirm what I have just said in regard to Davis, that the opinions are rather transferred, second-hand as it were, from the brain of another person, than the result of original intuition through the agency of clairvoyance: in other words, that the patient, in a spiritualised state, is *reading the mind* of the Mesmeriser, and nothing else.

A young girl, who had been brought up by her parents in an unbelief and great ignorance of Scripture, had been Mesmerised on account of her health. She had been Mesmerised by four different individuals, two of whom are friends of my own, without any remarkable effects of a mental character resulting. At last, she is Mesmerised by a gentleman of strong religious feelings, whose knowledge of Scripture is most profound and accurate, and whose theological tenets are somewhat peculiar. Religion is, in fact, the uppermost occupation of his mind; and mark the effect at once on the patient. She

* The reader is referred back to page 82, for remarks on Transference of Thought.

straightway becomes in her sleep most conversant with the Bible;—she compares one text with another;—she interprets the Old Testament by the New;—she discovers the deepest meaning in most abstruse chapters; she is 'an expositor of what she declares are the *real* doctrines of the Gospel. That a girl, almost ignorant of Scripture, should accomplish all this, is regarded as supernatural;—she is considered as inspired,—called a prophetess;—and for a time no one could say what turn the delusion would take.* The girl is next placed *en rapport*, with a gentleman whose studies are of an astrological character; and her talk is straightway of the "stars." She speaks, with accuracy, of central suns,—of Jupiter and Herschel,—sees butterflies in Sirius, and orange-trees in Andromeda. She is next placed *en rapport* with several ladies, who declare that their innermost thoughts are laid bare by the patient; and these parties know not what to think. Like Davis, our prophetess, though only eighteen years of age, *is ignorant of nothing*. Ask her any question on any subject, and she answers with rapidity. Of course great hubbub is raised, and the neighbourhood all stirred up; those who have a tendency towards religious novelties, look for fresh revelations from the magical maid; those who adhere to the Evangelical section of the Church, raise a cry of Satanic agency; while simple nature is forgotten, and both sides overlook the fact that the patient is sympathetically united with the mind of the Mesmerist.†

These transcendental revelations of E. A—— were on the point of being published by the enthusiastic clergyman before alluded to, when the affair fortunately sobered down. Our

* Meric Casaubon, speaking of some past wonders of an incredible character, said, "Had we not seen the like in these latter days, upon the same ground of divine revelations, acted and revived, it cannot be expected that any man should have belief to credit such relations."— *Treatise on Enthusiasm*, cap. i.

† Of course, this supposed prophetess not only reads the mind of the Mesmeriser, but is farther gifted with that enlargement of the spiritual faculties, which is so usual in the Mesmeric state, and which gives the additional marvel to the whole transaction. It is this exaltation of soul that stamps her "revelations" with the semblance of the miraculous. A description of this case may be found in the "Family Herald," in a criticism on Zadkiel's Almanack.

prophetess, (who in her waking state is an amiable girl, and knew nothing of what she had uttered in her sleep,) had described so much that was contradictory and impossible, that a faith in the miracle materially abated. Her powers have been since turned to a more practical purpose. E—— is a first-rate introvisionist. Her clairvoyant faculty of investigating disease, through an inspection of a patient's physical structure, is so great, and has been so tested by experience, that she is much consulted. A physician of large practice in her neighbourhood has often called in her diagnostic aid, as it is said, with the happiest results. This is one of the wisest methods of making Mesmerism of service; and if other prophets and prophetesses would employ their clairvoyant talents in the same useful direction, the prejudices against the art, on the score of its praeternaturalism and nonsense, would in great measure pass away.

Sufficient evidence has been now adduced to identify the condition of an ecstatico-prophetic somnambulist with that of a mesmeric patient, and to test the truthfulness of each in turn; and a still further number of instances will be found in the Appendix. Baron Feuchtersleben, in his "Principles of Medical Psychology," calls Mesmerism a "half-philosophical, half-medical, system," [*] and the appropriateness of the description must be acknowledged. Aided, therefore, by the light of this system, the Religionist and the Philosopher need no longer repeat the old, but not exploded, blunder of crying out "miracle," or "impostor," at every anomalous extravagance, when a slight physiological examination will explain the mystery. The sameness and spontaneity of the symptoms in all countries, in all ages, and under all conditions of life, is the great argument. A young and most ignorant peasant girl, in some secluded hamlet, has equally, with the most practised sleepwaker, developed certain phenomena; and the question is, *where* and *how* she learns her cunning? There has been but one school for all, the school of untaught, but misrepresented, and self-acting, nature!

---

[*] In his Chapter on the History of Psychology, p. 60. The Baron's learned work is edited by Dr. Babington for the Sydenham Society.

One or two other instances of a somewhat different character, though of the same family, may be also mentioned, which will assist in illustrating the philosophy of the subject.

The Sloane manuscripts, in the British Museum, give the history of a man who used to work hard in his sleep, and perform a number of strange antics. A few extracts will be amusing.[*]

"Jonathan Coulston, of the county of York, in the twentieth year of his age, and servant in husbandry, hath for about two years and a half last past frequently fallen asleep in the performance of his work, and *then* will do as much as *two or three men ordinarily do*, and very near as well.[†] In this state he is excellent in all parts of haymaking, as strewing, raking, cocking, &c. One day when he was spreading hay, a lusty man sat upon a haycock to try what he would do; when he came to him, Jonathan took him by the shoulders, and grumbling, gave him such a toss that he tumbled two or three times over; a cur-dog being asleep on another haycock, he took him by the legs and flung him as high as an ordinary house. He fodders his master's cattle, binds them up in the barn in their respective places, and unlooses them into the pasture. He delves in the garden, digs turf on the common, runs very fast, and climbs over stone walls near two yards high, without any harm. Once he got up into a tree about eight yards high, and hooped and hallooed as if he had been hunting a pack of dogs: his master was in great concern to get him down, but shouting to him to go to his work, he nimbly came down again. He plays at Put, but often names the cards falsely, and holds the wrong side towards him: he Puts every time, and takes up all the tricks: he has several times stood upon his head, leaning his hinder parts to the side of the room, and in this posture he always whistles.

---

[*] Sloane Collection, 403, 404, 406. The MS. has no date, and is anonymous, but probably drawn up by Sir Hans Sloane, as it is like his handwriting.

[†] The Mesmeric reader, who possesses Elliotson's "*Numerous Cases, &c.*" will find a similar story, at p. 45, respecting Samuel Chilton, the Sleeper at Bath,—a story which Sir B. Brodie once brought forward as a proof that Mesmerism were not a truth in nature! Is Sir Benjamin of the same opinion still?

"Having been to spread dung one day last Christmas, he came home, got his supper, and talked with the family over the fire; all this was whilst he was awake. About eight o'clock he went out of the house from among them: as he returned not in the time expected, they imagined he might be asleep, and went to seek him, with a candle and lantern, in the field, where they had wrought that day, and found him spreading dung, in his shirt, at a furious rate, and in a most profuse sweat, as he always is in this case, and suffers much by catching cold. At first, he might have been awaked by shouting and pulling him by the ears and nose,—but now, if *they were to be cut off*, 'tis the opinion of the family he would not awake. They have several strings or pieces of riband, given by his godmother, and as soon as he is *touched with them*, he falls as if he were knocked on the head, and about two or three minutes lies as if he were dead; then begins to rub his eyes, and complains of great pain in them; if he sees any *stranger about him when he awakes*, he is troubled. He tells every thing he knows in his dream, which troubles him still more.

"All his motions in sleep are quick and vigorous, and his countenance is more lively. When awake he is heavy and stupid, and, as to his intellect, he may be said to be betwixt one of common sense and an idiot. He was brought up a Quaker till ten or twelve years old, and *may still seem to have the light within.*[*] I have had a relation of these things amongst many others from my tenant, J. Reston, and his mother, and two of his brothers, who are all sensible, honest, cautious persons, and twenty others, have been eye-witnesses. How these things (the ribands) should produce such appearances in an instant, 'tis difficult to account. Be these things as they will, 'tis certain there is no contrivance in the case. He answers any question, if spoke to very loudly. Several other strings have been tried, but to no purpose."

The Mesmeric characteristics of this case are clearly discernible, and help us towards its unriddling.

[*] We see here the tendency to find something of a religious character in these anomalous occurrences.

1st. Coulston's great increase of strength in the sleep, "doing as much work as two or three men ordinarily do," lifting up and flinging men so easily and so high. I have seen a very little girl, in the Mesmeric sleep, carry a stout man of six feet high across a room with ease.

2d. The insensibility to pain,—a point at this present hour not necessary to dwell upon.

3d. The touch of certain bits of riband from one person instantly producing a deep coma, but not any other pieces.

4th. Distress at the presence of a stranger on being awakened.

5th. Coulston mentioning facts in his sleep that he did not wish to have known, and would not tell when awake.

6th. The improvement and liveliness of face and intellect: at other times being nearly an idiot.[*]

These phenomena all show the source from where they sprang: but inasmuch as the accidents of Coulston's condition did not take a religious turn, nothing was said about the miraculous nature of their origin; and the sleeping Yorkshire boy was simply the nine-days' wonder of his neighbourhood,—and a perplexity for Sir Hans Sloane and his philosophical acquaintance.

Military annals record one or two occasions, on which some poor fellows have been sharply dealt with by the martinets of their regiment, for what, in the phraseology of the Horse Guards, is called "Malingering,"—and in commoner parlance, a pretence of sickness. A knowledge of the Mesmeric symptoms may lead to more caution in future.

Dr. Hennen, in his "Principles of Military Surgery," mentions the case of a soldier, which at one time made much noise in the south-western part of England. He was called in his regiment the "Sleeping Man,"—and was placed under Dr.

[*] Gauthier quotes from Dr. Choron, physician at the Hospital of the Val-de-Grâce, a Mesmeric fact illustrative of the text. He had mesmerised a girl, aged 30, who had been an idiot from her birth. In her sleep-waking state, she became so intelligent, that no one would have supposed her to be the same person. Her parents were amazed, and cried with joy, "Oh, why is she not always a Somnambulist!"— *Gauthier*, p. 878.

H. in Hilsea Hospital, who describes it as a case of "somnolency combined with mental hallucination," and adds that "there can be no doubt that *grief and terror* had a share in the production of his disease." Many of the officers, and other parties, who came to study the symptoms, considered the condition feigned, for this reason, — that some of the experiments to test its truthfulness were successful to a certain extent; but the experiments simply proved the particular stage of the somnium, and that the sleep was not so deep as to leave the man in an utter state of unconsciousness. Dr. H. himself says, that "there is a *difference* between *this man's sleep* and *real sleep*," — and therefore leads the reader to infer that it was all assumed. The soldier smiled, I believe, and blushed in his sleep, according as certain observations were made in his presence; — and Dr. Hennen, who knew nothing of the *sleepwaking* state, in which far stranger incidents are constantly developed, concluded from thence that it was not all genuine nature. Much, however, remained inexplicable. The man bore "a *great many severe* shocks from the electrical machine,"[*] —and "the *injection* of hartshorn into his nostrils." "He was in a state of torpor: he lay without motion in bed; his eyes remained, during the day, immoveably open, unless when roughly touched." Dr. Hennen closes the narrative in giving one lesson to the profession; the man *gradually improved through gentle treatment.*

Dr. Beck, in his Medical Jurisprudence, furnishes a similar case, — that of Phineus Adams, a soldier in the Somerset Militia, aged 18, who was confined in gaol for desertion. This man was constantly lying in a state of insensibility, resisting a variety of remedies that were employed to rouse him, such as thrusting snuff up the nostrils, electric shocks, powerful medicines, &c. When any of his limbs were raised, they fell with a leaden weight of total inanimation. Pins were thrust under his finger-nails to excite sensation. The operation of scalping

[*] The shock of an electrical machine was applied to Elizabeth Okey, and of the electric eel to another patient, without an evidence of sensation. See Elliotson's Pamphlet, p. 30. The reader should also turn to p. 42, for the explanation of the sleep-waking condition, and the rationale of the phrase.

(to ascertain whether there was not a depression of the brain) was performed: the incisions were made, — the scalp drawn up, and the head examined. During all this time Adams manifested no audible sign of pain or sensibility, except when the instrument, with which the head was scraped, was applied. He then, but only once, uttered a groan.[*] How similar is all this to the case of Wombell, which chloroform has proved to be no longer alien to the laws of nature!

There is a passage in Carlyle's Sartor Resartus, in the Chapter on *Natural Supernaturalism*, so cleverly expressed, and so pertinent to much that has been stated, that a few extracts must be offered.

"But is it not the deepest law of nature that she be constant?" —cries an illuminated class: "Is not the machine of the universe fixed to move by unalterable rules?" Probable enough, good friends; nay, I too must believe that nature, that the universe, does move by the most unalterable rules. And now, of you too I make the old inquiry: what those same unalterable rules, forming the complete statute-book of nature, may possibly be?

"They stand written in our works of science — say you: in the records of man's experience. Was man, with his experience, present at the creation, then, to see how it all went on? Have any deepest scientific individuals yet dived down to the foundations of the universe, and gauged *every thing* there? These scientific individuals have been nowhere but where we also are; have only seen some hand-breadths deeper than we see into the deep that is infinite, without bottom, as without shore.

"System of nature! To the wisest man, all experience thereof limits itself to some few computed centuries, and measured square miles.

"Volume of nature! And truly a volume it is, whose Author and Writer is God. To read it! Dost thou, does man, so much as know the alphabet thereof? With its words, its sentences, and grand descriptive pages? It is a volume written in celes-

[*] Beck, p. 12. A similar case occurred with a soldier in the Prussian army.

tial hieroglyphics, of which even Prophets are happy that they can read, here and there, a line!"

. To return, however, to the question of mental and Mesmeric sympathy, there is every probability that the modern miracles in Egypt, which Lord Prudhoe witnessed, and which have so perplexed the learned of this country to explain, have some connection with this "transfer of thought," of which we have been speaking.[*] Dr. Collyer has written an able work on the subject; he supposes that a vital electricity is the medium of communication from *mind* to *mind*; causing an "embodiment of thought" on the brain or mind of another.[†] By this embodiment of thought the prophetess reads the mind of her Mesmeriser, and transfers his Scriptural acquirements into her own brain; and by the same embodiment the Arabian boy became acquainted with the likenesses of Nelson, of Shakspeare, and of the brother of Major Felix, and so perplexed the noble traveller and his numerous critics. It has been said by recent travellers that this Egyptian boy has lately failed. A hundred failures cannot upset one positive fact. The probability is, that the brain has been overfatigued by too much work: this is constantly the case in clairvoyance, and then the cry is raised of imposture:—for example, with Alexis.

In short, we are but in the infancy of our Mesmeric knowledge. Not only may the oracles of old, those for instance of Delphi, be explained by the responses of a magnetic somnambulist in the highest state of lucidity, but it may even be suggested to the philosophic inquirer to pursue the topic into a wider field. It may be possible that the sympathy of Mes-

[*] "Numerous experiments seem to show," says Mr. Lloyd, "that the Mesmeric influence is capable of reflection from polished surfaces, and some acquaintance with this fact, or others resulting from the same general law, may probably have led to the employment of mirrors in various forms of magic, from the engraved mirrors of the Etruscans, to the mirrors of the middle ages, such as that in which Lord Surrey was said to have beheld a vision of the fair Geraldine, and to the globule of ink in the palm of the Egyptian boy at the present day."—*Zoist,* vol. iii. p. 313. A good deal more to the same purpose will be found in the paper from which the above is extracted.

[†] See "Psychography, or the Embodiment of Thought," by Dr. Collyer. See also "The People's Phrenological Journal," No. XLIV.

meric action may throw a light on the hysteric excitement, by which large multitudes of men are stirred up into a strange contagious enthusiasm. Dr. Bertrand, in his well-known work, contends strongly for this opinion. The prophets of the Covennes, the nuns of Loudon, the convulsionaires of St. Medard, are cited by him as instances of proof. We might add to this list the strange sect of the Flagellants of Hungary and Bohemia, in the fifteenth century. L'Enfant, in the "History of the Council of Constance," gives a curious account of this heresy; and states that this love of self-flagellation became a perfect "furor," and so contagious was it, that some contemporaries deemed it as "supernatural, and the inspiration of Heaven;"—others "regarded it as the suggestion of an evil spirit."[*] The enthusiasm of the Quakers at their first establishment,—of the Methodists in their early days,—and in our own time the wildness and madness of the "unknown tongues," may all fall under the same class. A panic on board a ship, excitement in the field of battle, applause in a crowded theatre, make some approach to the same character. And when in these and similar cases we add the principle of imitation to the contagious influence of Mesmeric power,—we catch a clue that unravels much that is mysterious in the conduct of man; we see how intimately we are all united [†], physically as well as morally; sympathy and the force of attraction are called into being where it is little suspected,

"Striking the *electric chain* wherewith we are darkly bound"

one with another! Maxwell, whom we have before quoted, speaks of a "*vital or universal spirit,*" by virtue of which "wonders may be performed;"—and which was the "great

[*] This is so exactly a counterpart of what occurs at every other strange appearance, that the words should be quoted:—

"Elle avait un air surnaturel qui faisait juger aux uns que c'était une inspiration du ciel, pendant que les autres la regardaient comme une suggestion du mauvais Esprit."—*Histoire du Concile de Constance,* liv. v.

[†] "Without being mesmerised by special manipulations, how often do we think of persons who are approaching before they come in sight! How often do we simultaneously write or start the same ideas in conversation! &c. All such occurrences have been explained upon the principle of coincidence or mere chance,—*but, &c.*"—*Spencer Hall,* p. 13.

secret of witchcraft." [*]   Our illustrious Bacon seems also to
have known somewhat of the Mesmeric principle, when he says
that it "certainly is agreeable to reason that there are some
light effluxions from spirit to spirit, *when men are in presence
one with another*, as well as *from body to body*." He adds, that
there is "a *sympathy* of individuals, so that there should remain
a *transmission of virtue* from the one to the other ;" and he also
wrote on "experiments touching the emission of immateriate
virtues from the minds and spirits of men, either by affections
or by imaginations, *or by other impressions*." All this is very
remarkable language from the great father of instructive philosophy; and Bacon, who considered the knowledge of man to
man as the most important of all knowledge, adds this useful
caution, as a rule for every inquirer: "We have set it down as
a law to ourselves, to examine things to the bottom, and not to
receive upon credit, or *reject upon improbabilities*, until there
hath passed a due examination." "Much," he says again, "will
be left to experience and probation, whereunto indications cannot fully reach." [†]   And in accordance with these great principles of instructive philosophy by experiment and observation,
the statements related in this chapter are presented to the consideration of the student.

* Maxwell, *De Medicinâ Magneticâ*. Frankfort, 1679. "Spiritum uni-
versalem, si instrumentis hoc spiritu impregnatis usus fueris, in sextilium vocabis :
magnum Magorum secretum."—*Aphorismus*, lxxviii. p. 182.

† See Bacon's "Natural History." Century 10.

CHAP. VIII.

GENERAL RULES FOR MESMERISING. — DOMESTIC MESMERISM. — SLEEP NOT
NECESSARY. — DIFFERENCE OF EFFECTS. — CAN ANY ONE MESMERISE? —
MODES OF MESMERISING. — PATIENT NOT TO BE AWAKENED. — LENGTH-
ENED SLEEP NOT DANGEROUS. — METHODS OF DEMESMERISING. — EXER-
TION OF THE WILL. — WARMTH. — BENEFIT FROM EXPERIMENTS. — GOOD
SLEEP AT NIGHT. — ABSENCE OF MESMERISER AND CONTACT OF THIRD
PARTY. — CLASS OF DISEASES AFFECTED BY MESMERISM. — EPILEPSY. —
ORGANIC DISEASE. — PARALYSIS. — DIFFERENT STAGES OF MESMERIC
CONDITION. — FREEDOM OF MANNER. — CLAIRVOYANCE. — CONCLUSION.

AND now, after all, what is the process by which this peculiar
condition of the human frame is most easily induced, or maintained or managed ? in other words, what is the right method
of Mesmerising ?

In giving instructions under this head, my object is to
encourage DOMESTIC MESMERISM ;—to enable fathers or mothers, husbands or wives, brothers or sisters, to relieve the
sick members of a family through its soothing influence, and
assist nature in her work.[*] Not that, by any means, am I
setting up this treatment as a rival to the medical art,—as some
charm or specific that is to supersede every other appliance,
and at once to dispense with the contents of the Pharmacopœia.
Such notions would only foster a disappointing quackery. It
is true, indeed, that on several occasions the mesmeric power
has so "revolutionised the whole system,' and wrought with
such extraordinary efficacy upon a diseased habit of body, that
the patient has been enabled to discard every other item of
medical treatment, and to rely, in his progress towards recovery,
upon this power alone. It is true, also, that in certain con-

* I would also add *Parochial Mesmerism*, by a clergyman, for his
parishioners. I quote from a popular periodical : "It strikes us very
forcibly, that, on many of these occasions (a visit to a sick-bed), a minister
of the gospel would find the composing treatment of Mesmerism a useful
ally. He might, through its means and with the blessing of God, allay
many a sharp pain, assist a feverish and sleepless sufferer, &c."—*Church of
England Journal*, vol. ii. No. 92. See my own experience, p. 165, of this
work. See also *Vital Magnetism*, by Rev. T. Pyne.

stitutions there would appear to exist some repellant principle between medicine and Mesmerism, through which the latter will not always act harmoniously with the former. But these are exceptions, on which experience can alone instruct the student. My wish is rather to recommend the adoption of Mesmeric practice, *conjointly* and in strict accordance with medical advice;—to have magnetism thrown in, as it were, supplementarily to every thing else. If this plan were constantly pursued in families, by its own members, and at their own time, the amount of human relief that would be afforded would be incalculable. What is generally required in a sick-room is either something that shall assist a feverish patient in obtaining a remission of cerebral activity,—something that shall tranquillise the nervous system,—something that shall relieve pain or render it endurable,—something that may check inflammation without weakening the constitution. For all these purposes the "healing hand[*]" of the magnetiser acts repeatedly with promptness and success. It is, indeed, my firm persuasion, that if Mesmerism were extensively used by the healthy members of a household for the benefit of its sicklier portion, many an illness would be cut short at its commencement,—many a disease abated of its intensity and shortened in its duration,—many an organic and incurable malady receive palliation and respite, and many a life prolonged with comparative comfort to the sufferer. Mesmerism works no miracles,—but it often effects great wonders; it sometimes assists the action of medicine when its power has become all but dormant, and gives tone, sleep, and ease, when every other remedy has failed or lost its virtue.

Dr. Esdaile, who has employed Mesmerism so largely for surgical operations, declares that its power as a remedial agent is still more efficacious and useful.[†] Dr. Elliotson has said the

---

* Virgil speaks of the "manu medica Phœbique potentibus herbis."—*Æneid.* xii. 402.

† "The great field for a display of its usefulness is in the treatment of medical diseases, where it often comes to our aid when all other resources have failed."—*Letter from Dr. Esdaile. Zoist,* vol. v. p. 191. "The inestimable blessings of Mesmerism in the alleviation of diseases are of greater extent than its application in operations, &c."—*Dr. Elliotson. Zoist,* vol. iv. p. 590.

---

same thing. And when we know that this influence is capable of inducing the very same insensibility to pain that is procured by such formidable agents as ether and chloroform, we may well believe that its action on the human frame must be most searching and transforming, so much so indeed as oftentimes to bring on an actual "revolution" in the system. This is the phrase, indeed, that Dr. Esdaile himself employs.[*] And thus it is, that, in more ways than one, chloroform and ether confirm the usefulness of Mesmerism.

Before, however, that we enter upon directions for its use, there are two preliminary points, with which it is desirable that the learner should be impressed.

1st, That sleep is by no means indispensably necessary in proof of an effect. The ordinary notion on this head is, that sleep is the secret of the whole system. "I am sure you cannot send me to sleep," is the vulgar cry of the supercilious opponent; and if no somnolency be induced, his conclusion is, that no influence has been imparted. Now, in the first place, it is any thing but a correct inference, that because a person in health may not have been rendered somnolent, the same party would not be easily affected when in a different habit of body. Mesmerism, as Mr. Newnham says, is the "Medicine of Nature," and it is the sick and the suffering that nature has predisposed and fitted for its influence.[†] But, secondly, even with the sickliest patient, the absence of coma is no proof of the absence of action. Essential benefit may be communicated, and the invalid remain as wakeful and conscious as ever. Sleep is, in truth, a satisfactory symptom, from the intelligible evidence that it affords that some action has commenced; but Mesmeric annals record numerous cases of alleviation and cure, where

---

* "Mesmeric coma revolutionizes the whole system, and every other constitutional affection is for the time suspended."—*Dr. Esdaile's India,* p. 170.

† Gauthier says, "Out of a hundred persons in good health, two thirds will perceive no effect, and the other third a very slight effect."—*T. P.* p. 19. Dr. Esdaile says, "Debility of the nervous system predisposes to the easy reception of Mesmerism," p. 26. Preface. Mr. Newnham observes, that "susceptibility is greatly increased in emaciated persons, who have been enfeebled by chronic disease,"—and he adds, that "women are more susceptible than men, because of the much greater mobility of their nervous system." Chapter vii.

little or no somnolency has been imparted. Miss Martineau's is a striking instance. "I longed," she says, "to enjoy the Mesmeric sleep: *the sleep never came*, and except the great marvel of restored health, I have experienced less of the wonders than I have observed in others." (p. 14.) Mr. Townshend, speaking of a foreign Mesmeriser, says, "Many of his patients got well under *daily Mesmerising*, without having experienced any drowsiness or extraordinary symptom whatever." (Preface, p. 24.) Dr. Elliotson had a patient, whom he Mesmerised for four months half an hour daily, before he could send her to sleep for more than a minute or two, and then she became extremely susceptible. (*Zoist*, vol. ii. 197.) I know several other instances of the same kind, and have myself removed sharp local pain without inducing any somnolency whatever. Let, therefore, the inexperienced Mesmeriser be not disheartened at an *apparent* failure from the absence of sleep.[*]

2dly, In naming the different methods of Mesmerising, we can only touch upon the *general characteristics* of the condition induced. No certain effects can be predicated or depended upon. Nature is infinitely various, and the various complexities of the human constitution, of course, give out the most various operations for their result.[†] Exceptions and idiosyncrasies must be looked for. For instance, Mr. Snewing, in his interesting letter, says, that "so far from the passes bringing on a sleepy influence, they seemed to *banish sleep*; when, in ordinary circumstances, he should have been asleep in a few minutes." A curative effect was, however, equally obtained: "he was better, and the pain in his head relieved."[‡] Medical men bring this want of uniformity in Mesmerism as a charge against the art, and a proof of its uselessness, as if their own systems of treatment, their etherisation, and their opiates, did not occasionally induce the very opposite effects to these

intended. To mention one instance, I have seen creosote, which is repeatedly given to counteract sickness, nay, even seasickness, actually bring on the most violent retching and nausea. This would be no argument against its value for common use, any more than the anomalies of Mesmerism are any evidence against its more general facts: but these anomalies are now alluded to by way of caution to the young Magnetiser, that he may remember that in presenting these instructions for his guidance, I only pretend to offer some broad and general rules,— those salient points in the practice which observation has shown to be most applicable to the largest number of patients, and that his own judgment and experience must assist him in supplying all the rest.[*]

The first question that presents itself is, Can any one Mesmerise? Is it a gift appertaining to some few and favoured individuals,—or a property common to the whole human race? My answer is, any one in good health can Mesmerise: nay, persons of a weak and even sickly constitution can Mesmerise: but it is not to be recommended either for themselves, or for their patients. Teste says that "facts have conspired to prove to him that there exists in *man*, and *probably in all organised beings*, a subtle agent, a *cause* or product of life, transferable from one individual to another[†];" and this I believe that additional observation will affirm. The conclusion, then, is, that every member of a family, who is in the enjoyment of an equable state of health, and free from pain or sickness of body, is qualified to Mesmerise. "The stronger and healthier a person is," says Elliotson, "the greater, other things being equal, is his Mesmeric power." He adds again, "I am inclined to believe that, besides the difference of health, strength, activity, and bulk, very little difference of Mesmeric power exists

---

[*] In the Critic Journal for March, 1845, is a case of a severe attack of gout cured by Mesmerism, though no "somnolence appeared," p. 402. The reader is also referred back to Chapter III. for cures effected by Captain Vallant and Mr. Thompson without the induction of sleep. Dr. Ashburner and Mr. D. Hands can offer evidence on the same point.

[†] See Chapter I. p. 75. on this want of uniformity in Mesmerism.

[‡] *Zoist*, vol. v. p. 237.

---

[*] "No two constitutions are alike; and the nervous system exhibits a separate character in every separate person. It is of importance to remember that the variability of the recipients does by no means prove the agent itself variable."—*Townshend*, p. 290.

[†] Teste's Magnetism, p. 180. He says, in another place, "I think that this influence is constantly exerted, though in a latent way, in such a manner that all men, and probably all the beings of nature, are reciprocally and incessantly magnetised." (p. 85.)]

amongst us; and that the great difference of effects is referrible to the person Mesmerised.* At the same time, observation would seem to show that different Mesmerisers suit different patients; and that some have a peculiar power for controlling and removing certain peculiar diseases.† On the other hand, some Mesmerisers produce an unfavourable effect with particular parties, or while they are very successful with one disorder, can hardly touch another. Teste says, "There sometimes exists between the Magnetiser and the individual who submits himself to him, a certain moral *antipathy*, which nothing can dissipate. This circumstance is unfavourable." (p. 44.) Dr. Elliotson says, "There appears to be a difference in the character of the Mesmeric influence of different persons; for some patients experience comfort from one Mesmeriser, and discomfort, head-ache, &c. from another." (*Zoist*, iii. 52.) As a general rule, however, it may be shortly stated, that any person in good health is capable of Mesmerising.‡

Certain moral qualifications have been referred to in a previous chapter: it may be desirable to repeat that *patience*, *gentleness*, and *firmness*, are among the most essential.§

We will now suppose that a member of a family is prepared

* *Zoist*, vol. iii, p. 49. This whole paper by Dr. E. is particularly recommended to the Mesmeric student for its various information.

† Gauthier, who considers these points very fully. — *Traité Pratique*, p. 64. and p. 316.

‡ Deleuze says, " I ought to mention, as a condition essential to the success of every treatment, that the Magnetiser should be in the enjoyment of good health, &c."— *Instruction Pratique*, p. 239.

§ "Henzler (a great German physiologist) asserts, that, in magnetising, everything depends on the harmony of the original magnetic disposition in the magnetiser and magnetised. Henzler divided all men into four classes: those who have no magnetism, — those who have a fiery one, — those who have a cold moist one, — and those who have a mixed one; proving, from example, that when the magnetiser possesses the same magnetism as the patient, the cure will follow, as certainly as it will be prevented, if the magnetism on both sides do not correspond."— *Wolfgang Menzel's German Literature*, vol. iii, p. 66.

How far the above description be fanciful, I pretend not to judge. The Germans have deeply studied the subject, though they are sometimes more visionary than practical, and their opinions deserve consideration. Speaking of Mesmerism, Menzel himself says, "This discovery is certainly one of the most important that has ever been made, and one which redounds to the glory of our country." Vol. iii.

to commence the Mesmeric treatment with a sick relative, and that the latter is able to sit up in an easy chair. An hour should be selected at which the sittings could be renewed as nearly as possible, each day, at the same time; for with many patients punctuality in this respect is found to assist the influence. Silence of course is necessary: and it is better that not more than one or two persons be present; and the patient should be particularly recommended to be passive and easy, to banish all fears* and indulge every hope, and to trust in the mercies of a benevolent Providence.

The Mesmeriser, being seated opposite to, and a little higher than, the patient, and having concentrated his thoughts on the business before him, may begin by placing his hand gently on the head of the other. After a few moments, he will draw it slowly down the forehead, point the fingers, slightly separated, at the eyes, without touching them; and then make some passes downwards, at the distance of one or two inches over the face and chest to about as far as the pit of the stomach. On each occasion of raising the hand to repeat the movement, he must be careful to remove it by an easy sweep to the outside of the body, or at least to close the fingers up, so as not to produce a counter-current in ascending. He will continue these passes for some minutes, always remembering to carry the action *downwards*, gradually to the knees, and ultimately to the feet.

The above is the method that I consider most pleasant and most generally efficacious: some patients, however, cannot bear to have the head touched; with them it would be necessary to begin in a different way.

Deleuze, who had enjoyed more than thirty-five years' experience, recommends "you to take the thumbs of the patient between your own fingers, so that the inside of your thumbs may touch the inside of his, and to fix your eyes upon him. You are to remain in this situation from two to five minutes,

* "I have always found," says Mr. Townshend, "*fear* to be in Mesmerism a disturbing force." (p. 76.) Mr. Newnham says, "*Disbelief* of the patient is always an obstacle to successful magnetisation, like want of confidence in a medical man is an obstacle to medical treatment." (p. 112.)

until you perceive that there is an equal degree of warmth between your thumb and his; — that being done, you will withdraw your hands, one to the right, and the other to the left, moving them so that the interior surface or palm be turned outwards; you will then raise them as high as the head, place them upon his shoulders, leave them there for a minute, and then draw them along the arm to the extremity of the fingers, touching gently. You will, then, commence the passes or downward movements of the hands, at a little distance from the body (as before described), and continue this sort of process during the greater part of the sitting.[*]

Dr. Elliotson, in a paper in the *Zoist*, has quoted some instructions of his own, which are here repeated for their clearness and easiness of application. "I showed his wife how to make *very slow* passes from opposite his forehead to opposite his stomach with one hand, held at the distance of a few inches from his face, both parties looking at each other in perfect silence, and all in the room being perfectly still, for at least *half an hour*, and at least once a day. I told her she might change her hand when it was tired, and that she must either stand before or at one side of her husband, or sit a good deal higher than she was, or her hand would soon tire; that, if he should go to sleep, she had better continue the passes till the sleep was deep, and then contentedly allow it to expend itself, as it was sure to do sooner or later. At the same time, I begged him to omit all medicine, and live just as had always been his habit. This was done; and he obtained a complete recovery."[†]

I have great opinion of the efficacy of resting the hands upon the patient's shoulder, at the commencement of a sitting; and I fancy that I have seen, on some occasions, still further success by the Mesmeriser crossing his arms and placing his right hand upon the right shoulder, and his left on the left of the patient. With some parties, however, the very reverse would succeed best. Polarity has probably much to do in the matter.[‡]

---

[*] Deleuze, chap. ii. p. 35.
[†] *Zoist*, vol. v. p. 235. Cure of intense Nervous Affections, &c.
[‡] The student is particularly referred to Reichenbach's Chapter on

If none of these methods seem to succeed, the points of the fingers may be held steadily to the eyes, about an inch off, for some little time.[*] The patient is not required to stare at the Mesmeriser, nor even to open his eyes: though, if he do, a quicker action may be anticipated; but "staring" is an unpleasant process, and one that I am far from suggesting. It is not sufficiently composing to the nervous system, is an uncomfortable exertion for an invalid, and has a tendency to distress the brain; but the pointing the fingers near to the eyelids, when they are closed down, is a most efficacious method, though not one with which I like to *begin* a sitting, especially if it be a patient's first trial. It is an excellent plan for *seconding* the introductory manipulations, after the influence has a little circulated into the system, and especially for deepening the coma, if the patient has only dropped off into a light slumber.[†]

After that these various methods have been pursued for a little time, with some patients for only five minutes, with some for fifteen or more, and with the average for about ten, the first symptoms of an influence will probably develop themselves. The eyes will begin to wink, — the eye-lids to quiver and droop, — the patient will sigh gently, — sometimes swallow a little saliva, and sometimes yawn, — at last the eyes will close, and the patient be asleep. The operator should then continue the passes downwards [‡], slowly and without contact

---

Dualism, p. 93. "With the cross hands (of the healthy) all action was arrested; whereas, with the sick, the author's force was overwhelming." See also again, p. 105. of the same work.

[*] "I found," says Dr. Elliotson, speaking of a particular case, "that pointing the fingers towards the eyes at the distance of an inch or two had more effect than making passes." — *Zoist*, vol. ii. p. 49.

[†] "The modes of inducing the sleep are endless; and just as an operator may have accidentally met with persons more affected by a particular method, or may have accustomed them to it, or may have acquired the habit of operating in a particular method with more ease and energy, he will praise this method or that. Steady perseverance day after day, be it for weeks or months, for at least half an hour, is the greatest point. It is best to try all ways in turn, till an efficient way is found." — *Dr. Elliotson, Zoist*, vol. i. p. 312.

[‡] I have mentioned, at p. 174., the evil effects of making upward passes. Gauthier, at p. 109., gives quotations from Mesmer, Puysegur, D'Eslon, and Deleuze to the same effect. If they do no other harm, they would probably awaken a sleeper.

(unless some local Mesmerisation be needed), carrying the influence towards the knees and the feet.

After a time, if the patient remain quiet, and exhibit the common indications of slumber, you may speak softly to him, and ask, "if he be asleep?" If he answer in the affirmative, he is what is called "somnambulist," and you may regard his condition as at once distinct from that of common sleep. Somnambulism must not be generally expected at the first sitting: Gauthier says, "in not more than ten cases out of a hundred;" (*T.P.* p. 70.); other magnetists will, perhaps, scarcely allow of so great a disproportion.

Do not Mesmerise the head too much: it has a tendency to produce a head-ache, which will be felt, after the patient is awakened.

If the patient become hysterical, or begin to laugh or to cry, stop it at once with firmness but gentleness; take hold of his hand, or place your own upon his chest, and require him to be composed. A quiet and serious manner on your own part will gradually induce quietness with him.

The passes may be continued for about half an hour; a longer time is not necessary, as a general rule; some even say, for only a quarter of an hour; and if at the expiration of that period, the patient has not exhibited impressionability to the influence of sleep, the operator should leave off, and renew the manipulations the next day, as nearly as possible, at the same time. The absence of sleep, it has been already shown, is no proof of the absence of action or of a beneficial influence.

The question, that now presents itself, is whether the patient should be awakened, when the time is come for the Mesmeriser to return home? As a general rule, *most certainly not*. There are some patients, indeed, who cannot bear the absence of the Mesmeriser, and whom, therefore, it would be imprudent for him to leave asleep; and these, of course, must be awakened: but the longer that the sleep continues, the greater generally is the benefit, and I would *always* recommend the Mesmeriser to retire, if possible, without disturbing the patient. The latter will probably wake up in a quarter of an hour; but if not, the longer he sleeps, the better for him. Elliotson says, "If I have

my own way, and have no special reason for deviating from a general rule, *I would never wake a patient.*"

There is an idle notion abroad, that persons may never awake again from a Mesmeric sleep, and great alarm is sometimes felt at the prolongation of the slumber. A more erroneous opinion never existed: they are *sure to wake up one time or other*; and the less that they are disturbed or troubled by efforts of awakening in these long trances, the sooner will the influence wear itself out. The attempts at arousing a sleeper often seem to have the effect of deepening the coma;—but if we wait patiently, let it be even for twenty-four hours or more, we shall be rewarded by the result. In a previous chapter[*], I have referred to some instances of this lengthened slumber, and showed its harmlessness. At any rate, we must not employ any strong measures towards awakening the sleeper. Dr. Elliotson says, "It is in truth highly improper to use violent means to rouse persons in sleep-waking, whether spontaneous or induced by Mesmerism. The mere state is free from danger, and expends itself sooner or later. If the patient is still, the repose is harmless; and if he is moving about, he will at length be still or awake, and care should only be taken that he do not hurt himself. To wake persons suddenly and roughly, even from common sleep, is improper."[†]

If, however, when the half-hour or hour be expired, it be expedient to awaken the patient, a few gentle methods will usually succeed. But, first, we should always give him notice that we are going to arouse him, otherwise he may awake distressed or startled. Sometimes, the mere telling the sleeper to wake up is sufficient: it is better, however, in this case to give him a little leisure for preparation, and to require him to rouse up in two or three minutes.

The best methods for demesmerising are the opposite to those of Mesmerising. The application of cold instead of warmth, *rapid transverse* or upward passes across the face and eyes,— blowing upon the eyes,—touching or drinking cold water, raising a current of fresh air by waving a handkerchief, and opening the door,—cold steel, as, for instance, the fire-irons,

applied to the forehead,—are the plans most generally adopted. Some succeed best with one case, and some with another. The sleeper on awakening should always have time given him to recover, before he be addressed.

It is a good regulation, in cases of a serious or unpleasant illness, for the Mesmeriser to wash his hands immediately after the *séance* is over, both to avoid the retaining any bad effects himself, or communicating the same to others. Allusion has not been made to the necessity of cleanliness, as preliminary to the manipulations: it is so obvious and indispensable, that reference would appear idle. I mention it, however, because I believe that ablution actually *assists* the transmission of the influence,—that a well-washed hand will communicate the power both more readily as well as more pleasantly.

The above are those general rules, that apply to the young practitioner's first essay with Mesmerism. Gauthier and other French writers from thence proceed to the most minute instructions,—turning a simple process into a wearisome study. Without denying the correctness of their views, I shall confine myself to those further points in the practice, which the most experienced magnetists appear to regard as most important.

Among the first, is the exertion of the will. Many Mesmerists attach the greatest value to the power of the will towards effecting an impression, and some have produced the greatest marvels by its means. In two small pamphlets in the British Museum, published in 1790, and written by practical men, the greatest stress is placed on willing. "Let there be a constant *intention* within you: keep up an idea of the complaint that you wish to remove." "Constant intention is a great promoter of success, strange as it may seem." "Exert the will,—*determine to do good.*" "Exert all the *volition* you are possessed of." This point is pressed over and over again by both writers with the greatest earnestness; and later Mesmerists use the same language. In the fifth volume of the *Zoist*, are two very striking letters from Dr. Ashburner, and Mr. Thompson "On the Power of the Will"[*] Deleuze says, that "the first condition of magnetising is to will,—that the

[*] Page 253.

will is necessary to conduct the fluid, and to maintain a proper action;" and Mr. Townshend, in his chapter on the "Mesmeric Medium," enters at length on the subject. "When attention remits," he says, "there is a remission of Mesmeric power:" and he mentions an instance of a patient, who, although he had his eyes closed and his limbs paralysed in the torpor of the Mesmeric slumber, was not slow to perceive the wanderings of his attention, and called out to him constantly and coincidently with the remission of his thoughts,—"You influence me no longer—you are not exerting yourself."[*]

Another valuable adjuvant is Warmth. Jussieu stated in his report that Warmth (chaleur animale) was a principal source of magnetic success. Gauthier says that the communication of Warmth is one of the causes of magnetic somnambulism. Dr. Esdaile has pointed out the great importance of Warmth for the happy termination of surgical operations in the Mesmeric sleep; and Dr. Elliotson observes, "This is an opportunity for stating the greater Mesmeric susceptibility of persons, and the greater power of Mesmerisers, if the respective party is warm. The apartment, the two parties, and the Mesmerising hand should be comfortably warm. Patients have frequently assured me that the effect of my passes was much less when my hand was cold, though I felt elsewhere warm and comfortable. All the susceptibilities and powers of a living frame, even the power of thinking, are lessened by cold."[†]

Experiments are also very useful, and rather to be encouraged than otherwise. When the brain of the sleeper has become to a degree active, and he has passed from the stupor into what is called sleep-waking, the more a cheerful conversation is carried on the better; some patients, indeed, do not like to be spoken to, or to answer; some, on the contrary, are

[*] Townshend's Facts, p. 310.

[†] Zoist, vol. vi. p. 6. Maxwell, in the old Treatise so often referred to, considers that disease and health are communicated from man to man, and mentions various ways: among them he mentions the insensible perspiration. "Sudor, igitur, et insensibilis dicta a medicis perspiratio, non mere emanationis sunt, verum etiam resolutae corporis particulae aereum vehere continentur. Hinc fit, ut in Medicina Magnetica maximi sunt usus," &c.—Liber ii. cap. 16.

annoyed if they are not addressed; with the majority, I should say, that it were desirable to converse a little. If, however, the patient has not passed into the sleep-waking state, "the deeper the sleep can be made by breathing, continued passes, laying the fingers over the eye-balls, or the hand upon the head, or by experiments made with traction, rigidity, &c., the greater the good. Not, however, always," (adds Dr. Elliotson): "I have seen a few patients who suffered if the sleep was made so deep that they could not converse." [*] Experiments, also, with metals, and with mesmerised water, are also very useful. The application of gold to a joint stiffened by rheumatism, or disease, often brings on a quasi-galvanic action, and is most serviceable. Too deep a sleep, however, "produced by metals, or water, or in any other way, may overpower the system, and greatly exhaust the strength."

Experiments with crystals are useful. Several of my patients have declared that when they have held in their hands, or on their lap, a piece of quartz, or of carbonate or sulphate of lime, they have found the Mesmeric influence act more rapidly, and their sleep rendered more deep. If traction can be induced, by the application of a crystal, so much the better.

The notion with inexperienced persons is, that experiments do harm, and fatigue the sleeper. The very reverse is the fact, provided that they are not pushed to an extravagant length. The patient, on awakening, feels rather refreshed and strengthened than otherwise.[†]

It may here be appropriate to allude to a fact, which is one of the most convincing proofs of the truth of Mesmerism, and one at which medical men seem always staggered,—I mean *the good sleep at night* that so generally succeeds the Mesmeric slumber. If an invalid, who is but an indifferent sleeper, dozes in the evening for about an hour, or obtains repose during the day through the influence of narcotics, we too generally hear that the sleep at night has suffered in consequence. This is so common an occurrence, that many sick people exert themselves of an evening to avoid sleep. It is the very opposite with Mesmerism. I have very rarely known (so rarely, indeed, that it amounts to an exception) a patient say that his sleep at night had not been improved by the previous Mesmeric slumber. Some most disturbed sleepers have often declared that they have enjoyed a most refreshing night's rest after their magnetic trance; and that the more lengthened was the Mesmeric sleep, the sounder and better was the one that followed. Now, how is this remarkable point to be explained, but by the fact, that Mesmerism is a condition *sui generis;* that its sleep is distinct from common sleep, and that its influence on the human frame is of a peculiar and abnormal character?

The effect of the presence or absence of the Mesmeriser is a point for observation. "When a patient can be left asleep, it is a happy circumstance, and we ought always to *attempt it the first time.*" [*] And I would add, that if you succeed the first time, you will rarely find any difficulty at a subsequent sitting. And here it will be as well to notice by the way the importance of not "*humouring*" a patient unnecessarily at the commencement of a treatment. Somnambulists are very encroaching and *exigeant*, and the more that their fancies are complied with, the more will they require.[†] Many sleepers imagine that they cannot be left, especially if they are asked about it, by whom, if the Mesmeriser retires cautiously and gently, no inconvenience is felt. "When it is found that the patient cannot be left without distress, we must remain. In some instances this will wear off." "I have a patient who dashes violently after me if I attempt to go to another part of the room; another holds one or both of my hands all the time I am with her, and cannot be

---

[*] *Zoist*, vol. iv. p. 472.

[†] "This is one of the most striking things in Mesmerism: that persons very weak, perhaps exhausted by previous exertion, shall be thrown into the Mesmeric sleep-waking, and be kept in constant muscular action, perhaps extending their arms and legs, or in a state of rigid flexion, forced into and retained in the most awkward, and one would think painful attitudes, such as they could not support a hundredth part of the time in the natural state, and on being awakened, know nothing more than that they feel much stronger and better than before you sent them to sleep."—*Elliotson. Zoist*, vol. i. p. 382.

[*] Elliotson. *Zoist*, vol. iv. p. 472.

[†] Deleuze says, "If your somnambule be capricious, you must oppose him, in expressing your own will, without discussion. Never suffer yourself to be managed by him. If he have fancies that you disapprove, employ your ascendancy over him to conquer them." (p. 126.)

prevailed upon to let me retire." [*] On these occasions, the Magnetiser must act with kindness and judgment.

Another point for consideration is, whether a sleeper can bear the touch or proximity of a third person. To some sleepers, the near approach of even their dearest relatives is most painful and distressing, and ought, therefore, to be avoided. If, however, contact be for any reasons necessary, a *rapport* should be gradually induced between them, by the Mesmeriser holding each party by the hand, and placing them in communication gently, and by degrees.[†]

A sitting should not commence immediately after full eating, while digestion is first proceeding either with the patient or the operator. Deleuze says, however, that it is sometimes desirable for the Magnetiser to eat a little, to avoid exhaustion or fatigue. Temperance and moderation are valuable qualifications in a Mesmeriser.

If Mesmerism be applied locally, and pains shift themselves and descend, it is an admirable sign. "The displacement of a malady," says Deleuze, "proves the efficacy of the magnetism." If pains even increase, there is no cause for alarm. They often do at first; and it proves that an action has commenced in the system. The Mesmeriser should endeavour to attract them downwards, and out at the feet.

If the eyes of the patient be unpleasantly closed after he is awakened, or his eyelids feel stiff, or his limbs or jaws rigid, relaxation may be obtained by the Mesmeriser breathing upon them. This is an important fact for a young Mesmeriser to remember. His breath may release himself and his patient from many an embarrassment.

I have already spoken, in a previous chapter, of the value of firmness and patience, should any thing unusual arise. Calmness and perseverance will always carry a Mesmeriser through every crisis. Nothing serious has ever been known to result

from any change, when the Magnetiser has not given way to the apprehensions of others.

If a sleeper be only partially awakened, or if a disturbing effect remain after he is demesmerised, the patient should be thrown back into a deep sleep again, and allowed to remain so for some minutes; the evil effects will then generally pass off, and the sleeper will probably wake up again, unconscious of their former existence. In all likelihood there had been some little mismanagement.

Some patients of extreme susceptibility are disturbed by the touch of gold, or other metallic substances; and many Mesmerisers, on that account, take off their rings or jewellery, and remove their keys or purses from their pocket. If the patient moves anxiously, and exhibits pain when the Mesmeriser touches or approaches him, the latter has probably some irritating material about his person. This, however, is a point on which no rule can be given; with my patients, the touch from metals has been almost invariably efficacious.

Mesmerism, however, does not always produce sensible effects; and one of our next questions is, how long must it be before we abandon the hope of experiencing real benefit from the treatment? In acute attacks, it will be soon seen whether Mesmerism be likely to render service; but, in chronic cases, the time is uncertain. Gauthier says, "that *generally* fifteen days are sufficient to show whether any real effects are likely to arise [*], though oftentimes an influence is not perceived till at the end of several months." The pages of the Zoist corroborate this latter statement. Much must depend upon the feelings of the patient, as to the prolongation of the treatment; but innumerable instances of ultimate relief obtained, could teach the sufferer *not to be discouraged too soon.*

On the other hand, Dr. Esdaile gives a caution, which it is desirable for the convalescent to bear in mind. "The fewer liberties we take with nature the better, the rule being *never to do more than enough.*" "To practise on the system," he again says, "*more than is necessary for the cure of disease,* appears to me to be a danger to be avoided in the use of Mes-

---

[*] Elliotson. Zoist, vols. v. and ii.

[†] The meaning of being en *rapport,* says Deleuze, is when "one individual acts upon another by the existence of a physical sympathy between them,— and when this sympathy is well established, they are said to be en *rapport.*" Gauthier calls it, "the communication of the vital principle, and a uniformity of movement between two persons."

merism." In the soundness of this advice, I fully concur. When the patient is fully restored to health, it is expedient that the treatment should be discontinued. *Dr. Elliotson* says, "I have noticed, that as recovery advanced, Mesmerism required to be performed less frequently; as in a tonic medicine, patients, as they improve, require a gradual diminution." [*]

Another question often asked, is, what is the class of diseases, which Mesmerism most usually deals with? The medical man has his answer ready: "nervous cases." He will tell you, "hysterical and fanciful women, these are the subjects for Magnetism, and the patients on whom imaginary cures have been wrought." As Miss Martineau, however, observes, "No mistake about Mesmerism is more prevalent than the supposition that it can avail only in nervous diseases. The numerous cases recorded of cure of rheumatism, dropsy, and the whole class of tumours, cases as distinct, and almost as numerous, as those of cure of paralysis, epilepsy, and other diseases of the brain and nerves, must make an inquirer cautious of limiting his experiments to the nervous system. Whether Mesmerism acts *through* the nervous system is another question." [†] The index of the Zoist will confirm this statement; and without enumerating the cures there recorded, it will be sufficient to repeat the language of the accomplished lady, before quoted, that "Mesmerism is successful through the widest range of diseases that are not hereditary, and have not caused disorganisation."

Epilepsy is one of the diseases for which Mesmerism is considered almost a specific; in its treatment, however, there is a caution which it is desirable to give to the inexperienced Magnetist.

Teste says, "an *increase* in the *number* and *severity* of the fits constitutes *almost always* the first effect of the treatment." I think that he has stated this opinion far too strongly; it ought rather to be said, that an increase in the number and severity of the fits, is a not uncommon result of the Mesmeric influence, and a most favourable prognostic of a successful issue.

But this increase in the fits is a distressing commencement for a young Mesmeriser; he not unnaturally apprehends that he is doing harm rather than good, and would be apt to suspend his operations at the very moment that he has received the best promise of a cure. Teste adds, "These crises soon diminish in frequency and severity, and ultimately disappear altogether;" [*] and he gives a case or two in illustration of the fact. One of them was reported by Dr. Koreff, a physician, in which a "frightful succession of fits" came on, which the patient described as "a *stormy explosion* necessary to terminate the disease," after which she was perfectly restored and enjoyed excellent health. (*Spillan's Teste*, p. 269.) Dr. Elliotson mentions a case in which "*for three weeks* the patient had a fit *almost as soon* as the process was commenced; and when the fit was over, the process was recommenced, and so on several times at each sitting. The process then produced only a shaking for a month. She continued to be mesmerised for a twelvemonth, and *has not had a fit now for above six years.*" (*Zoist*, vol. ii. 76.)

Teste says, "These violent paroxysms do not occur constantly. M. Mialle's work contains a number of cases, in which the disease observed an inverted course,—i. e. began by exhibiting an amendment from the first days of treatment." (p. 269). Dr. Elliotson, says, "It occasionally happens at first that the process either excites a fit instead of the Mesmeric state, or a fit which passes into the Mesmeric state; or that the Mesmeric state so favours the disposition to an attack that it is interrupted by one, and sometimes continues when the fit is over, sometimes is perfectly broken up by the fit, and sometimes the process of waking a patient excites a fit. But, if the process is repeated, such a result ceases. When attacks occur from the Mesmeric process or state, they decline after a time, and at length cease, if the course of Mesmerism is persevered with. If a continuance of the passes during the fit clearly aggravates, it may be proper to desist till this is over; but in general the fit yields the sooner to a steady continuance of the passes, or to

passes down the chest and back with contact, transverse passes before and behind the trunk, or to what is often better, breathing very slowly and assiduously upon the eyes, nose, and mouth, or the bosom, and holding the patient's hands in our own; and the Mesmeric state may manifest itself in proportion as the fit is subdued."[*]

Another question that is often asked by medical men, and too generally with a sneer, is, Can Mesmerism cure *organic disease?* by which is meant, such an aggravation of disease in the part affected as amounts to an actual alteration of structure? For instance, Can Mesmerism cure an enlarged liver, or a uterine cancer? We might ask in return, can medical men cure it? and if not, why this sneer at the presumed impotency of Mesmerism?

Of course, on a question of this kind, I am not competent to offer an opinion. Some medical Magnetists assert, that Mesmerism does produce such a "revolution" in the system as occasionally to bring about a cure, where actual disorganisation has set in; and in confirmation of this view they present some very startling facts. Other Mesmerists, however, say, that the extent of this agency goes no farther than to palliate for a season, and to suspend the progress of disease. And if this be all, is this nothing? Well does Mr. Newnham observe, "It is, however, something gained, to get time,—to arrest the rapidity of the downward path,—to renovate strength for a while,—to induce sleep where narcotics fail,—to tranquillise the nerves,—frequently to discard pain, and generally to diminish suffering; and such effects we claim for magnetism over organic lesion."[†] But, (as Mr. Townshend observes,) "with most persons, not to cure is equivalent to doing nothing at all. Is mitigation of suffering nothing in this suffering world? Who are the persons who choose to deny the advantage of a remedy because it is not entirely curative? Certainly not those who are tortured by disease, nor their friends who witness that torture."[‡] Let us assume, that in the whole class

* Zoist, vol. ii. p. 159. Dr. Storer of Bristol has been very successful in treating Epilepsy by Mesmerism. See particularly, Zoist, vol. iv. p. 447.
† Newnham's "Human Magnetism." p. 194.
‡ Townshend's Facts. Preface.

of organic maladies, in cancers, or in diseases of the lungs or of the liver, no final cure can be obtained,—still it is something to mitigate symptoms, and procure a partial victory over pain,—most especially when the conventional arts of established practice have altogether failed to produce improvement. A cure, indeed, may not be obtained,—but

. . . "The salutary spell
Shall lull the penal agony to sleep."[*]

But, because Mesmerism may be insufficient to restore disorganised structure, this is no argument, as some employ it, against its application in functional disorders, or in partial derangements of the system. "We scarcely ever cease to hear of the curative effects of the system," says Mr. Allison, an opponent. "Let the reader seriously ask himself, whether Mesmerism is adequate to restore an altered composition, and a structural change? May Providence aid the afflicted, who trust in means so disproportionate to the object!" "Among the diseases, which are supposed to be influenced by the passes, paralysis occupies a prominent place. Paralysis must have a cause. That cause is a disorganisation of structure in the nervous matter; for every properly-conducted examination after death has demonstrated the existence of a structural change."[†] Whether paralysis be organic or functional, it is certain that Mesmerism has been of essential service to many afflicted with the disease;—and with all deference to the anatomists, it would scarcely seem to follow, because structural change had been detected in examinations conducted *after death*, that disorganisation had equally existed in the earlier stages of the malady. And it is for those earlier stages that I strongly urge this remedy. Like galvanism and electricity, which are constantly recommended by the faculty for the cure, Mesmerism will be found to succeed, when every thing else has failed; and even in cases of long standing, to produce essential, though gradual, benefit.

Deleuze, who wrote in 1825, and who is a most safe guide to follow, mentioned more than *sixty cures* of paralysis, that

* Thalaba, book v.
† "Mesmerism and its Pretensions," &c., by J. Allison, Surgeon, p. 50.

had occurred in France through Mesmerism, up to that time. Dr. Elliotson, Dr. Esdaile, and Mr. D. Hands record some cures in the *Zoist*. And in the seventeenth number of that periodical, there is a cure reported of a case of paralysis of thirty years' standing. The Rev. L. Lewis, the Mesmeriser, says, "The paralysed leg and foot which had been in a cold and withered state for thirty years, are now as warm as any part of the patient's frame, much larger in size, and strong enough to bear her weight. She can walk many miles."

Friction of the paralysed part is particularly recommended by Deleuze and Gauthier, after the patient is asleep, and when the *rapport* is well established.

Paralytics often *begin* to use their limbs in the sleep. "I have seen," says Dr. Koreff, "paralytics recover the full use of their limbs in somnambulism, which they lost, when awakened. Gradually, however, the cure has been completed."[*] Dr. Elliotson mentions a case in point, where by tractive passes he made a young paralytic elevate his head and walk after him. "The father and mother were petrified, and called in their people from the shop to witness the strange sight of their child with his head nodding in sleep, and slowly moving after me, though unable to raise his head an inch or move his legs at all a quarter of an hour before." Dr. E. adds afterwards, that "he is in perfect health."[†]

It is unnecessary, however, to recapitulate every disease to which Mesmerism is applicable. Let it be tried on every occasion, when circumstances render it convenient,—not, as was before remarked, in antagonism to the physician, but as subsidiary to his kind and practised care.[‡]

The student would probably be glad to know that modern writers divide the Mesmeric condition "into several states or stages, which are not always found to occur in the same in-

* Koreff, p. 445.   † Zoist, vol. i.
‡ Coleridge, in a note to Southey's Wesley, alludes to "the successful application of Animal Magnetism in four or five cases of suspended animation; in two of them, every known means had been used for six hours to no purpose, and for which the Emperor of Russia, who was present, and the King of Prussia, had a medal struck, one of which, in gold, was given to Dr. Wolfart." (p. 606.)

dividual,—sometimes one only appearing, sometimes another, and sometimes two or three in succession."[*]   Gauthier classifies the condition under four heads.   Some Mesmerists distinguish as many as seven degrees.

Perhaps the most accurate division may be as follows.

First,—the simple sleep, without phenomena of any description.

Secondly, — the deep sleep or coma, in which the sleeper speaks to the Mesmeriser, and exhibits attachment, or sympathy, or attraction, according to the passes, and insensibility to pain.

Thirdly, the sleep-waking state, in which the patient converses freely, and often noisily, with the Mesmeriser, and shows community of taste and sensation, &c.

It is this peculiar freedom of manner, that is exhibited by the sleep-waker in this stage, which is often so perplexing to the stranger and to the incredulous. The sceptic cannot understand it, and will not believe it to be genuine. In short, he deems it the most impudent part of the whole imposture, though, in truth, it is one of the most convincing points as to the reality of Mesmerism. Dr. Forbes, in a paper in the Medical Gazette, on his search for clairvoyance[†], speaks of a sleeper "waking up in the *brisk pert humour* common to the so-called somnambulists." This "brisk pert humour," however, is what I have seen manifested in the sleep-waking state, by all classes of patients, by the most ignorant and the most refined, — by those whose delicacy of taste would shrink from thus exhibiting themselves, and by those who had never seen or heard of Mesmerism. Mr. Townshend says, "Mesmerised persons speak with a freedom, instances of which being related to them in their waking condition cause them surprise and even vexation."[‡] I have had patients apologise to me for what I told them they had said or done during their sleep, and evidently were more than half-incredulous as to its truth. Dr. Elliotson observes, "The generality of this striking effect is

* Professor Gregory, p. 7.
† "Notes of another Trial with the Mesmerists," by Dr. Forbes.
‡ Townshend, p. 202.

one proof of the reality of the Mesmeric state. This *happy feeling of equality* depends upon the cerebral character and education of the patient. Those, whose familiar conversation (when awake) is marked by levity, may, in the Mesmeric state, rattle and be rude, — and then, if there is a degree of delirium mixed with it, the conduct begets a suspicion of imposition."[*] Dr. Esdaile describes how the same freedom of manner developed itself among the Hindoos. He mentions a case, where (to use his own language), "those who did not see the somnambulist, may imagine how little the poor fellow knew what he was about, when they are told that he took the "longitude" of the Judges of the Supreme Court with the *cool impudence* and precision of a cabman.[†] But the most striking instance is that recorded by Mr. Eliot Warburton, of what occurred at Damascus, with a black slave, whom he Mesmerised. The sleeper, with a fearful howl, suddenly started to his feet, flung wide his arms, seized a large vase of water and dashed it into fragments, smashed a lantern into a thousand bits, and rushed about the court-yard. All this was done by a slave in the presence of his master! When awakened, he was quite unconscious of all that he had done, but described his sensations as having been delightful, that of *perfect freedom*, of a man with all his rights, such as he had never felt before in his life.[‡]

The fourth stage is that of clairvoyance and of the ecstatico-prophetic, in which the sleeper appears to acquire new senses, and obtains with the vulgar the reputation of the miraculous. Clairvoyance has several degrees, and various powers. Mental travelling, thought-reading, prevision, introvision, pure clairvoyance, are the terms most generally employed to describe the highest phenomena. Of these, introvision, by which the clairvoyant is enabled to see the structure of the human frame, and

report the condition of a diseased organ, would seem to be the most useful.[*]

Clairvoyance is a fatiguing and exhausting condition. The presence of sceptics has a disturbing effect[†]: it is not always the same on all occasions, (most especially, it is said, with women;) and if the faculty be overworked, it will fail altogether.

Clairvoyants are very vain of what they can perform, and are fond of creating wonder. If the Mesmeriser encourages display, their vanity will increase and their wonders also. This has been the source of much imposture, and of discredit to Mesmerism.

In short, — to be useful should be the first study with the Mesmerist. Man does not live for himself alone. Man must be reared by man; must be taught by man; must be comforted and healed by man. We are all necessary the one to the other; we are all formed from the same clay, and are hastening to the same end; — and while our sojourn continues on this earth, are all intimately identified with each other's happiness. As that wild, but powerful writer, Thomas Carlyle, — in one of the wildest and most powerful of his writings, — "The French Revolution," — speaking on the very subject of this work, says: "And so under the strangest new vesture, the *old great truth* begins again to be revealed, — that man is what we call a miraculous creature, *with miraculous power over men;* and on the whole, with such a life in him, and such a world round him, as victorious Analysis, with her physiologies, nervous systems, physic and metaphysic, will never completely name; to *say nothing of explaining.*"

The task to which I have so anxiously devoted myself, is now completed; and my readers must judge with what success.

---

[*] Zoist, vol. iii. p. 356.   [†] Esdaile's India, p. 113.

[‡] See "Crescent and Cross," vol. ii. p. 290. Dr. Radclyffe Hall, speaking of a curious instance of the effects of ether on a lady, says, "Her manner of expressing her opinion during her ether-dreaming, though free from the slightest immodesty, was far removed from the reserve which a knowledge of the presence of those around would have occasioned."— *Lancet*, March, 1847. When this absence of reserve occurs in Mesmerism, it is called imposture.

---

[*] See Appendix I. for instances of Clairvoyance unconnected with Mesmerism.

[†] Baron Feuchtersleben observes, "The presence of an indifferent or incredulous spectator excites their antipathy, and they produce their most astounding wonders only before believers, a fact of which I have often convinced myself."— *Medical Psychology*, p. 309.

I have endeavoured to show that there is in Mesmerism the existence of a power which, if properly directed and controlled, may be found eminently serviceable in increasing the happiness of human kind.

I have endeavoured to prove this position by numerous instances confirmed by observation and experiment.

I have respectfully invited the attention of the medical world to a philosophic consideration of the uses of this power.

I have shown that the vague charge of Satanic action is one which has been renewed at every fresh and mysterious discovery,—that it is a charge, too, which often proceeds less from the grossest ignorance than the interested motives of the inventor.

I have endeavoured to prove that our knowledge of Mesmerism does, in no degree, affect our belief in real miracles, and in the doctrines of Scripture, though it may throw light upon many of those secrets respecting the relationship of mind and matter, which have hitherto appeared miraculous or perplexing, according as the priest or philosopher have respectively regarded them.

And, lastly, I have given a few plain rules in mesmerising, for those who wish to employ the art for the benefit of their family and of their sick friends.

And now nothing remains but to congratulate the friends of truth, at the marked and steady progress that the great cause is making. The adversaries may be numerous and influential,—but their number is diminishing daily. The established leaders of the medical profession, who have fixed the principles of their practice, and desire no disturbance in their views from the detection of a fresh and unknown law in nature;—a decreasing proportion of the Evangelical clergy, whose unfortunate love of popularity and power tempts them to uphold their otherwise well-deserved eminence by fanatical denunciations of the first object that perplexes them;—every weak and nervous woman, who deems it one of the privileges of the sex to surrender her reasoning faculties into the guidance of some favourite and spiritual adviser;—and, lastly, the large portion of the public that hates to think for itself,—that loathes every

thing which is new,—that calls reformation revolution,—and prefers a vapid uniformity of existence, to the animating pleasures of knowledge and discovery; these are the opponents of Mesmerism; and with these any controversy is worse than useless. How cheering is the opposite side of the picture! The friends of the art are those of whom any cause might be proud. Men of science,—men of philosophy,—men whose benevolence is as wide and practical as their intellects are clear and commanding; these are our guides and champions in this glorious field of Christian usefulness, and under their banners a day of complete success cannot be far distant. But they are not merely a few select and leading minds that rank among its advocates; large bodies of men are taking up the question. It is a fact that a numerous portion of the junior members of the medical profession are alive to the truths of Mesmerism, and only biding their time till the ripened mind of the public gives them a signal for its more general adoption. It is a fact that very many individuals among the younger portion of the clergy, are conscious of the medicinal value of the science, and are introducing its practice as one of their means of parochial usefulness.[*] Nay, the two extremes of the great social pyramid are both exerting their energies in the same direction. Mechanics' Institutes are taking the subject up; and many of the operatives in the North, and in the manufacturing towns, have experienced a sense of its domestic benefit.[†] But it is among our haute noblesse itself that the strongest division of supporters may perhaps be found. Some of the leading members of the aristocracy are practising the art for the benefit of their poorer brethren; and very many are giving to the subject a patient and anxious investigation. It is, indeed, one of the most favourable signs of the times—in spite of the fearful storms that seem to cloud the social horizon—this growing disposition on the part of all ranks of the community to devote

* See, for instance, an article in The Christian Remembrancer recommending the practice. This article, it is well known, was written by a near relation of one of our ablest bishops.

† In confirmation of the above, I see that Mr. Parker states, that "Mesmerism is resorted to in Exeter by the industrious classes as a most extraordinary remedial agent."—Zoist, vol. v. p. 145.

themselves most extensively to the useful and to the instructive. There is, perhaps, at this moment no single department of science or general literature which cannot boast amongst its followers one or two most accomplished members from out of the circle of the British aristocracy. And Mesmerism is no exception to the progressive character of their studies. In short, as Mr. Chenevix said a few years back, MESMERISM IS ESTABLISHED. Nothing but a general convulsion of society — a loss of the art of printing, and a return to the barbarous condition of those of old, can, humanly speaking, roll back that current of knowledge on the subject which is growing and expanding every year. Soon, very soon, will it be an acknowledged — an admitted branch of medical practice. And when that day shall at length arrive — when the mists of prejudice and bigotry shall be dispersed before the glowing splendours of the Sun of truth, and men shall look back in wonder at that hardened incredulity which checked its onward progress — let it never be forgotten who it was that in this country first placed the question on its legitimate footing, — who it was that first took the practice out of the hands of the charlatan, and added its multiplied and profound resources to the former stores of the healing art, — who it was that, risking the loss of friends, the loss of income, the loss of elevated standing in his own profession, stepped out manfully and truthfully from the timid crowd, and asserted the claims of this great discovery to a place within the circle of the medical sciences: and when the question is asked who it was that so boldly ventured on this untrodden ground, a grateful posterity will respond with the name of JOHN ELLIOTSON. But it will also be added, that he lived to see his calumniated art acknowledged and pursued; that he lived to see the stream of professional success flowing back to him with the full tide of popular support; that he lived to see every statement which he had advanced, every treatment which he had adopted, established and confirmed; and that as one of the first physicians of the age, first in practice, and first in reputation, he was classed with the proudest names of that honourable band,

" Qui sui memores fecere merendo."

APPENDIX.

No. I.

INSTANCES OF CLAIRVOYANCE UNCONNECTED WITH MESMERISM.

THE great use to which Clairvoyance may be turned, — is the detection of disease through intro-vision, or, in other words, the inspection of the inner and vital portions of the human frame, such as the lungs, the heart, the liver, &c., and the report of their condition for the guidance of the practitioner.

The question, however, that first presents itself is this, — does such a faculty exist in nature?

Mr. E. Fry's "Report of an Examination of a case of Clairvoyance at Plymouth before a Committee," as given in the fourth volume of the *Zoist*, — is one of the most convincing statements that I have ever read.

Dr. Ashburner's letter, in the twenty-first number of the *Zoist*, narrating some experiments, made by himself and others, is startling in the extreme. His high character, and his competency for an examination, place the question in a strong light.

The case of Alexis Didier was genuine. Unfortunately, he was so overworked on his visit to England, through the mercenary activity of his employer, — that frequent failures attended the exhibition, and a report spread everywhere, that "Alexis was an impostor." I saw him, on four different occasions, upon his first arrival in London, and am satisfied as to the realities of his power.

An ably written article in the "Critic" for February, 1844, says, — " We have no hesitation in asserting as the result of accurate experiment, that there *is a state of human existence*, in which the mind perceives external objects through *some other medium than the*

A A 3

wonted media of the senses, and that in this state the mind perceives things imperceptible in its natural condition." Startling as this position is, — there is no escaping from the fact. Long before Mesmer appeared, or Mesmerism was practised, — have such facts been stated on the most unquestionable authority. What is the manner, by which these effects are produced, is another and difficult question, — for the solution of which, in the present state of knowledge, — we are little prepared. Whether it be, as the writer in the "Critic" suggests, "by a sixth* sense of which in our ordinary condition of existence we are not conscious, and which is developed only under certain circumstances;" — or whether, "by an extraordinary quickening of the senses, so that they catch sights and sounds invisible and inaudible to us;"—whether, "by the partial severance of the immaterial mind from its material tenements, and its perception of things directly without the intervention of those senses through which only it is usually permitted to hold intercourse with the material world;" or whether it be "by a mysterious or unexplained sympathy;" whatever be the hypothesis, — the fact is certain, and cannot admit of contradiction. The useful point, however, to be borne in mind, is this, — that these phenomena have occurred without the action of animal magnetism. In a useful little work by Mr. Edwin Lee on Clairvoyance †, — which, all who are interested on the subject should read, — there is a quotation from a German work on practical religion, which is corroborative of the opinion. "Nevertheless, it is not to be denied that we are but learners in our investigations into the secrets of nature, and that what appears to us to be incomprehensible, is not, on that account, to be denied altogether. We now know, for instance, that the human soul, which employs for its instrument as regards earthly things the nervous system more particularly, can also feel and perceive beyond the sphere of the nerves. We know that in certain conditions of nervous disorder, man may possess increased powers, may perceive distant things, which are separated from him by an interval of many miles. We know that in some states of the nervous system, persons can see with firmly closed eyes, — can hear with closed ears. We have examples of this in somnambulists (natural sleep-walkers) — who during the complete sleep of their bodies, perform things which in their waking state they were unable to accomplish. Thus, herein shows itself very

* Wienholt, who has written so ably on the subject, altogether rejects the sixth sense. See Colquhoun's Translation, p. 126.

† "Report on the Phenomena of Clairvoyance," by Edwin Lee, Esq. (Churchill, Prince's Street, Soho.)

clearly an activity of the human soul altogether independent of its outward senses. But, in point of fact, it is not the eyes which see, nor the ears which hear; it is the soul which sees, hears, and perceives by means of the nerves, which are distributed over the whole surface of the body, and the powers of which are almost redoubled in the apparatus of the senses, smell, feeling, &c.*

A few instances of Clairvoyance, occurring spontaneously in a natural state, shall be here adduced in confirmation of the above statement. The case of Somnambulism, which is reported on the authority of the Archbishop of Bordeaux, was alluded to in the Third Chapter. There the young ecclesiastic wrote and read with his eyes closed, and when an opaque body was interposed by the archbishop between them and the paper.

Here is a case of hysteria, with extraordinary acuteness of some of the senses. It was communicated by Sir G. S. Mackenzie, Bart. to the Editor of the Edinburgh Phrenological Journal: —

"Dear Sir,

"The following copy of a letter from a clergyman was sent to me nearly six years ago, at a time when Mesmerism had not attracted my notice. The case referred to in it was evidently one of natural sleep-walking; and it is to be regretted that so little of it is known, as it appears to have been one of great interest. Now that the subject is better and more generally understood, we may hope that such cases, when they occur, will not be concealed.

"Yours faithfully,

"24th October, 1843.   G. S. Mackenzie."

"'Dear Sir,   "'24th January, 1838.

"'It is perfectly true that our poor friend, who has now been some months with us, presents one of those singular and almost incredible cases of hysterical or nervous affection which are at distant intervals witnessed under the dispensation of the Almighty.

"'The overthrow of the regular functions of the nervous system was occasioned by the almost sudden death of her father, to whom she was most fondly attached, who was seized with illness during her absence from him, and died a few hours after she returned to her home. I cannot enter into any longer details of the case, which has been attended with all those varieties which have long characterised the complaint, among medical men, as the Protean disorder. The extraordinary powers communicated to the other senses by the temporary suspension of one or two of them, are beyond credibility to

* Mesmer has remarked, that the "whole system of nerves becomes eye and ear."—See Gauthier, p. 515.

all those who do not witness it; and I really seldom enter into any of the details, because it would be but reasonable that those who have not seen should doubt the reality of them. All colours she can distinguish with the greatest correctness by night or day, whether presented to her on cloth, silk, muslin, wax, or even glass —and this, I may safely say, as easily on any part of the body as with the hands, although, of course, the ordinary routine of such an exhibition of power takes place with the hands, the other being that of mere curiosity. Her delicacy of mind and high tone of religious feeling are such, that she has the greatest objection to make that which she regards in the light of a heavy affliction from God, a matter of show or curiosity to others, although to ourselves, of course, all these unusual extravagances of nervous sensibility are manifest for at least twelve out of every twenty-four hours. She can not only read with the greatest rapidity any writing or print that is legible to us, music, &c., with the mere passage of her fingers over it, whether in a dark or light room (for her *sight* is for the most part suspended when under the influence of the attack or paroxysm, although she is perfectly *sensible*, nay, more *acute* and *clever* than in her natural state); but, within this month past, she has been able to collect the contents of any printing or MS. by merely laying her hand on the page, without *tracing* the lines or letters; and I saw her, last night only, declare the contents of a note just brought into the room, in this way (when I could not decipher it myself without a candle), and with a rapidity with which I could not have read it by daylight. I have seen her develop hand-writing by the application of a note to the back of her hand, neck, or foot; and she can do it at any time. There is nothing unnatural in this; for, of course, the nervous susceptibility extends all over the surface of the body, but use and habit cause us to limit its power more to the fingers. Many, even medical, men take upon themselves to declare that *we are all* (her medical attendants as well) under a mere delusion. We ask none to believe any thing if they prefer not to do so, and only reply —The case is equally marvellous either way; either that this our poor patient should be thus afflicted, or that eighteen or nineteen persons of my family and friends, in the daily habit of seeing her, should fancy she is, for every twelve hours out of twenty-four, doing, at intervals, that which she is *not* doing. There are many exhibitions of extravagant powers which she possesses, that we talk of to no one; for, finding it difficult to acquire credit for lesser things, we do not venture on the greater. *Her power ceases the moment the attack passes off.* A considerable swelling has at times been visible at the back of the head, which has yielded to the treatment.

"'It is certainly a case which would be an instructive one in the consideration of the physiology of the human frame; but she, poor thing! is most averse to experiments being purposely made on her: but in her every-day life among us, we have no lack of proof for all we believe and *know*.

"'Between the attacks she is as perfectly in a *natural* state as ever she was in her life. There is but one *paradox* in her state, and that is, that she can at such times hear *some* sounds and not *others*, though very much louder,—and see some things and not others, though placed before her. She could hear a tune whistled, when she would not hear a gun fired close to her. It is certainly the absorption or absence of mind that occasions this: *absent* to some things, though *present* to others, like any absent man; and thus Dr. Y—— accounts for it.

"'In making this communication to you, in part to vindicate the testimony of my friend Mr. M——, I have really exceeded my usual custom and resolution; for I do not think it fair to the poor sufferer herself to make her too much the talk of others. Very few believe what we tell them, and, therefore, we are in no degree anxious to open our lips on the subject. All I know is, that I should not have believed it myself, had I been only *told* of it. I must beg, therefore, that you will not make any undue use of this communication, by handing my letter about to any one. The friend for whom you ask the information is perfectly welcome to read it, or I should not have written it. If the case were my own, the world should be welcome to it; but a young female of much sensibility might be much embarrassed, by finding the world at large in possession of all particulars on her recovery, should God so please to permit.

"'I am, &c.'"

Mr. Colquhoun, in the "Isis Revelata," has collected several similar cases.

One is the case of a boy, named Divaud, residing at Vevey. The Philosophical Society of Lausanne examined into this case, and reported the facts. The committee testify, that the boy read, *when his eyes were perfectly shut*;—that he wrote accurately; "*though we put a thick piece of paper before his eyes*, he continued to form each character with the same distinctness as before." "He has told the title of a book, when there was a thick plank placed between it and his eyes." Many other singular circumstances are narrated of this natural somnambulist.

Another instance of clairvoyance, is that of a student, who, during a severe nervous complaint, experienced several attacks of somnambulism. Professor Feder of Gottingen is the authority for this

case. Several facts are given, from which it is evident that this somnambulist saw distinctly without the use of his eyes.

The "Transactions of the Medical Society of Breslau" mention the case of a ropemaker, who was frequently overtaken by sleep,—whose eyes were then firmly closed, and in this state he would continue his work with as great ease as when awake. But this somnambulist "*could not see when his eyes were forced open.*"

Dr. Knoll gives the example of a gardener, who became a somnambulist, and in that state performed a variety of occupations, requiring light and the use of the eyes, with which he dispensed. Among other things, he *put the thread through the eye of a needle*, and sewed his clothes.

Lord Monboddo has recorded a curious case of somnambulism, in which a girl in his neighbourhood performed a variety of acts *with her eyes shut.*

Dr. Schultz of Hamburgh mentions a patient, who wrote, and distinguished colours, and recognised the numbers of cards, and cut figures in paper, with her eyes fast closed. "In order to *be certain,* that upon these occasions she made no use of her eyes, they were bandaged upon the approach of the convulsions which preceded the somnambulism."

Moritz's "Psychological Magazine" gives an account of a boy, who frequently fell asleep suddenly; and although his eyes were completely closed, was *able to see* and discriminate *all objects* presented to him.

Dr. Abercrombie in his "Intellectual Powers," and Dr. Dyce of Aberdeen, in the "Edinburgh Philosophical Transactions," have described cases of a very similar character; but they have been so often quoted, and are so familiar to the reader, that further reference is unnecessary.

Those who are anxious to pursue the subject, should consult the "Isis Revelata," (in which these cases are more fully detailed,) and Dr. Wienholt's Lectures on Somnambulism.

Several other instances of Clairvoyance, independent of, and previously to, Mesmerism, may be adduced.

Glanvill, in his Sadducismus, mentions a boy, Richard Jones, who described the clothes that people at a distance wore; the constable and others often tried, and "found the boy right in his descriptions." (p. 120.)

Lebrun, in his "History of Superstitions," mentions that towards the end of the fifteenth century there was a man who *saw through all stuffs,* except those whose colour was mixed with red. (Liv. i. chap. 6.)

In Chambers's Journal (vol. iv. N. S.) is an account of Zschokke,

a Swiss, who possesses this faculty, which he calls his "inward sight." Some remarkable instances are given.

In Forbes's "Oriental Memoirs" is the description of a Brahmin, who possessed the Clairvoyant power in a marvellous degree. (*Zoist,* vol. v. 130.)

In the *Zoist* (vol. v. p. 344. and 347.) are two other striking instances of Clairvoyance, independent of Mesmerism,—one, that of Goethe's grandfather; the other, that of Swedenborg.

Teste, quoting M. Mialle, speaks of a Polish Jew, named Denemark, who sees through opaque bodies in his natural sleep. "He reads fluently a shut book." His son, ten years old, possesses "the same faculty, but in a higher degree." (p. 404).

My friend Mr. Ashhurst Majendie tells me of a well-known case of natural Clairvoyance, at St. Malo. M. Eugene Gilbert, after a dangerous illness, fell spontaneously into somnambulism, and became Clairvoyant. He described accurately the plan of the citadel of Antwerp, its being taken, &c. Several other instances of his power are notorious at St. Malo.

The above facts, and others that are recorded by Pététin in his *Electricité Animale,* and by Wienholt in his Somnambulism,—might surely cause the unbeliever to hesitate, before he pronounces that Clairvoyance is impossible, and not a fact in nature! Let it be again repeated, to prevent mistake,—that Mesmerism had nothing to do with any of the above instances. [*]

No. II.

ECSTASY AND SLEEP-WAKING, AND INSENSIBILITY TO PAIN, INDEPENDENT OF MESMERISM.

An accomplished writer in the Dublin University Magazine (to whom I take this opportunity of confessing sundry obligations) has observed that Mesmer and his disciples "have thrown light upon one of the darkest chapters in the history of man; they have solved, at least partially, the riddle of those wild accusations, and still wilder confessions, in virtue of which so many thousand of human beings were delivered to an appalling death." * * * "It is

---

[*] In Colquhoun's Wienholt, pp. 89. 109. and 182, and in the Introduction, p. 17, are various observations on Clairvoyance of so philosophical a nature, that they will well repay the student for their perusal.

impossible to compare the appearances observable in a modern Mesmeric patient with those presented by a witch or a devil-possessed Nun of the period referred to, without being led to the conclusion that it is *one* influence which affects both; — that *their states are identical*; that either the Mesmeric patient is a witch, or the witch was nothing more than a Mesmeric patient. And this recurrence of phenomena so similar, under circumstances so widely diverse, is the strongest of all arguments against the supposition that the phenomena are the result of imposture. If we find insensibility to pain in the witch, or the demonopathic, we have the less reason to believe the insensibility to pain, shown by the Mesmeric patient to be simulated. If we find Clairvoyance, or a perception of things without the ordinary range of the senses, in the witch or the demonopathic, we have the less ground for supposing the Clairvoyance of the Mesmeric patient to be a hallucination or a pretence. If we observe that very strange state of things which, in the language of the Mesmerists is termed *rapport* — a community of sensation, thought, or will, between the witch and the victim of her sorceries, or between the demonopathic and the exorcist, we are the less warranted to assume that such *rapport*, as subsists between the Mesmeric patient and the Mesmeriser, is a chimera, or a trick sustained by collusion. And these are but a few of the points in which the two classes of phenomena we speak of *correspond*. In the hundreds of Mesmeric cases that have been treated, &c. * * — and in the thousand cases of diabolism in its thousand forms, &c. &c. a *unity of character*, a *constant reproduction of the same leading features*, is to be recognised, wholly inexplicable, unless on the hypothesis of a common origin, of one principle operating throughout."

After narrating the most curious phenomena of the demoniacs, &c. the writer asks, "Is there no where a reality corresponding to all this?"

"No doubt there is such a reality: and we think that the Mesmeric phenomena yield a clue, by which we may advance some one or two steps, in the direction in which it lies. Whatever the psychic state of the witches and demonopathics of the middle ages was, into the same state does the agency of Mesmerism throw the person on whom it is brought to bear. It is a state *sui generis*, — a state of great nervous disturbance, but of which no familiar form of nervous disease supplies us with a definition." *

The above clearly-expressed remarks accord with much that has been stated by myself in the Seventh Chapter. This writer has,

* From "An Evening with the Witch-finders." Dublin U. Magazine, July, 1847.

however, rather referred to the presumed demoniac possession of the bewitched, than to imaginary miracles and divine revelations. This, however, is indifferent. Accident and education determine the name. What is a miracle with one people, or age, is a demoniacal visit with another.

Several additional facts are herewith appended in continuation of the argument of the Seventh Chapter. The points, in the respective cases, only are alluded to, — which will throw light upon Mesmerism.

It has been shown that long and serious ill-health has been an almost invariable precursor of the ecstatic condition, when the latter has been induced by Mesmerism.* If we turn to the lives of those Saints among the Catholics and Methodists, in whom ecstasis developed itself spontaneously, — we shall equally trace the preparatory stages of disease. Severe abstinence also strongly predisposes for the same condition.

Ribadeneira tells us that St. Catherine of Sienna, who died in 1380, had been a dreadful martyr to ill health. The evil spirit afflicted her, he says, with such cruel maladies and pains, that none but those who witnessed them could credit the full amount. "She was nothing but skin and bone, — and was a very skeleton and anatomy of death." St. Catherine, it is well known, was regarded as a miraculous ecstatic in her church: her dreams were most frequent and lasting: often in her divine trances her body remained in as motionless a state as if she were dead; — she was insensible to pain, and unconscious of all that was done to bring her to herself.†

St. Elizabeth of France, the sister of St. Louis, was another ecstatic, — whose holiness of life is celebrated in the annals of French piety. This excellent but mistaken woman brought herself by fastings and austerities, which were so severe as to seem to surpass the power of nature, into the most fearful ill health. For six years she was unceasingly attacked by fevers and other maladies. The miraculous condition then came on. Sister Agnes one day called to see her at the monastery, and was astonished to find her in an an ecstasy. She summoned the chaplains and domestics, — who,

* A patient of Mr. Charles Child's, whom he cured of neuralgia, &c., and who had been long a great invalid, was a most exquisite ecstatic. Her countenance received an expression of devotional resignation that was beautiful. Henry W. (Mr. Spencer Hall's ecstatic patient) had been an invalid at an early age. His attitudes at the sound of music were extraordinary. The severe ill health of Anne Vials, — that of a patient of Mr. D. Hand's, and of another of Dr. Elliotson's, (all ecstatics,) are those that have come under my own knowledge.

† Ribadeneira, "Vies des Saints," vol. i. p. 404.

on their arrival, seeing Elizabeth sitting up on the bed, without motion, — her eyes and face fixed straight forward, — and her lips only slightly stirred, from whence proceeded the words in a low voice, "To him alone be honour and glory," waited some time to see what would happen. At last they made a noise, and tried to awaken her, but in vain: when after a time, her countenance became "resplendent as the sun." She continued in this state, until the evening, when she awoke, says Ribadeneira, like an infant in a cradle. Her ecstasy was the source of religious admiration and wonder.[*]

St. Mary Magdalen of Pazzi, "whose life," Bishop Lavington says, "was almost one continued ecstasy," was born in 1566, in Florence, and became a Religieuse of the order of our Lady of Mont Carmel. In consequence of some delay and disappointment in taking the "habit," or in making "profession," she fell sick and was so extremely ill, that her friends, supposing her to be at the point of death, carried her to the altar, where she was allowed to take the vows. She seems to have lain before the altar some time in a state of great bodily suffering. "Upon being carried back to the infirmary," says Ribadeneira, "she became wrapt in ecstasy, and her face appeared as beautiful and brilliant as the sun, and so much on fire that it resembled that of the Seraphim. She kept her eyes fixed on a crucifix; and this condition lasted for more than an hour, and recurred every morning after the holy communion, for the space of forty days. From the very commencement of her ecstacies, she spoke most profoundly on divine things." Our author adds, that so far from these ecstasies and raptures weakening or exhausting her, they actually (like Mesmerism) gave tone and strength to her system. She was able in her trances to walk from one part of the convent to another, — to converse and answer questions, and even to work with her needle, "with as much perfection as if she had been free and enjoying a perfect use of her senses." Some of her needlework was exhibited and preserved, as proofs of the miraculous character of her condition.[†] One day, she remained in a state of rapture twenty hours without coming to herself. This poor creature, who at times was in this state of exaltation and ravishment, and consequently the admiration of all around her, appears to have been a frightful sufferer. The least touch caused her at times as much torture as if she had been hacked by razors (hachée à coups de rasoirs), and she at last passed from this life

* Ribadeneira, vol. ii. p. 214.

† My friend, Captain James, had a mesmeric patient who was quite unable to work with her needle during her natural state, but who in the sleepwaking condition worked very beautifully.

worn out by the extremity of her agony. She appears to have been a patient and pious Christian, and an example of every virtue. But these ecstatic dreams caused her to be considered a saint, and she was beatified by Pope Urban VIII., and canonized by Pope Clement IX., in 1669.[*]

Lord Shrewsbury, in a second edition of his pamphlet, has referred to a third case of miraculous ecstacy, in which the Mesmeric characteristics are not less marked than in the two that I have quoted in the seventh chapter.

Domenica Barbagli, the Ecstatica of Monte San Savino, near Arezzo, in Tuscany, had been as a child remarkable for her pious feelings, and had suffered greatly from ill health. "She is now (1842) twenty-nine years of age." "About sixteen years since, she had a severe fall down stairs, which so terrified her, and otherwise affected her, as to bring on convulsions and lay the foundation of corporeal maladies." When Lord Shrewsbury saw her, she was "confined a cripple to her bed," from whence she looked through a grating into a small chapel fitted up for her especial service. "She was a perfect skeleton; — were her eyes shut, she would be like a corpse." "Her reputation for piety is such that persons come from a distance to consult her; — her ecstacies only occur during, and for a short time after, the mass," spontaneously; — but "*they are able to be excited at the desire of her confessor,*" when her prayers are requested on very particular occasions, for it is during her ecstacy" that she performs these devotional exercises, &c., which with the ignorant assume the semblance of inspiration. "When, therefore, the confessor sees occasion to require it, to satisfy some urgent case, she falls, *at his bidding,* into that state of intimate communion with God which is most propitious for the purpose." The confessor, it may be observed, unconsciously on his own part, exercises a Mesmeric influence over the *sympathies* of the entranced devotee. In this state, this poor bed-ridden sufferer, who is all but a corpse, *springs into a beautiful attitude,* in which she remains for a few minutes. While she was in this condition, says Lord Shrewsbury, "the chaplain desired me to *touch her head,* when the slightest pressure of my finger upon her made her arm fall several inches, and put her into a swinging motion from side to side. This movement was considerably increased by the same person *blowing at her gently with his breath,* so exceedingly aerial and unsubstantial is her frame." This swinging motion to and fro, in her insensible state, was "according to the direction from whence the breath came."

Meric Casaubon, in the Preface to his Treatise on Enthusiasm,

* Ribadeneira, vol. ii. p. 706.

speaking of a "Life of Sister Katherine of Jesus," — a work which was dedicated to the Queen of France, written by a Cardinal, and published with the approbation of an Archbishop and the Doctors of the Sorbonne, and made a sensation at the time, says, "I found the book to be a long contexture of several strange raptures and enthusiasms that had happened unto a melancholic, or if you will, a devout maid. In this I saw no great matter of wonder; neither could I observe much in the relation of the particulars, but what as I conceived rationally probable, so I might believe charitably true. I could observe, as I thought, a perpetual coherence of *natural causes*, in every particular, which gave me good satisfaction."

Casaubon afterwards mentions the case of a baker's boy at Oldenburgh in Germany, in 1581, who would fall into deep sleep or ecstasies, and "prophesie many things." His prophecies seem to have affected the people of Oldenburgh strongly.

Casaubon next mentions an entranced maid at Friburgh, in Misnia, who had "ecstacies and visions, and was full of religious discourses, most in the nature of sermons and godly exhortations, so that she was generally apprehended to be inspired, and her speeches were published under the name of divine Prophesies." On this occasion, the ecstacies were in favour of Lutheranism. The popular cry was loud in behalf of the maid's "inspiration," but Eberus, the clergyman, was much opposed to it, — but durst not against the *public voice*, affirm that there was nothing of God's Spirit in all she said." (Chapter iii. p. 72.)

The ecstatic cases among the Quakers and Methodists are of the same kind. Southey, in his Life of Wesley, in speaking of the "contagious convulsions" among the converts in Bedfordshire at the preaching of the Methodists, says that Wesley "recorded the things which occurred not as psychological — but as religious cases." Numbers fell into trances: one became "stiff like a statue — his very neck seemed made of iron." Many "began to doubt whether such trances were not the work of Satan; — with the majority, however, they passed for effects of grace. Wesley believed and recorded them as such." [*]

[*] Southey's Life of Wesley, vol. ii. chapter xxiv. To this Coleridge appended the following marginal note: — "I regret that Southey is acquainted only with the magnetic cases of Mesmer and his immediate followers, and not with the incomparably more interesting ones of Gmelin, Weinholt, Eschenmeyer, Wohlfart, &c. — men whose acknowledged merits as naturalists and physicians, with their rank and unimpeached integrity, raise their testimony above suspicion, in point of veracity at least, and of any ordinary delusion. The case Wesley saw is, in all its features, identical with that of the Khumeria, and with a dozen others in the seventh or ecstatic grade. The facts it would be now quite absurd to question; but their direct relation to

Wesley in his Journal says, "Mr. B. came and told me Alice Miller (fifteen years of age) was fallen into a trance. I went down immediately and found her sitting on a stool, and leaning against a wall with *her eyes open and fixed upward*. I made a motion, as if going to strike, but they continued immovable.[*] Her face showed an unspeakable mixture of reverence and love, while silent tears stole down her cheeks. Her lips were a little open, and sometimes moved. I do not know whether I ever saw a human face *look so beautiful*. Sometimes it was covered with a smile, as from joy mixing with love and reverence. *Her pulse was quite regular.* In about half an hour I observed her countenance change into the form of fear, pity and distress. Then she burst into a flood of tears, and cried out, 'Dear Lord, they *will* be damned, — they *will* all,' &c. Then again her look was composed, and full of love and joy. About seven her senses returned. I asked, 'Where have you been?' 'I have been with my Saviour, — I was in glory: I cried not for myself — but for the world,' &c., with much more of the same matter."

Wesley mentions several other of his disciples who fell into trances. "I talked largely with Ann Thorn and two others. What they all agreed in was, — that from the moment they were entranced, they were in another world, *knowing nothing* of what was said or done by all that were round about them."

Wesley at times was cautious of committing himself: still he says, that "God favoured several of his people with divine dreams, others with trances and visions, to strengthen and encourage them that believed, and to *make his work more apparent.*" This is much like what Professor Bush asserts of the lad Davis's testimony to Swedenborgianism, and of Lord Shrewsbury's view respecting the Tyrolese Ecstatica. The phenomena in each are of the same family: all, therefore, must be supernatural, — all or none! [†]

the magnetic treatment, as effect to cause, remains as doubtful as at the beginning. And these cases of the Methodists tend strongly to support the negative. And yet it is singular, that of the very many well-educated men who have produced effects of this kind, or under whose treatment such phenomena have taken place, not one should have withstood the conviction of their having exerted a direct causative agency: though several have earnestly recommended the suppression of the practice altogether, as rarely beneficial, and often injurious, nay, calamitous." — S. T. C.

[*] This I have seen constantly with Anne Vials in her mesmeric trances. Sennert, in giving the *Signa diagnostica* of Catalepsis, mentions among other things: "Æger apertos oculos habet, eosque fixos et immobiles, palpebris veluti rigentibus, quas ne ad minax quidem claudit." Vol. iii. p. 154.

[†] See Wesley's Journal, vol. ii. p. 464, &c.

In the Church Magazine, for 1839, is a sneering account of a "Methodistical servant-girl, who some thirty years back, in the neighbourhood of Lynn and Wisbeeh, acquired the art of suspending her faculties for hours together, and of lying in a state of complete stupefaction, her eyes glazed as in death, and her breath every thing but imperceptible. The *drawing of a feather across her eye-balls*, and burning of feathers near her nostrils, produced no effect. She pretended to see visions and receive revelations." The writer, in his ignorance, charges the poor girl with having been an impostor,—and takes occasion of indulging in some offensive observations on Methodism. [*]

George Fox, the celebrated Father of Quakerism, at one period of his life lay in a trance for fourteen days,—and people came to stare and wonder at him. He had the appearance of a dead man; but his sleep was full of divine visions of glory and beauty, and his followers believed that his "revelations" were the result of spiritual agency working supernaturally by dreams. [†]

Job Cooper, a weaver in the state of Pennsylvania, became, in the year 1774, like Rachel Baker, a sleeping preacher, and attracted the usual attention. People came from considerable distances to hear him. "He was insensible,"—says an eye-witness,—"of all that passed in his room during the paroxysm: and his articulation during his preachings was remarkably distinct, and his discourses were delivered with a fluency far *superior to any thing he could perform when awake*." [‡]

In the Gentleman's Magazine for May 1760, is an account of Joseph Payne, a lad of sixteen, who in his trances delivered a series of regular theological discourses at Reading. He had formerly lived servant to a farmer, who had educated him strictly in religious knowledge. He attended constantly at church,—and while living as post-boy with a Captain Fisher at Reading, began to preach. Dr. Hooper, a medical man, ordered a candle to be lighted, and the flame applied to the boy's hand while he was preaching, till a blister was raised,—but no sensation was manifested.

Bishop Lavington, having quoted Bodin, a French lawyer, who, in a work on Dæmonology, produced a variety of ecstatic cases that had occurred before the Christian era,—observes, "Ecstacies are by no means peculiar to religion, much less to the Christian." [§] In

[*] Church Magazine, June, 1839, p. 178.
[†] See "Popular Life of Fox, compiled from his Journal," &c.
[‡] "Statement of Job Cooper's Somnial Devotion," by Andrew Eliot, Professor at West Point.—January, 1815.
[§] Lavington's Enthusiasm, p. 245.

corroboration of this remark, we shall find ecstasy and sleep-waking among the Hindoos.

Ward, in his history of that people, gives a description of the Philosophical Sects, and of the religious austerities that they practised. One school was that of Patunjulu. Its leading feature was "the restraining of the mind, and the confining it to internal meditations." This was called Yogu. The effect was analogous to self-induced Mesmerism. The method was this. The Yogee, in preparing his mind for intense meditation, "first, gradually suppresses the breath,"—i. e. he retains his breathing for twenty-six seconds, and enlarges this period till he is perfect. The ascetic then endeavours to fix his thoughts upon some act of the senses; for instance, "*he places his sight and thoughts on the tip of his nose*." "He must practise these exercises daily,—as often and for as long a time as he can. By continued action and meditation of this kind for a period, the mind of the half-starved fanatic will "become truly fixed,"—says the treatise,—"fixed, like that of a person *in a state of deep sleep*, who, without any union with the senses, partakes of perfect happiness." "By withholding the mind from wandering, the organs are turned from their accustomed objects inwards. The Yogee, who has perfected himself in all this," or in other words, has induced the ecstatic or Mesmeric condition, "obtains a knowledge of the past and of the future,"—"discovers the *thoughts* and hearts of others,"—"becomes acquainted with the *anatomy of the human body*,"—"sees all visible objects,"—"renders his body invulnerable,"—"will no longer feel the inconveniences of heat or cold, but acquires a victory over pain," &c. [*]

The above is a very curious passage. Here are all the higher phenomena of Mesmerism, Clairvoyance, Prevision, Introvision, Thought-reading, and Insensibility to pain, said to be brought on, with a sect of religious fanatics, by intense meditation acting on a body emaciated with fasting.

Salverte, in his Occult Sciences, in observing upon the above fact of certain among the Hindoos falling into ecstasy, adds, that it is a condition "to which the Kamschatdales, the Jakoutes, and natives of North and South America, are very prone. It has been observed that since the persecutions exercised by Europeans in the countries of Tahiti and the Sandwich Islands, the *imagination* of the adherents of the old religion has been much excited," and ecstasy brought on.

Volney (whom Salverte alludes to) says, that it is a "physiological problem very interesting to solve, to know what was the singular

[*] Ward's "History of the Hindoos," vol. ii. p. 208.

state of nerves, or what was the movement of the electrical fluid in the system, through which the North American Indians were brought to such a state of ecstasy as to be enabled to endure the most frightful torments with the most extraordinary courage. This question deserves to be considered in the schools of medicine."[*]

Physiological facts, indeed, decidedly show that the Mesmeric-ecstatic condition is induced by many causes independent of Mesmerism. We have seen that in religiously-excited minds, intense contemplation of a subject may be one cause. Other influences may act on other natures. I again quote from the Dublin U. Magazine.[†] "Horst relates that a merchant of Silesia, named Löhnig, was condemned, under the government of the Emperor Paul, to receive a hundred and seventy-five blows of the knout. At the same time another criminal received thirty blows, and a third fifty: the former of whom Löhnig saw die before him, and the latter he saw kicked out of the way like a lifeless log, after his punishment. At last Löhnig's turn came, and *from that moment he lost all consciousness and sensation*, yet without falling into a swoon. He received the full tale of stripes, his nostrils were slit up, and his forehead branded, and of all this he afterwards declared he felt nothing." Heim reports a somewhat similar case. A soldier received fifty lashes, which were administered by two corporals. During the punishment *he gave no sign of pain*, neither groaned or winced, but bore the whole without a stir. When it was over, he said to the commanding officer, with a confused air, "I beg pardon for falling asleep in your presence."

In the year 1461 a noble Hussite was tortured at Prague. He was so insensible under it, that the executioners believed him to be dead, and threw the carcass, as they thought it, on the ground. After some hours he came to himself, and wondered at the state he was in, and related a pleasant dream he had had during the torture.

Of a similar character to the above is a story told by T. Heywood in his History of Women. Heywood said, "Of the several sorts of jugglings with which the devil deludes his scholars, I will nominate some few." . . . "An honest citizen in the Delphinate, calling for his maid servant one day, and hearing no answer, searched the rooms and found her lying all along by a fire which she had before made in a private chamber; which seeing, he kickt her with his foot, and bid her arise, and get about her business, but seeing her not to move he took a rough wand, and belaboured her soundly;

but perceiving her neither to stir or complain, and finding all the parts of her body insensible, took fire and put it to such places of her body as were most tender; but perceiving her to have lost all feeling, was persuaded she was dead, and called in his next neighbours, telling them in what case he found her, but concealing the blows he had given her." The body was then laid out as dead. In the morning, hearing somebody groan, they went in and found her alive, and suffering sorely from the wounds the master had inflicted. This poor woman was burnt alive, as a witch![*] Physical insensibility, as Salverte observes, being always considered a certain sign of Sorcery.

The ecstatic condition was most strikingly developed at the tomb of the Abbé Paris, through the religious excitement of the devotees. A Report describes the terrific blows and weights, which the convulsionists endured, not only without pain, but even with pleasure, crying out at times, "Oh, how delightful,—what good it does me!" The details furnish a curious exemplification of what religious enthusiasm can affect.

Hoffman, physician to the Elector of Brandenburg, who wrote a treatise on Catalepsy, mentions the case of a young woman, who, hearing at church the word of God on the nature of sin, dropped down, like a statue, with her eyes open and raised to heaven, and remained in that condition an hour. The attacks continued for more than forty days, and always came on at the utterance of any words expressive of the love of Jesus Christ for a sinful world. Hoffman says, that some thought that the visitation was miraculous and divine, "others referred it to the devil; for his part, he referred it to *disease*."[†]

Baker, in his "Reign of Henry VIII.," mentions one "William Foxely, potmaker for the Mint of the Tower of London, who fell asleep, and could not be waked with pinching and burning *for fourteen days*; and when he awaked, was found, as if he had slept but one night, and lived forty years after."[‡]

Wanley, in his "Wonders," mentions several cases of long and deep sleep, and of men who worked in their sleep, particularly of a boy, William Withers, who remained in a (Mesmeric) sleep for ten days.

In "Magnetism before the Court of Rome," and in the Chapters on "the Middle Ages and on Antiquity," will be found much curious matter illustrative of the subject. Teste also contains some

---

[*] Volney, tom. vii. p. 449.
[†] Number for June, 1846. In Miscellanea Mystica, p. 692.

[*] T. Heywood's "Historie of Women." 1657.
[†] Dissertatio Hoffmanni de Affectu Cataleptico.
[‡] Baker's Chronicle, 296. Folio.

striking quotations from early writers: and the "Isis Revelata" abounds with information that every Mesmerist will peruse with pleasure.*

No. III.

LIGHTNESS OF BODY, ETC.

When the sceptic shows his contempt for the wonders of Mesmerism, and for the credulity of Mesmerists, we reply that no phenomenon has ever yet developed itself under magnetic treatment, for which we cannot find something correspondent, or similar in the spontaneous workings of nature. Some things, however, are recorded of natural ecstatics, and sleepwakers, for which I have not yet met with any thing parallel in Mesmerism; and of such are the statements in the Seventh Chapter, relating to Martha Brossier being lifted up above the heads of several strong men, who were pulling her downwards; to Maria Mori, the Tyrolese, *miraculously* resting on the tips of her feet, when unequal to *any* effort; and to John Evans *demoniacally* resting the whole weight of his body on the point of his toes; now can such things be true? Dr. Arnold gives us a useful caution, before we positively reject them.

"Being wholly ignorant of the nature and object of wonders, and being ignorant of a great many natural laws, by which they may be produced; the question of their credibility resolves itself into little more than a question as to the credibility of the witnesses. A man may appear ridiculous if he expresses his belief in any story of this sort, and yet, to say that all such wonders are false, would be an extravagant boldness of assertion. The accounts of wonders, then, from Livy's prodigies downwards, *I should receive*, according to Herodotus's expression when speaking of one of them, οὔτε ἀπιστέων, οὔτε πιστεύων τι λίην: sometimes considering of what fact they were an *exaggerated or corrupted representation*, at other times trying to remember *whether any, and how many other notices occur of the same thing*, and whether they are of force

* I have made no allusion to the transcendental views of Mrs. Crowe in her "Night-side of Nature," touching a Mesmeric rapport, &c., with the spiritual world; though my attention has been called to her statements by more than one party. I have advanced nothing in this work relating to Mesmerism, which has not been based on my own personal observation, and for which I have not seen something analogous, or the same, though perhaps differing in degree. With Mrs. Crowe's far loftier theories I have no experience whatever.

enough to lead us to search for some law, hitherto undiscovered, to which they may all be referred, and become hereafter the *foundation* of a new science."*

Are there, then, according to Arnold's canon, any "other notices" of such incredible facts as these related of Martha Brossier, and Maria Mori, occurring in any other writer?

Glanvill, in his "Saducismus Triumphatus," gives an account of a boy, named Richard Jones, "who, more than once, was *found* in a room by himself, his hands flat against a beam that traversed the ceiling, and his body suspended in such a manner, that his feet were about a yard from the ground. At such times, he was in a profound stupor, and would hang there as if held on by a *magnetic force*, to the beam, a quarter of an hour together. Nine people at a time saw the boy so strangely hanging by a beam." (125.)

This boy, says Glanvill, was bewitched by Jane Brookes, who was executed for it, in Somersetshire.

In Pitaval's *Causes Célèbres*, vol. xii., there is a report from four Bishops, and four Doctors, assisted by M. Morel, a physician of Châlons-sur-Saone, respecting eighteen Religieuses, of the town of Auxonne, who were troubled by an evil spirit. Among the phenomena developed, according to the report, were knowledge of the thoughts of others, knowledge of languages, insensibility, rigidity, &c., and *that of holding their bodies almost in the air, only the ends of their toes touching the ground.* M. Morel and the Bishops appeared to have examined the symptoms with attention, and to have had no doubt as to the facts, only pronouncing them demoniacal.

In Mr. Heaton's "Dæmon," published in 1822, in addition to the case of John Evans, is an account of a child of Mr. Kennard's, of Lodderwell, near Kingsbridge (Devon), aged eleven, who "ran up the side of the room to the ceiling, impossible as it may seem, where she remained immovable on her feet for several minutes, her clothes being unaltered in their usual position, as if, by some supernatural law, she had the power of changing the centre of *gravity*." (p. 22.) This was witnessed by numerous spectators.

Mr. Heaton then quotes from "a narrative of some extraordinary things that happened to Mr. Lawford's children, Bristol, supposed to be the effect of witchcraft," and which was published at Bristol, in 1800. Among other things, "these children were *pulled towards the ceiling* with great force, that they were all tired with holding them, though above a dozen were there. Sometimes they *seemed suspended in the air.* They were convinced that nothing but a preternatural power could pull with such force against so many. Four stout men could scarcely hold a child from being pulled away."

* Arnold's Lectures, p. 129.

Ward, in his "History of the Hindoos," speaking of the phenomena, which the half-famished ecstatic would develop in his trance, says, that "the body of the Yogee, who meditates, will become light as wood, and able to walk on the fluid element, and able to ascend into the air." (203.)

Salverte, in his "Occult Sciences," mentions a sorcerer who, in his sleep, performed various movements, and struck out even as though he were on the wing.

Now, as to all these facts, the question (as Arnold observes) "resolves itself into the credibility of the witnesses," though at times I feel with Hume that no testimony could satisfy me as to the reality of such improbable occurrences; but the coincidence between these various statements must not be thus dismissed, especially when it is remembered, that the different parties are not likely to have heard of the corresponding performances of their ecstatic brethren and sisters. What, also, gives interest to the inquiry, is the fact that at this moment, in the Tyrol, the elevation of Maria Morl on the tips of her toes, is regarded as a proof of miraculous intervention.

Baron Feuchterleben, in his work on Medical Psychology, says, "The obscure ideal images which exert their influence, even in ordinary dreams, have evidently become so vivid in the somnambulist, under repressed spontaneity, that they become invested with a *motor power*, and consequently take the place of spontaneity altogether, so that we might here certainly apply to the effect produced, the familiar expression of a "*reversion of the poles.*" Thus the walking on the roofs of houses, &c., &c., which it would be impossible for a man to accomplish in a state of waking, may be, in a degree, explained." (p. 203.)

Do the above observations of the learned Baron go any way towards assisting us in our belief? Perhaps we may say, with Arnold, that these different statements are "*an exaggerated or corrupted representation*" of a real fact.

No. IV.

SPEAKING STRANGE LANGUAGES, ETC.

In the History of Martha Brossier, I have mentioned that one of the phenomena in her case, was the power of speaking foreign languages (Greek and English), of which, when she was awake, she knew nothing.

This is another point, in the ecstatic condition, respecting which more curious evidence can be adduced than may be generally suspected.

If we analyse the different statements, the faculty would appear to fall under three very different heads, though they are apt to be confounded together; viz.—

1. Imitation of the voice of another in a most surprising degree.

2. Understanding the thoughts of another when addressed in a foreign tongue.

3. The actual speaking in a foreign tongue, of which the party, when awake, is said to be ignorant.

I. In regard to the faculty of "Imitation," instances are very numerous in the Mesmeric world: perhaps one of the most surprising cases is that of the imitation of Jenny Lind's voice, by one of Mr. Braid's patients at Manchester. The narrative will be found in the "Medical Times" for September, 1847.

A patient of Mr. Braid, "though ignorant of the grammar of her own language when awake, when asleep would prove herself competent to accompany any one in the room in singing songs in any *language*, giving both notes and words correctly: a feat which she was quite incompetent to perform in the waking condition." A "Mr. Schwabe played and sang a *German* song, in which she accompanied him correctly, giving both notes and words simultaneously." The same was done in Swedish with another gentleman. The somnambulist next accompanied Jenny Lind "in the most perfect manner, both as regarded words and music. Jenny now seemed resolved to test the powers of the somnambulist to the utmost by a continued strain of the most difficult roulades and cadenzas, for which she is so famous, including some of her extraordinary *scala-auto* notes, with all their inflections, from *pianissimo* to *forte crescendo*, and again diminish to thread-like *pianissimo*; but in all these fantastic tricks and displays of genius, by the Swedish nightingale, even to the shake, she was so closely and accurately tracked by the somnambulist, that several in the room occasionally could not have told, merely by hearing, that there were two individuals singing—so instantaneously did she catch the notes, and so perfectly did their voices blend and accord. Next, Jenny having been told by Mr. Braid that she might be tested in some other language, this charming songstress commenced 'Casta Diva,' and the 'Alla Bella,' in which the fidelity of the somnambulist's performance, both in words and music, was most perfect, and fully justified all Mr. Braid had alleged regarding her powers: she was also tested by Mlle. Lind in merely imitating language, when she gave most exact imitations;

and Mr. Schwabe also tried her by some difficult combinations of sound, which he said he knew no one was capable of imitating correctly without much practice, but the somnambulist imitated them correctly at once."

In the Critic (No. 145.), is a further account from Mr. Braid himself of the same patient imitating Greek and Celtic, — and of another patient singing songs in Latin, Italian, and French, after her mistress, with the utmost accuracy.

Mr. Howitt has also given a similar account of a patient of Mr. Spencer Hall's. "His faculty of imitation being tested, he threw back any sound issuing from the company as the most perfect echo would do. He was addressed in various languages, and threw back every sentence with the most perfect pronunciation, and generally without the omission of a single syllable." *

Dr. Esdaile has made his Hindoo patients speak Greek. An East India paper says, that Dr. Esdaile uttered words and sentences in the learned languages, which were repeated with wonderful exactness by the poor ignorant Bengalee.†

In the third volume of the Zoist (p. 222.), is a letter from Mr. Jago of Bodmin, describing a similar scene with a lady in the Mesmeric state, when her organs of imitation and language were influenced.

Mesmeric experience could produce sundry instances of the same kind.

II. We next come to a higher phenomenon, where the patient not only repeats and mimics foreign languages, but even *understands* them, and often understands them, without having the faculty of repeating or imitating them. This power, I should say, was only transference of thought appearing under a different guise.

Mr. Jago's patient above mentioned is one instance of this power. Miss Martineau's patient is another. Parties spoke to her in German, Italian, and French, and she understood them. Miss M. observes, that, "provided the ideas conveyed to the girl were within *her scope*, it mattered nothing *in what language* they were uttered." (Appendix.)

Some of the Ursulines of Loudun understood any orders given to them in Latin, provided that they were in a state of somnambulism. In the *Démonomanie de Loudun* we are told that M. de Bouillé, who had resided in America, bore testimony that he spoke to the nuns the language of certain savages of that country, and that they

* Spencer Hall's Mesmeric Experiences, p. 31.
† See also Dr. Esdaile's India, p. 113. for another case.

answered him very readily. Sister Clara understood Turkish, Spanish, and Italian, and others understood Greek.

In the History of the eighteen nuns that I referred to from Pitaval's *Causes Célèbres* (in the last Appendix), it is mentioned in the report, that among the phenomena which the Religieuses developed in their sleep, was a knowledge of languages, of which, when they were awake, they were quite ignorant.

My friend, Mr. A. Majendie, has mentioned to me the case of an ignorant peasant girl of Normandy, Marianne ——, aged 22, who was magnetised by Mr. Marie, manager of the Gas Company at Caen, on account of her health. She soon became somnambulist, and readily answered questions. Mr. Marie, has spoken to her in English, German, Italian and Latin: Madame Marie in Spanish: the somnambule answered in French to the questions with perfect accuracy. The Curé de Ranville asked her questions in Greek, to which she answered pertinently, and with an occasional exaltation of thought that was very remarkable. Mr. Majendie gives some interesting statements on this point.

More cases under this head could be brought forward.

III. The last point to notice is that, where the ecstatic is said to *speak* in a language of which, when awake, he is utterly ignorant. Of this power I have myself seen not the most distant indication; but names of such eminence have made allusion to the assumed facts, — that I cannot altogether dismiss their evidence, — as too trifling and absurd. Again, let us remember Arnold's canon of criticism, and hear what they offer.

Sennertus, a name of authority, in his treatise on Madness, (vol. iii. of Works), says, "There are some who deny that the melancholy or the mad can speak in foreign languages. * * * But of the truth of these facts we cannot doubt."

Forestus, in his tenth book, (in Sckol. p. 340.), mentions the son of a sailor, whom he himself saw, who having received a wound in the head and become delirious, made syllogisms in "the German language," which he was unable to accomplish when he was cured.

Forestus also mentions a woman that he attended, who, during her illness and melancholy, sang Latin hymns, which she had never learnt. Forestus adds, that she may have heard them in church and remembered them.

Erasmus, in his declamation in praise of medicine, mentions a case which fell under his own knowledge, — of a native of Spoletum — who, during an illness, spoke the German language admirably. When he recovered, adds Erasmus, he neither spoke it nor understood it.

Melancthon, in an epistle to Hubert Languetus, says that, twelve years before, there had been a woman in Saxony that never learnt letters, and yet when she was influenced by the devil, she spake Greek and Latin, respecting the Saxon war. *

Some of the ecstatic nuns at Loudun are said to have spoken in Greek and German, of which, when in a normal state, they were ignorant.

Dr. Brigham, in his " Remarks on Health," refers to similar instances, — particularly the case of a child "twelve years of age, who knew only the first rudiments of the Latin language, but during a fever spoke it with fluency."

Mr. Colquhoun, (vol. ii. p. 23, 24.) refers to divers learned writers, who state similar facts.

The Seeress of Prevorst, in her sleep-waking state, frequently spoke in a language that had some resemblance to the Eastern tongues. Mr. Jago, and other Mesmerisers, also record instances of the power in question.

Now, how is the above to be explained? Are the statements pure invention? — or were the writers misinformed?

Baron Feuchterleben cannot deny some of these facts: he admits that somnambulists do "speak in a more refined dialect, and frequently in a language with which they are not otherwise familiar," (p. 206.) — but he explains it afterwards by adding, that " *Foreign languages are reproductions of dormant recollections.*" (p. 208.) Probably this view would meet the majority of cases, — but scarcely all. Would the conveyance of such a mental acquisition as the knowledge of a foreign language to a brain in a high state of exaltation and impressionability be a much more incredible fact, than a transfer of thought and of ideas, and the communication of theological and philosophic learning? I offer this suggestion to the cerebral physiologists. " The *History of Errors*," says Sir Joshua Reynolds, " properly managed, often shortens the road to truth." †

---

* Melancthon, Epist. l. 2. p. 550.   † Second Discourse.

THE END.

London:
Spottiswoode and Shaw,
New-street-Square.

The borrower must return this item on or before
the last date stamped below. If another user
places a recall for this item, the borrower will
be notified of the need for an earlier return.

*Non-receipt of overdue notices does **not** exempt
the borrower from overdue fines.*

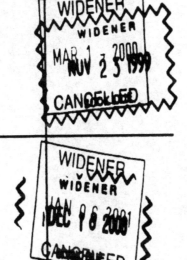
Please handle with care.
Thank you for helping to preserve
library collections at Harvard.

Check Out More Titles From HardPress Classics Series In this collection we are offering thousands of classic and hard to find books. This series spans a vast array of subjects — so you are bound to find something of interest to enjoy reading and learning about.

Subjects:
Architecture
Art
Biography & Autobiography
Body, Mind &Spirit
Children & Young Adult
Dramas
Education
Fiction
History
Language Arts & Disciplines
Law
Literary Collections
Music
Poetry
Psychology
Science
…and many more.

Visit us at www.hardpress.net

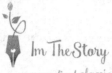
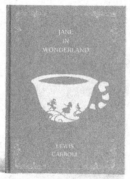